PHARMACOLOGY - RESEARCH, SAFETY TESTING AND REGULATION

ANTIHYPERTENSIVE DRUGS

PHARMACOLOGY, MEDICAL USES AND POTENTIAL SIDE EFFECTS

PHARMACOLOGY - RESEARCH, SAFETY TESTING AND REGULATION

Additional books in this series can be found on Nova's website under the Series tab.

Additional e-books in this series can be found on Nova's website under the e-book tab.

PHARMACOLOGY - RESEARCH, SAFETY TESTING AND REGULATION

ANTIHYPERTENSIVE DRUGS

PHARMACOLOGY, MEDICAL USES AND POTENTIAL SIDE EFFECTS

SCOTT CALDWELL
EDITOR

New York

Library of Congress Cataloging-in-Publication Data

ISBN: 978-1-63463-829-6
Library of Congress Control Number: 2015935506

Published by Nova Science Publishers, Inc. † New York

Contents

Preface

Arterial hypertension is one of the most important preventable contributors to disease and death, and is commonly treated with antihypertensive drugs combined with appropriate changes in life-style. The first chapter focuses on the options in the enantioseparation of antihypertensive drugs, the synthesis of single enantiomers and chiral aspects of their action and dispositions. The second chapter of this book examines the potential genotoxic effects of five Angiotensin II receptor blockers, analyzed in vivo and in vitro in human peripheral blood lymphocytes (PBLs). The third chapter includes a general description about polymorphism and some techniques used in polymorphism characterization. Then, the specific description of some antihypertensive drugs that present polymorphism phenomena are introduced. Finally, hypertension is by far the most important modifiable risk factor for cardiovascular disease in sub-Saharan Africa. In this book, the authors discuss the ethnic/racial peculiarities in the incidence, pathophysiology and management of hypertension in the black hypertensive patient.

Chapter I – There are many classes of antihypertensive drugs which decrease blood pressure using different mechanisms. The most important and most widely used drugs are the diuretics, the beta- adrenergic blocking agents (β-blockers), renin-angiotensin system inhibitors, calcium channel blockers (calcium channel antagonists or calcium antagonists). Many of these drugs have one or more chiral atoms in their structure. Chirality can affect their pharmacological, pharmacokinetics and toxicological properties. In many cases enantiomers have different activity and for these reasons it is essential to study chiral aspects in these compounds. In this chapter, antihypertensives as chiral agents will be divided to several groups: β-blockers, diuretics and alfa2 adrenergic agents, ACE inhibitors, angiotensin II receptor antagonist, renin inhibitors, and calcium channel blockers. Chapter pays attention to the ilustration of methods for enantioseparation of clinically used drugs such as chromatograhic methods (HPLC, TLC, LC-MS, GC-MS), capillary electrophoresis and capillary electrochromatography. Methods for stereoselective syntheses are also mentioned. In addition, the pharmacodynamic and pharmacokinetic differences of enantiomers in each group of compounds are described.

Chapter II – Arterial Hypertension is one of the most important preventable contributors to disease and death, and is commonly treated with antihypertensive drugs combined with appropriate changes in life-style. The large majority of hypertensive patients need long-term therapy and because of the long duration of the pharmacological treatment, documentation of safety and efficiency is required, including sensitive indices of genotoxic damage. In this study, the potential genotoxic effect of five Angiotensin II receptor blockers (ARBs: Candesartan, Telmisartan, Eprosartan, Valsartan, Olmesartan) was analyzed *in vivo* and *in vitro* in human peripheral blood lymphocytes (PBLs) by means of the cytokinesis-block micronucleus (CBMN) assay in combination with fluorescence *in situ* hybridization (FISH) with a centromeric probe, and by the analysis of structural chromosomal aberrations (sCA) and expression of fragile sites (FS). The *in vivo* study was carried out in 55 hypertensive patients while the *in vitro* study was performed in 10 control individuals by adding the drugs to the culture medium at a final concentration similar to the levels found in plasma in patients. In relation to the CBMN assay, our results showed a significant increase in the frequencies of MN and binucleated cells with MN (BNMN) *in vivo* and especially *in vitro*. FISH analysis revealed no significant differences between patients and control individuals in the frequency of centromeric signals. Regarding the incidence of sCA, the data revealed again a significantly higher rate of sCA *in vivo*, and mostly *in vitro*. Chromosomal location analysis pointed at chromosomes 16 and 17 as preferential targets for the clastogenic effect of ARBs drugs. Several FS emerged as specific; among them, the *locus* 17q21, recently proposed as a new FS, was only expressed in ARBs-treated patients, supporting the findings for a linkage between hypertension and a telomeric *locus* on chromosome 17. Therefore, these results are consistent with our previous studies of beta-blockers genotoxicity and provide evidence for an association among the antihypertensive therapy, arterial hypertension and DNA damage in human lymphocytes.

Chapter III – Polymorphism, which can be described as the ability of the compound to crystallize in different phases with different crystalline arrangement and / or conformation of the molecules in the crystal lattice, has become a very interesting focus of investigation in the last years. The main purpose of this kind of study is the strategic construction of distinct crystalline arrangements, and the complete comprehension of the connection between structure and physicochemical properties. In recent years, it is a topic of great interest to the scientific community and presents a great challenge for the pharmaceutical industry, since changes in the crystalline arrangement can alter the physicochemical properties of drugs. This chapter will first include a general description about polymorphism and some techniques used in polymorphism characterization. Then, the specific description of some antihypertensive drugs that present polymorphism phenomena will be introduced.

Chapter IV – Hypertension is by far the most important modifiable risk factor for cardiovascular disease in sub-Saharan Africa. Studies have documented the prevalence of hypertension to be highest in blacks and the incidence and progression of end-organ damage from hypertension are worse in black patients. For example the risk of stroke is double in hypertensive black patients compared with white hypertensive patients. Hypertension in blacks is strongly associated with a lot of other modifiable risk factors for CVD such as obesity, physical inactivity and reduced potassium intake. This observation also applies to black patients in USA and Europe. Consequently, effective treatment of hypertension is particularly important in black patients. Calcium channel blockers and diuretics are effective monotherapy in blacks. Beta blockers, alpha adrenergic blockers, angiotensin converting enzyme inhibitors and angiotensin receptor blockers are less effective as monotherapy. They are however effective as combination therapy which is particularly attractive for black patients. Medical education is important in hypertensive black patients because of the cluster of modifiable risk factors and socioeconomic considerations. Because of its clinical course, apparent lack of symptoms and association with complications, hypertension has emerged as a major public health concern. The International Society on Hypertension in Blacks in 2010 recommended antihypertensive therapy for blacks without target organ damage or concomitant cardiovascular diseases at blood pressures greater than 135/85 mmHg, or greater than 130/80 mmHg for those at higher risk. Current understanding of the underlying pathophysiology of hypertensive disease indicates that the pathophysiology of hypertension in the black is slightly different from those of other races. Black patients with hypertension have enhanced sodium retention, expanded plasma volume, low plasma renin activity and a higher incidence of salt-sensitivity. Consequently, there are differences in the appropriate drugs to use for optimal treatment of hypertension in black patients. Studies of black hypertensive patients in Africa have documented high prevalence of hypertension and low prevalence of control to target levels. Many factors are responsible including poverty, lack of access to health facilities, poor health seeking behaviours, cultural beliefs including myths and superstition. Attention to all these in addition to education and life style modification and not merely drug therapy will make the necessary change in the current state of hypertension in blacks. In this chapter, the authors will discuss the ethnic/racial peculiarities in the incidence, pathophysiology and management of hypertension in the black hypertensive patient. The authors shall also review the management of black hypertensive patient in resource limited setting emphasizing the race-related differences in the pathophysiology of hypertension and the need to stream line management taking cognizance of the cost burden of management of hypertension.

In: Antihypertensive Drugs
Editor: Scott Caldwell

ISBN: 978-1-63463-829-6

Chapter I

Antihypertensive Drugs As Chiral Agents

R. Čižmáriková*[*], *J. Valentová*, *A. Némethy and I. Pechová
Department of Chemical Theory of Drugs, Faculty of Pharmacy,
Comenius University in Bratislava, Bratislava, Slovak Republic

Abstract

There are many classes of antihypertensive drugs which decrease blood pressure using different mechanisms. The most important and most widely used drugs are the diuretics, the beta- adrenergic blocking agents (β blockers), renin-angiotensin system inhibitors, calcium channel blockers (calcium channel antagonists or calcium antagonists). Many of these drugs have one or more chiral atoms in their structure. Chirality can affect their pharmacological, pharmacokinetics and toxicological properties. In many cases enantiomers have different activity and for these reasons it is essential to study chiral aspects in these compounds.

In this chapter, antihypertensives as chiral agents will be divided to several groups: β-blockers, diuretics and alfa2 adrenergic agents, ACE inhibitors, angiotensin II receptor antagonist, renin inhibitors, and calcium channel blockers. Chapter pays attention to the ilustration of methods for enantioseparation of clinically used drugs such as chromatograhic methods (HPLC, TLC, LC-MS, GC-MS), capillary electrophoresis and capillary electrochromatography. Methods for stereoselective syntheses are also mentioned. In addition, the pharmacodynamic and pharmacokinetic differences of enantiomers in each group of compounds are described.

[*] Corresponding author: R. Čižmáriková. E-mail: cizmarikova@fpharm.uniba.sk.

1. Introduction

Several statistical indicators confirm that diseases of the cardiovascular system (CVS) are among the most widespread civilization diseases. Essential hypertension is the world's most prevalent cardiovascular disorder, affecting approximately 26% of the worldwide population and still rising [1]. A detailed analysis of CVS diagnoses suggests that essential hypertension is the most frequent diagnosis according to the number of prescriptions. A varied range of drugs with different mechanisms of action and different chemical structures are used for its effective treatment. Examples include β-blockers, diuretics, α-adrenergic agonists, calcium channel blockers, ACE inhibitors, angiotensin II receptor antagonists and renin inhibitors.

Many of these drugs are chiral. In their molecular structure, they contain a stereogenic centre and they form stereoisomers (enantiomers or diastereomers) which may differ in their pharmacological, pharmacokinetic, and toxicological properties. Many of the physical and chemical properties of enantiomers are identical and the evaluation of the chiral aspects of their action and metabolism requires stereospecific methodologies.

The most commonly used techniques for enantioseparation include chromatographic techniques, such as high performance liquid chromatography (HPLC), gas chromatography (GC), thin layer chromatography (TLC), methods of capillary electrophoresis and capillary electrochromatography. In addition to these, stereoselective synthesis is another alternative method of obtaining the enantiomeric forms.

Enantioselective analytical methods play an important role in the entire process of development and application of chiral drugs. They are used to obtain the single enantiomers of chiral agents, to examine the enantiomeric purity in stereoselective syntheses, to check the stereochemical purity and stability in the preparation of dosage forms, to evaluate the bioavailability, and in pharmacological, pharmacokinetic, and toxicological studies.

This chapter is focused on options in the enantioseparation of antihypertensive drugs, synthesis of single enantiomers and chiral aspects of their action and dispositions.

2. Beta-Adrenergic Antagonists (β-Blockers)

β-Blockers are among the most widely prescribed drugs in the treatment of hypertension and are also indicated in other cardiovascular diseases such as angina pectoris, arrhythmias, heart failure [2]. They proved useful in the treatment of patients with hyperadrenergic conditions such as thyrotoxicosis, essential tremor, glaucoma, and even in the prophylaxis of migraine. β-Blockers selectively bind to beta-adrenergic receptors and thus competitively and reversibly antagonise the effects of endogenous catecholamines – adrenaline and noradrenaline [3, 4]. β-Blockers have different pharmacodynamic and pharmacokinetic properties. Some β-blockers can be more selective for β_1-receptor (atenolol, metoprolol, acebutolol, bisoprolol, nebivolol) and some can be described to have a property of intrinsic sympathomimetic activity on the β_1-receptor (labetalol, acebutolol, pindolol). They can be vasodilating with α-adrenergic blocking activity (labetalol, carvedilol) or with an increased production of nitric oxide (nebivolol) [5]. In terms of chemical structure, they form a group of substances derived from aryloxyaminopropanols and arylaminoethanols. In both groups, the individual β-blockers contain a stereogenic carbon in the linking chain which is the origin of their optical activity. Due to the presence of a stereogenic centre, they are capable of forming two types of enantiomers which, in an achiral environment, differ in their ability to rotate the plane of polarised light either to the right (+) or to the left (-). Some β-blockers, such as labetalol, nadolol, and nebivolol, have multiple stereogenic centres.

The absolute configuration of the derivatives with one stereogenic centre in terms of the Cahn-Ingold-Prelog system is either (*R*) or (*S*). β-Blockers exhibit a high degree of stereoselectivity in relation to β-adrenergic receptors. In both groups, (-)-enantiomers are more active – with the (*S*) absolute configuration in the group of aryloxyaminopropanols and (*R*) in the group of arylaminoethanols (e.g. labetalol, pronethalol) [6] (Figures 1, 1a, 2).

Carvedilol is marketed as the racemate for treatment of hypertension and congestive heart failure. Like other β-blockers, the (*S*)-(-)-enantiomer of carvedilol is more potent as an antagonist of β-receptors. However, both the (*R*)- and the (*S*)-enantiomer, are also effective in blocking of the α-adrenergic activity [7]. Labetalol is administered as mixture of four stereoisomers. (*RR*)-labetalol is responsible for the β-blocking activity of the drug, on the other hand (*SR*)-isomer is the most potent in α-receptor blocking activity.

Both the *RS* and *SS* isomers display weak alpha and β- receptor actions [8]. Stereoselectivity in antagonism of β-receptors has been reported for nadolol [9] and nebivolol [10], other β-blockers with four stereoisomers.

In the therapeutic practice, β-blockers are mostly used as racemates or enantiomers combination. Only penbutolol and timolol are used as pure enantiomers.

Stereoselectivity in different pharmacokinetic properties of β-blockers has been documented [11]. However, it could not be generalized, because it depends on the individual structure. E.g. propranolol showed stereoselective binding to the plasma albumin opposite to acebutolol, pindolol and sotalol, which have relatively high free fraction in plasma, the binding appears to be nonstereoselective. It was also demonstrated that the uptake and release of atenolol from the adrenergic nerve ending are stereoselective, favoring the more active (-)-enantiomer. In contrast to atenolol, the uptake of propranolol, a more lipophilic β-blocker, into adrenegic nerve cell appears to be via passive diffusion and therefore is not stereoselective [12, 13]. While the more hydrophilic β-blockers, such as atenolol and nadolol, are almost excreted unchanged in urine, the lipophilic β-blockers such as propranolol, are eliminated mostly by metabolism. In humans, propranolol is metabolized by three pathways: glucuronidation, ring oxidation and side chain oxidation. Oxidation by human CYP2D6 enzymes mainly into 4-hydroxypropranolol (4-OH-PL), followed by 4-OH-PL and N-desisopropylpropranolol were observed to be an enantioselective substrates: (*S*)-PL > (*R*)-PL [14]. Stereoselectivity was also confirmed in the study of propranolol side chain glucuronidation by human UDP-glucuronosyltransferase (UGT) 2B7 and 1A9. UGT1A9 preferred catalysing (*S*)-enantiomer to (*R*)-enantiomer. UGT2B7 catalysed slightly less (*S*)-enantiomers than (*R*)-enantiomer [15]. It has been reported that UGT prefers metabolism of (*S*)-carvedilol to (*R*)-carvedilol stereoselectively.

Stereoselectivity of carvedilol glucuronidation by UGT was different between in human liver (*S*>*R*) and intestinal microsomes (*R*≈*S*), it was supposed that the differnce is due to the tissue –specific expresion of UGT isoforms involved in the glucuronidation of carvedilol [16]. Seeringer et al. [17] studied enantioselective pharmacokinetics of metoprolol after 100 mg racemic metoprolol was administered. A slight enantiopreference towards metabolism of (*R*)-metoprolol was observed.

Except for metoprolol and propranolol, the stereoselectivity in the plasma concentration of other studied β-blockers (acebutolol, atenolol, pindolol, sotalol) was relatively modest.

The stereoselectivity in the plasma concentration of metoprolol and propranolol mostly related to the stereoselective metabolism and first-pass effect favour (*R*)-enantiomers [11].

For pharmacokinetic study and therapeutic drug monitoring the analytical methods for separation and quantification of the isomers in biological samples are desirable.

2.1. Stereoselective Analysis of β-Blockers

In this group of chiral agents, many enantioseparation methods have been used such as biocatalysis, crystallization, chromatography (HPLC, TLC, GC), and capillary electrophoresis (CE). In addition to the above-mentioned methods and biocatalysed reactions, stereoselective synthesis is another alternative method for obtaining the enantiomeric forms.

The chromatographic separations of enantiomers are characterized according to the method as direct and indirect. Indirect methods of enantioseparation are based on the derivatization, with an optically active reagent, of the enantiomers to be separated.

This leads to stable diastereomers which have different physical properties and can be separated on non-chiral stationary phases. Direct methods of enantioseparation use the formation of diastereomeric complexes between the chiral selector and the enantiomers to be separated. The selector is part of the chiral stationary phase (CSP) or of the chiral mobile phase (CMP) [18].

Chromatographic enantioseparation on chiral stationary phase has appeared as the most effective and convenient way of determining the enantiomeric composition of chiral drugs.

Different structural types of CSPs including the π-donor/acceptor phases (Pirkle phase) [19, 20], derivatized polysaccharides [21, 22], proteins [23, 24], β-cyclodextrin [25, 26], macrocyclic antibiotic [27, 28] and molecular imprinted phases [29] were utilized for enantiomeric separation of β-blockers. The following molecular interactions with CSP are supposed to play role in chiral discrimination of enantiomers: H-bonding, π-π interaction, hydrophilic, dipole-dipole and steric interactions [30, 31].

The possible interactions between analytes depend on type of CSP and mobile phase selection, which determines that enantiomers fits into the three-dimensional structure of sorbent [32].

2.1.1. High-Performance Liquid Chromatography

Pirkle CSPs

These include various dinitroaryl phases which were the basis of the first commercially available chiral columns. E.g., *N*-3,5-dinitrobenzoyl-α-aminophosphonate as a chiral selector was used for the enantioseparation of propranolol, metoprolol, oxprenolol, pindolol, bufuranol, metoprolol, oxprenolol, pindolol, and pronethalol without prior derivatization [33, 34]. (*R*)-1-naphthylglycine and 3,5-dinitrobenzoic acid as CSP were applied to enantiseparation of metoprolol and bisoprolol [35].

With other columns of this type, there is a strong interaction of the separated compounds with a chiral selector. It is therefore necessary to reduce the reactivity of the amino and hydroxy groups by suitable derivatization. A series of β-blockers were thus separated in the form of urea derivatives after derivatization with 1-naphthyl isocyanate or in the form of the N-acylated derivatives.

Most of the CSPs of this type use a mixture of hexane with propan-2-ol and modifiers – acetic acid and diethylamine – as the mobile phase for the separation [36]. New Pirkle type CSP such as Chirex (π-acceptor and π-donor phase) were used for enantioseparation of underivatized atenolol and propranolol in pharmaceutical formulation [37].

Protein CSPs

From this group of CSPs, the first phases used for the enantioseparation of β-blockers were phases based on serum albumin. Acidic α_1-glycoprotein is the basis of a commercial chiral AGP column and was used for the enantioseparation of metoprolol and its metabolite [38] as well as of β-blockers with multiple stereogenic centres: nadolol and labetalol [36]. One of the advantages of protein-based CSP column is possibility using an aqueous mobile phase and the fact that analyte derivatization is unnecessary.

Enantiomers of propranolol and oxprenolol were also separated on CSP based on chicken α_1-acid glycoprotein (c-AGP)-immobilized silica particle column [24]. Barbato et al. [39] investigated the enantioselective retention of thirteen β-blockers on CSP with human serum albumin (HSA) and with α_1-acid glycoprotein (AGP). Eight β-blockers were enantiomerically resolved on the AGP column whereas only four β-blockers were resolved on the HSA column. Analyses performed on AGP with eluent containing dimethyloctylamine as the displacer demonstrated that enantioselective sites bind to both (-)-forms and (+)-forms, but the binding to (-)-forms is stronger. Successful enantioseparation of β-blockers was also achieved with other protein CSPs containing ovomucoid [40] or cellobiohydrolase I (chiral-BSH column) [41].

The most progressively evolving stationary phases are CSPs based on glycoprotein antibiotics such as vancomycin, teicoplanin and their analogs. These are used in organic or reversed phase mode and mobile phase is mostly consisted of acetonitrile, alcohols and amines [42].

Lehotay et al. [43] evaluated the enantioseparation ability of the vancomycin CSP and the effect of different solvents, modifiers (aliphatic carboxylic acids) in a series of potential β-blockers of the aryloxy aminopropanol with substituted piperazine in basic part of molecule. In addition to ionic interactions and hydrogen bonds between the macrocyclic antibiotic and the analyte, enantioseparation was also influenced by steric effects.

Enatioseparation of more than 62 of new potential β-blockers with various modifications in the lipophilic and hydrophilic moiety of the molecule was studied on teicoplanin CSPs The significant resolution were observed in derivatives with substitution of *ortho* position on benzene ring [44-46].

The vancomycine-based CSP (Chirobiotic V) in reversed mode was utilized in LC-MS method for enantioselective determination of propranolol and atenolol in biological matrices (urine, plasma) [47, 48] and in nano-liquid stereoselective chromatography for resolution of propranolol, metoprolol and oxprenolol enantiomers. The method was applied to the analysis of drugs in human plasma [49]. The latest application of vancomycine based CSP are stereoselective analysis of β-blocker in environmental samples (natural and waste water) [50].

Ribeiro et al. [51] used Chirobiotic V under reversed mode in LC-MS/MS with a triple quadrupole analyser for identification of β-blocker enantiomers beside other chiral pharmaceuticals, β_2-adrenergic agonists, selective serotonin reuptake inhibitors) in the effluents of wastewater treatment plants (WWTP).

Bagnall et al. [52] presented first chiral liquid chromatography quadrupole time-of-flight mass spectrometry (LC-QTOF-MS) for analysis of enatiomers of propranolol and other drugs in river water and sewage eluent using separation on Chirobiotic V and CBH (cellobiohydrolase) column.

Teicoplanin as a chiral selector (Chirobiotic T) found application for enantiselective quantification of atenolol in plasma during pharmacokinetic study [53]. Similarly the LC-MS/MS method using Chirobiotic T CSP was utilized for enantioselective pharmakokinetic study of carvedilol [54].

Polysaccharide CSPs

The chiral selectors comprise various carbamates of cellulose and amylose which have higher separation efficiency in comparison to native polysaccharides. For β-blockers, the most widely used CSPs include commercially available phases such as cellulose tris(3,5-dimethylphenyl carbamate) – Chiralcel OD, and amylose tris(3,5-dimethylphenyl carbamate) – Chiralpak AD, whose separation efficiency is mainly based on the formation of inclusion complexes [31, 55].

Chiralcel OD was used for direct separation of metipranolol and its major degradation product, desacetylmetipranolol. A mixture of hexane and propan-2-ol was used as the mobile phase. In both compounds, the (*R*)-(+)-enantiomer was eluted before the (*S*)-(-)-enantiomer [56]. Chiralcel OD was also used for enantiomeric separation of atenolol [57].

Antunes Nde et al. [58] realised stereoselective determination of metoprolol and its metabolite α-hydroxymetoprolol in plasma by LC-MS/MS using Chiralpak AD column. The method was applied to the study of kinetic disposition of metoprolol in plasma after the administration of single oral dose. The clinical study showed, that pharmacokinetics of metoprolol is enantioselective, with observation higher AUC for (*S*)-metoprolol.

Nebivolol was enantiomerically separated using Chiralpak AD and Chiralpak AD-RH columns in normal and reverse mode with a mobile phase comprising ethanol and propan-1-ol. The separation coefficient was the same on both phases and the resolution of the enantiomers was more effective on Chiralpak AD-RH [59].

In the study Valentova et al. [60] enantiomers of propranolol and some of novel aryloxyaminopropanol derivatives with β-adrenoceptor antagonist activity were separated on Chiralpak AD CSP with final composition of mobile phase: hexane:ethanol:methanol: dimethylamine (85:3.75:11.25:0.1%). The enantiomeric elution order was determined to be *R*-before *S*-enantiomer following semipreparative isolation and induced CD spectrum of complexes formed in situ with molybdenum tetraacetate.

Chiralpak AD stationary phase was used also for rapid determination of biologically active enantiomers of nebivolol [(+)-*RRRS* and (-)-*SSSR*] in dosage formulation. The mobile phase used was heptane:ethanol:diethylamine (85:15:0.1) and the chiral separation occurred within 12 min [61].

Ribeiro et al. [62] performed enantiomeric separation of the four nadolol stereoisomers on Chiralpak AD at both analytical and preparative scales. β-Blockers belong to the group of active pharmaceuticals, which presence in waste and in surface waters becomes a major concern in envirometal pollution.

This could be due to excretion from human and veterinary use, an inappropriate disposal of unused pharmaceuticals, and due to an incomplete elimination in waste water treatment plants [63, 64]. During the last years, new analytical methods for enantiomeric determination in enviromental waters were developed. Morante-Zarcevo et al. [65] developed method for simultaneous enantiomeric determination of propranolol, metoprolol, pindolol and atenolol in natural water using different new commercially CSP: Lux, Cellulose-1/Sepapak-1 based on cellulose tris(3,5dimethylphenylcarbamate).

The stereoselective analysis of these β-blockers was also performed on four different type CSPs: polysaccharide CSPs (Chiralpak AD-H, Lux Cellulose-1), vancomycine-base CSP (Chirobiotic T) and Pirkle type CSP (Sumichiral OA-4900) using polar organic elution mode and normal phase. The mixture of the four enantiomeric pairs could not be separated with none of the four CSPs tested in polar organic mode. In normal phase elution mode with Lux Cellulose-1, the four pairs of enantiomers can be separated in the same run in gradient elution mode. The method was applied to determine the propranolol enantiomers in natural water samples [66]. Recently new immobilized CSPs have become commercially available based on tris(3,5-dimethylphenyl carbamate) of amylose and cellulose - Chiralpak IA, Chiralpak IB and and tris(3,5-dichlorophenyl carbamate) of cellulose - Chiralpak IC.

Enantioseparation of β-blockers involving propranolol on immobilized CSP (Chiralpak IA) was compared to the enantioseparation on coated CSP (Chiralpak AD). The coated phase showed a higher resolution power than the immobilized phase [67].

The enantioseparation of celiprolol was achieved also on a new phase based on amylose tris(3-chlorophenylcarbamate) -Chiralpak ID using capillary LC under normal phase condition [68].

Cyclodextrin CSPs

Cyclodextrins (CD) are cyclic oligomers formed of 6 to 8 α-D-glucopyranose units linked at the C1-C4 carbons and referred to as α-CD, β-CD, γ-CD. Derivatization of the hydroxyl groups results in a change in the molecular structure which in turn is reflected in a change in the size and hydrophobicity of the cavity and new possibilities of stereoselective interactions with the analyte. In the group of β-blockers, β-cyclodextrin is the most useful in view of its availability and the appropriate dimensions of the cavity [36, 69].

β-CD was used for the enantioseparation of a range of clinically used β-blockers using a mobile phase consisting of acetonitrile and methanol with additives (acetic acid and triethylamine) [70, 71]. Guillarme et al. [72] used cyclodextrines as chiral mobile phase additive for enantioseparation of several β-blockers (propranolol, pindolol, acebutolol, metoprolol, atenolol). However this strategy suffered from drawback linked to column lifetime and low enantioseparation efficiency.

Better resolution of enantiomers was obtained by indirect mode after derivatization of analytes with Marfey´s reagent and 2,3,4-tri-*O*-acetyl-α-D-arabinosyl isothiocyanate. New prepared β-CD-based silica monolithic capillary column were investigated for enantioseparation of celiprolol in nano-liquid chromatographic separation [73]. Modified cyclodextrins were used as chiral stationary phase for stereoselective analysis of propranolol and alprenolol by the gas chromatography method [74]. Cyclodextrins as chiral selectors are frequently used for enantioseparation in capillary electrophoresis.

Indirect Chiral Separation

A variety of derivatization reagents is used for indirect separation of β-blockers. After reacting with individual enantiomers, such reagents allow separation on a non-chiral column.

Most commonly, this involves a reaction with a basic amino group or a hydroxy group attached to a stereogenic centre. The derivatization agents used include acid anhydrides and chlorides, cyanides, isocyanates, and isothiocyanates [74].

One of new derivatization reagents were prepared by substitution of the fluorine atoms in 1,5-difluoro-2,4-dinitrobenzene (DFDNB) with three optically pure amines [(*R*)-(-)-1-cyclohexylethylamine, (+)-dehydroabietylamine and (*S*)-(-)-α-4-dimethylbenzylamine], by amino acid amides and amino acids. The formed diastereomers with six β-blockers (atenolol, propranolol, bisoprolol, metoprolol, salbutamol, and carvedilol) were separated by RP-HPLC [75]. Enantioseparation of five racemic β-blockers, namely, atenolol, propranolol, bisoprolol, metoprolol and carvedilol, was achieved as their diastereomers were prepared with chiral derivatizing reagents (CDRs) synthesized on a cyanuric chloride platform (6-methoxy derivative with amino acids or their amides).

Separation of diastereomers was carried out on a C18 column and gradient eluting mixtures of methanol with aqueous trifluoroacetic acid with UV detection at 230 nm [76].

2.1.2. Thin Layer Chromatography (TLC)

The methods used to separate enantiomers include TLC which can be used for both direct and indirect separation. Its advantages include simplicity, speed of separation, and low cost. The direct separation of enantiomers either uses a chiral stationary phase or a chiral selector which is added to the mobile phase. Chiral selectors for direct separation include, as part of the mobile phase, mainly (+)-camphorsulphonic acid or ammonium-(1*R*)-(-)-camphor-10-sulphonate and *N*-benzoxycarbonylglycyl-L-proline [77].

In the group of β-blockers, laboratory prepared cellulose-derivative-based CSPs have proven useful, among others [78, 79]. Enantioseparation of propranolol, atenolol and metoprolol were achieved by using different amino acids impregnated into silica gel plates: optically pure L-lysine (0.5 %) and L-arginine, L-glutamic and L-aspartic acids [80-82].

Beside L-aspartic acid also L-tartaric acid was used as a chiral selector for enantioseparation of propranolol and its derivatives. Different combinations of acetonitrile–methanol as mobile phase were found to be successful in resolving of the enantiomers and spots were usually detected using iodine vapour [83].

Bushan et al. [84] used TLC plates impregnated by (-)-erythromycin, pure L-tartaric acid, and (*R*)-mandelic acid for enantioresolution of atenolol and propranolol.

TLC enantioseparation of propranolol was also conducted on molecularly imprinted stationary phases. Several molecularly imprinted polymers were prepared using the enantiomer of (*R*)-propranolol as a print molecule [85]. Suedee et al. [86] used molecularly imprinted polymers by α-agonists: (+)-ephedrine, (+)-pseudoephedrine, (+)-norephedrine as chiral stationary phase.

2.1.3. Capillary Electrophoresis (CE)

Recently, the use of CE as a reliable method in enantioseparation has increased. The advantages include simplicity, speed, varied separation mechanisms, and low cost. The direct CE method employs various chiral selectors added to the basic electrolyte, incorporated into the gel, bound to a carrier, or immobilised on the capillary walls. Depending on the type of the chiral selector, various types of interactions may take place, such as, for example, the formation of inclusion complexes, affinity interactions, formation of micellar systems or microemulsions [87-89]. The most commonly used chiral selectors used for enantioseparation of β-blockers include different types of cyclodextrins. Cyclodextrins (CDs) and their derivatives as chiral selectors are frequently used for enantioseparation due to their good solubility in aqueous buffers and wide availability [90, 91].

Enantiomers of propranolol were successfully separated using native CDs [92] and their derivatives, namely hydroxypropyl-β-CDs [93], methyl β-CDs [94], and sulfated cyclodextrin [95]. Heptakis-2,6-di-*O*-metyl-β-CD as a chiral selector was used for enantioseparation of atenolol [96], and non selective β-blocker oxprenolol and pindolol [97].

CE method with carboxymethyl-β-cyclodextrin (CM-β-CD) as a chiral selector was applied in enantioseparation of metipranolol and quantification of side products during its synthesis [98] and also for enantioseparation of novel β-blockers derived from 4-hydroxyacetophenone [99].

Matthijs et al. [100] investigated the highly sulfated CDs (α,β,γ-HSCDs) for the determination of chiral impurity in pharmaceuticals containing propranolol and atenolol. The best separation conditions were obtained using phosphate buffer containing 5 % m/v of HS-α-CD. Sulfated derivatives of CDs, heptakis (2,3-di-*O*-methyl-6-sulfo)-β-cyclodextrin (HDMS-β-CD), and heptakis (2,3-di-*O*-acetyl-6-sulfo)-β-cyclodextrin (HDAS-β-CD) were successfully used for enantioseparation of talinolol and propranolol in a nonaqueous CE system (NACE). The use of non-aqueous solvents in the background electrolyte enhances hydrophobic analyte solubility and the method selectivity [101, 102].

Among other chiral selectors in CE, human serum albumin [103] macrocyclic antibiotics, namely clarithromycin lactobionate [104], sulfonated polysacharide χ-carragenan, and its sulfobutylether derivative [105], polysaccharides [106] and β-lactam antibiotic [107], were investigated for enantioseparation of β-blockers.

CEC- capillary electrochromatography has also become an important mode of CE for separation of enantiomers. It is a hybrid of CE and HPLC and combines the high efficacy of CE and high selectivity of HPLC. Chiral separation by CEC can be performed in wall-coated open tubular, packed and monolithic capillary column. Many chiral analyses have utilized chiral selectors based on macrocyclic antibiotics mainly vancomycin [108-110] and teicoplanin [111], derivates of cellulose and amylose [112].

Indirect method of resolution of propranolol, oxprenolol, pindolol, metoprolol and atenolol enantiomers by CEC was conducted by Aturky et al. [113]. They used precolumn derivatization with (+)-1-(9-fluorenyl)ethyl chloroformate. The prepared diastereomers were resolved on octadecylsilanized silica-gel-based stationary phases.

A recent trend in chiral CE separation is the use of microfluidic chip devices as reported by Guo et al. [114] for the analysis of atenolol and metoprolol in human urine employing CM-β-CD as chiral selector. They fabricated a microfluidic chip system with ELC detection. Racemic propranolol was separated in two enantiomers by a built miniaturized CE system coupled to deep-UV fluorescence detection. The chiral separation was carried out in a fused-silica capillary containing S-α-CD and HS-α-CD [115]. Miniaturized system offers several advantages, such as short analysis times, the need of sample volume, reduces cost analysis and waste disposal.

2.2. Stereoselective Syntheses of β-Blockers

To convert a prochiral substrate into an enantiomerically enriched product, two types of chemical catalysts are used in stereoselective syntheses of aryloxyaminopropanols. In the process of catalysis by a metal – ligand complex, stereoselection takes place through the coordination of enantiomeric ligands to the metal atom. The substrate molecule binds to this complex. Another type of chiral catalysts comprises chiral organic molecules in the absence of metals.

In addition to chemical catalysts, the syntheses of single enantiomers of β-blockers involve enzymes and live cell cultures. The stereoselective synthesis can also employ the chiron approach, wherein the chiral centre is already built into one of the precursors [116].

In asymmetric reduction of α-sulfonyloxyketones, the synthesis of enantiomerically pure arylaminoethanols (*R*)-nifenalol and (*R*)-pronethalol used N-ethyl-N-isopropylaniline-borane complex and (*R*)-methyl-CBS-oxazaborolidine as catalysts [117].

The synthesis of (*S*)- or (*R*)-epichlorohydrin or epoxide precursors of aryloxyaminopropanols can be carried out using a stereoselective epoxidation of allyl alcohols (the Sharpless epoxidation). In 2001, K. B. Sharpless was awarded the Nobel Prize in Chemistry for this discovery. The enantiomeric selection is provided by a complex of titanium isopropoxide with (+) or (-) diethyl or diisopropyl tartrate [118].

A similar principle was used in the asymmetric dihydroxylation of allyl aryl ethers catalysed by osmium tetroxide. Using a chiral ligand, hydroquinidine phthalazine-1,4-diyl diether $(DHQD)_2$-PHAL and a co-oxidant, potassium ferricyanide $K_3[Fe(CN)_6]$, (*S*)-3-arylpropan-1,2-diols were synthesized as intermediates for the synthesis of seven β-blockers [119]. Another possible method of stereoselective synthesis is the hydrolytic kinetic resolution of terminal epoxides using the Jacobsen's catalyst, which, chemically, represents a chiral complex, *N,N'*-bis(3,5-di-*tert*-butylsalicylidene)-1,2-cyclohexanediaminocobalt(II) chloride, wherein the organic ligand may be in the (*R,R*) or (*S,S*) configuration. The epoxy group of the corresponding enantiomeric form of the substrate is hydrolysed during the process to a diol, water being an effective nucleophile for the opening of the epoxide ring. Another enantiomer remains in the epoxy form and is useful for the subsequent condensation with the appropriate amine to yield an aryloxyaminopropanol [120-124].

Another published method employing kinetic resolution of a key intermediate, α-naphthyl glycidyl ether, catalysed by $Zn(NO_3)_2$ and L-tartaric acid, was used in a simple "one pot" streroselective synthesis of (*S*)-propranolol [125, 126].

Stereoselective reduction of an aminoketone intermediate in the presence of chlorides of divalent metals was used to prepare (*S*)-propranolol. The divalent metal cation forms, in the transition state, a 5-membered ring with the ketone and ether oxygen atoms and increases the regioselectivity of ketone hydrogenation [127].

Another type of chemical catalysis involves the use of purely organic substances of low molecular weight not containing metals in the process of incorporating asymmetric information in the reaction products. In the synthesis of (*S*)-propranolol and (*S*)-naftopidil, L-proline was used for chiral catalysis [128].

An organic catalyst was also used in the preparation of (*S*)-betaxolol and (*S*)-metoprolol by non-enzymatic kinetic resolution of an aminoalcohol intermediate using derivatives of higher C12 saccharides derived from sucrose [129]. In chemo-enzymatic kinetic resolution of β-blocker enantiomers, the chemical catalyst allows the reaction to proceed, but the racemate is resolved using an enzyme, thereby allowing the formation of enantiomerically enriched intermediates. Enzymatic resolution on the principle of enantioselective hydrolysis of a methyl ester intermediate or its enantioselective acylation yielded (*S*)-propranolol and (*S*)-alprenolol.

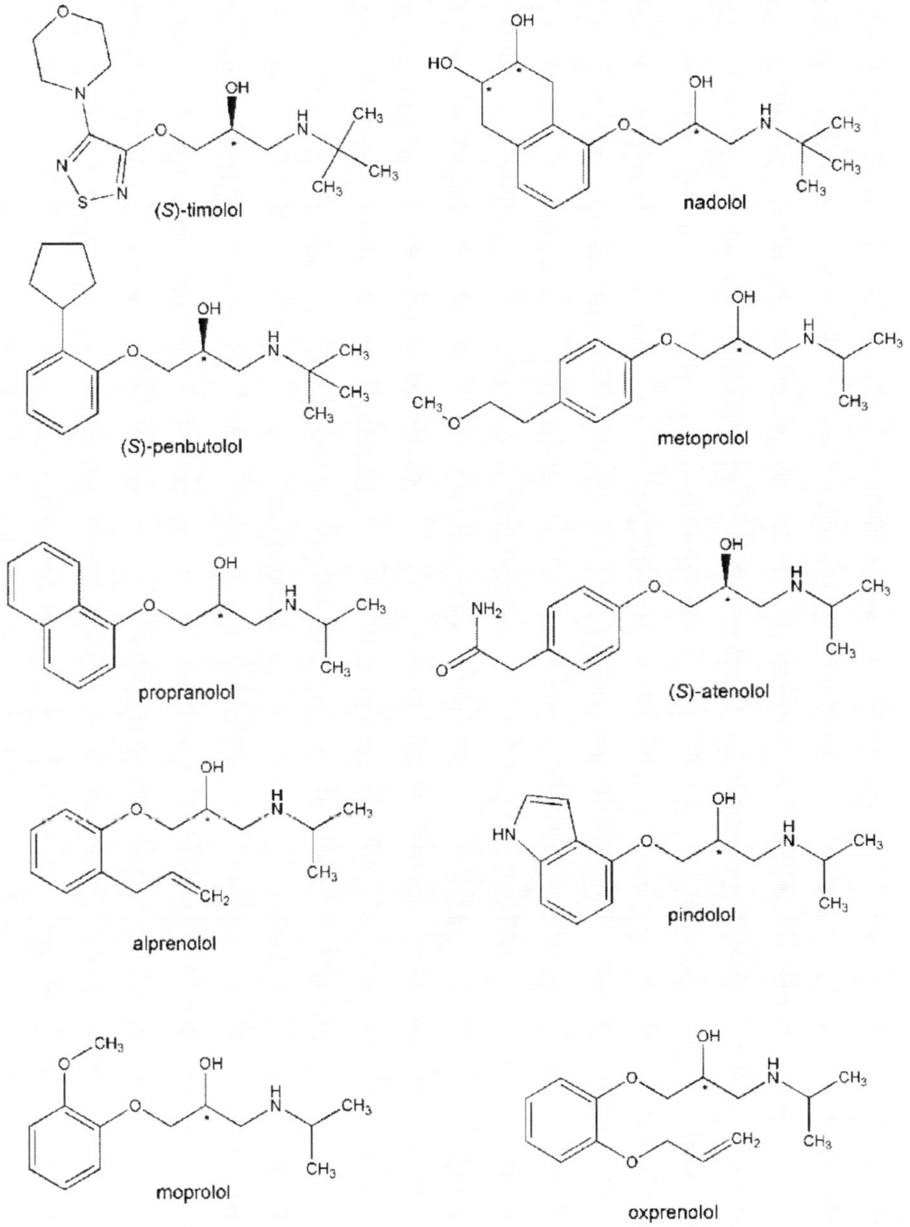

The asterisk denotes the stereogenic centre.

Figure 1. Chemical structure of major β-blockers derived from aryloxyaminopropanol.

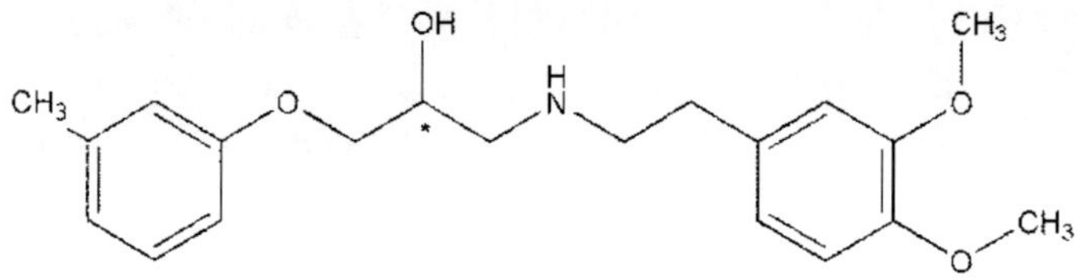

bevantolol

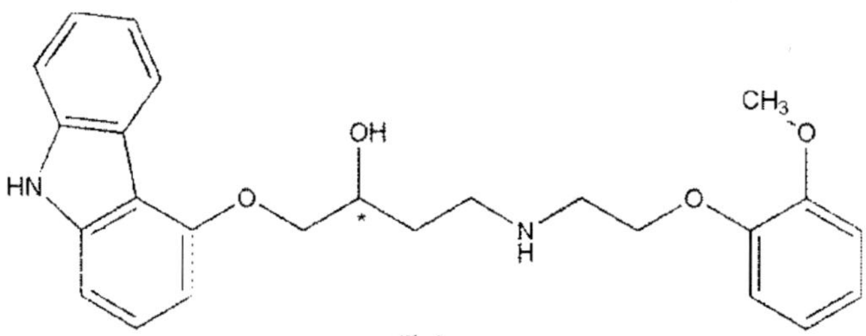

carvedilol

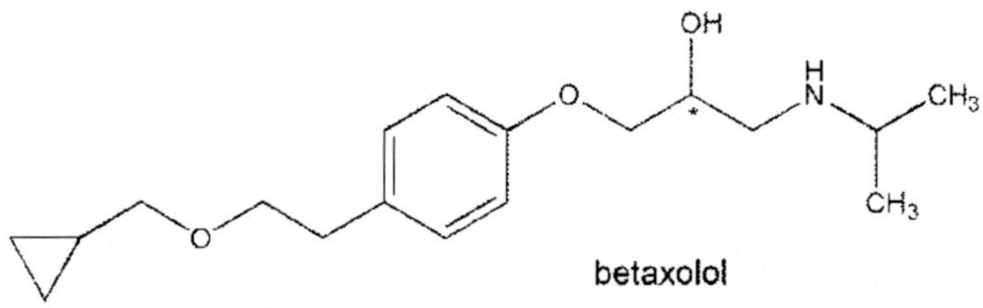

betaxolol

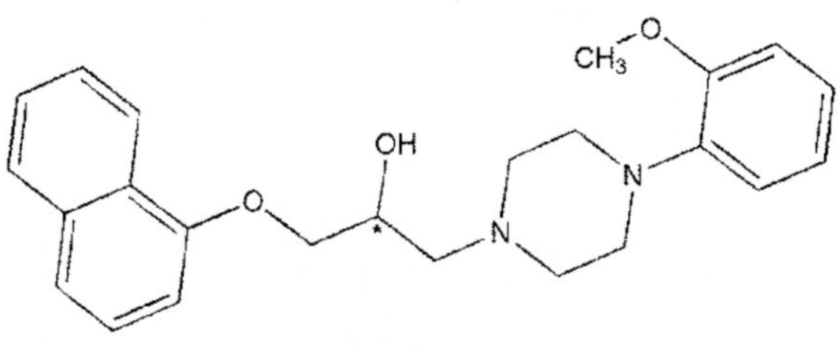

naftopidil

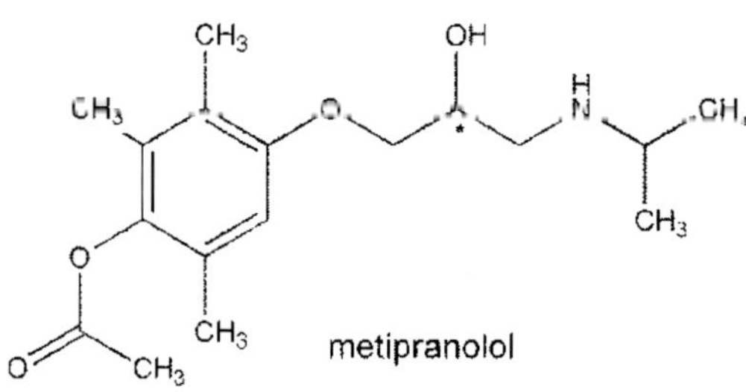

metipranolol

The asterisk denotes the stereogenic centre.

Figure 1a. Chemical structure of major β-blockers derived from aryloxyaminopropanol.

A higher enantiomeric efficiency and shorter reaction time were observed for the use of a lipase from Pseudomonas cepacia as compared to lipases isolated from porcine pancreas, Candida rugosa, Chromobacterium viscosum, and Rhizomucor mieheia [130].

A chemo-enzymatic kinetic resolution using lipases of a yeast of the Candida genus, Candida rugosa, was used for the synthesis of an (S)-enantiomer of a non-benzodiazepine anxiolytic, enciprazine, with an aryloxyaminopropanol scaffold [131].

A Pseudomonas cepacia lipase immobilised on ceramic plates was used for the enantioselective transesterification of precursors of propranolol, alprenolol, and moprolol with shorter reaction time as compared to the free (non-immobilised) lipase [132].Dynamic kinetic resolution combines the enzymatic kinetic resolution of racemic precursors and *in situ* chemical racemisation of a distomer. The newly formed racemate is again involved in the enzymatic kinetic resolution [133]. The process of dynamic kinetic resolution was also applied to the azido alcohol precursor of propranolol. It was resolved using an enzyme lipase B of *Candida antarctica* (Novozyme 435); a ruthenium-based catalyst was used as the racemisation agent [134].

Cell cultures can be used instead of isolated enzymes in resolutions of racemic substrates. In the synthesis of β-blockers of the arylaminoethanol type, a variety of microorganisms have been investigated; in addition to the most frequently used baker's yeast, *Saccharomyces cerevisiae*, these included, e. g. *Rhizopus arrhizus*, *Merulius tremellosus*, *Geotrichum candidum*, *Rhodococcus ruber* and *Trichothecium sp.* Stereoselective synthesis of (*R*)-nifenalol was performed using *Rhodotorula* sp. AS2.2241 [135].

The Chiron approach to the stereoselective synthesis of aryloxyaminopropanols comprises the use of substrates that have the specific chirality already incorporated in the structure. Such syntheses are based mainly on natural substances such as D-mannitol, (*R*)-glyceraldehyde, and L-ascorbic acid. The catalysts used in these syntheses function regardless of the chirality of the substrate [136, 137].

3. Diuretics

Diuretics are recommended as first-line drugs for the treatment of hypertension. Thiazide-type diuretics, whose mechanism of action is based on the effect in the proximal tubule, where prevent sodium reabsorption, are the most commonly prescribed diuretics. They are administered either alone or in combination with potassium-sparing diuretics, optionally with other antihypertensive agents [138].

Many of thiazide diuretics have one or more stereogenic centres in their structure. Their enantiomers may differ in the intensity of the biological activity but this has not yet been published in view of the non-specific effect of their action which is little affected by the stereochemical arrangement (Figures 3, 4). The differences in the pharmacological effects of the enantiomers have been described only for a loop diuretic, indacrinone. The (R)-enantiomer showed diuretic-natriuretic activity and the (S)-enantiomer exhibited uricosuric activity. By manipulating the enantiomeric composition, it was found that the optimal diuretic effect with a low uricosuric effect was achieved in a mixture with an enantiomer ratio of S/R 4:1. Although the development of the drug was stopped, the study of indacrinone served as the basis for the concept of adjusting the enantiomeric composition to improve the therapeutic profile of chiral drugs [139].

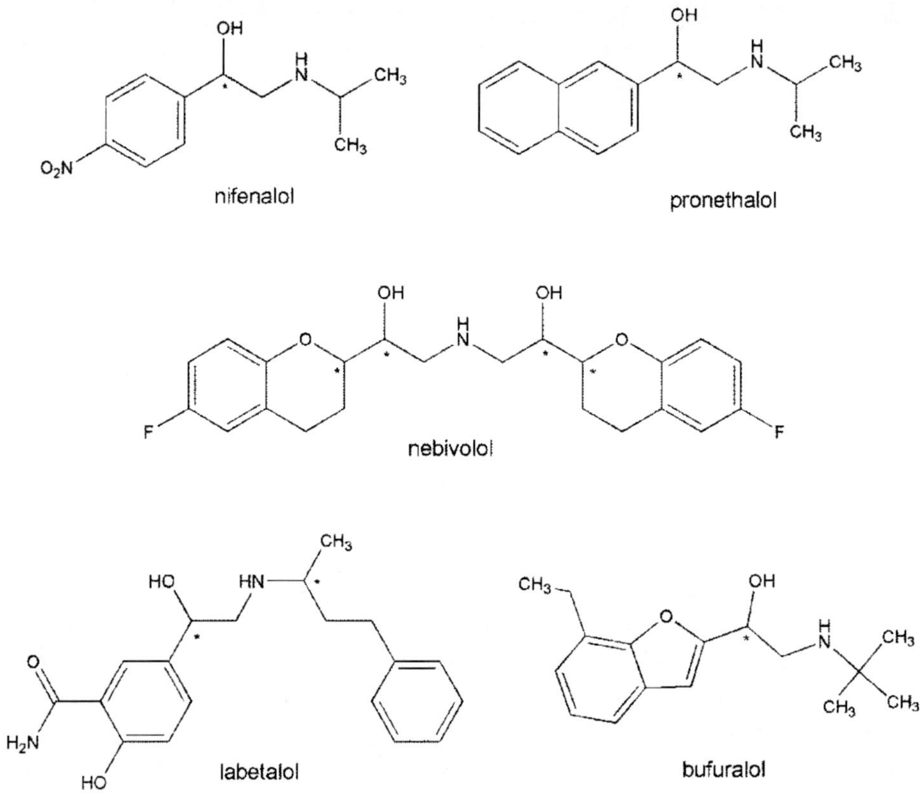

The asterisk denotes the stereogenic centre.

Figure 2. Chemical structure of major β-blockers derived from arylaminoethanol.

3.1. Stereoselective Analysis of Diuretics

Various analytical methods are described for the separation of chiral diuretics, the most commonly used one being HPLC. Most of the HPLC separations of chiral diuretics were performed on polysaccharide chiral stationary phases – derivatives of cellulose and amylose.

Visegrády et al. [140] observed the enantioseparation of a series of thiazide diuretics (butizide, polythiazide, bendroflumethiazide, chlortalidone, cicletanine, mefruside, and bemetizide) on three chiral columns, Chiralcel OD-RH with cellulose tris-3,5-dimethylphenyl carbamate as the chiral selector, Chiralcel OJ-R with cellulose tris-4-methylbenzoate, and Chirobiotic T with teicoplanin CSP. The columns used exhibited a good chiral resolving power. Most of the diuretics were resolved to the baseline on at least one of the columns used.

For example, bemetizide, which has two stereogenic centres, was resolved to the baseline into all four stereoisomers on a Chiralcel OD-RH column. The mobile phase used in the enantioseparation consisted of acetonitrile and water (35:65 v/v). Changing the ratio of acetonitrile/water to 40/60 (v/v) reduced the retention and the resolution was poorer. On Chiralcel OJ-R column, chlortalidone and polythiazide could not be separated and for bemetizide, only two enantiomers were resolved, similarly as on teicoplanin column.

The enantioseparation of diuretic etozoline, was performed on two substituted cellulose phenylcarbamate columns with an electron donor (methyl) and an electron acceptor (chlorine) attached to the phenyl group, namely on cellulose tris-4-chloro-3-methylphenylcarbamate and on cellulose tris-3-chloro-4-methylphenylcarbamate.

On both columns, the two enantiomers of etozoline were successfully separated to the baseline [141].

Chankvetadze et al. [142] compared the enantioseparation of etozoline on four types of polysaccharide CSPs in polar organic mode using acetonitrile and methanol as the mobile phase. The best enantioselectivity for etozoline was exhibited on a CSP Chiralpak AD column with both mobile phases. The lowest enantioselectivity was achieved on Chiralcel OJ.

Comercially available column Chiralpak IC (cellulose tris(3,5-dichlorophenyl)carbamate) was used for enantioseparation of indapamide in serum and was applied for pharmacokinetic study [143]. Ates et al. [144] tested the enantioseparation of chlortalidone on new chlorinated polysaccharide columns: Sepapak-2 (cellulose tris-3-chloro-4-methyl phenyl carbamate) and Sepapak-3 (amylose tris-5-chloro-2-methyl phenyl carbamate), in polar organic mode using acetonitrile, methanol, and ethanol as eluants.

Chlortalidone was resolved to the baseline on Sepapak-2 eluting with acetonitrile and ethanol with the addition of diethylamine and trifluoroacetic acid.

Enantioselective separations of diuretics were also obtained using β-cyclodextrin and its derivatives in both stationary and mobile phase.

Different β-cyclodextrins (β-CD, HP-CD, Me-β-CD) have been tested as chiral additives in the mobile phase for the chromatographic analysis of chlortalidone enantiomers in a C18 LiChrospher column. The best enantioseparation of chlortalidone was achieved by using β-CD. The method was applied for analysis of chlortalidone enantiomers in different pharmaceutical preparations [145].

β-Cyclodextrin as a chiral stationary was used for separation of enantiomers of chlortalidone [146] and bendroflumetiazide [147].

Zhong, Q. et al. [148] synthetised novel nitrophenyl-substituted β-cyclodextrin (DNP-*O*-β-CD) CSP´s and compared their separation efficiency in all three modes. Chlortalidone was successfully separated on five DNP-*O*-β-CD's in both the normal and reverse mode, the best resolution being achieved on CSP-5 (three dinitrophenyl substitutions on β-cyclodextrin).

Other chiral stationary phases used included Pirkle phases, proteins, macrocyclic antibiotics, and commercially unavailable chiral stationary phases.

Welch et al. [149] carried out separation of different drugs, including indapamide and bendroflumethiazide, on a Pirkle CSP using a chiral column, Whelk-O-1.

Hyun and Pirkle [150] studied enantioseparation of number of racemic thiazide diuretics and analogues on two diastereomeric chiral stationary phases prepared from (*S*)- or (*R*)-alpha-[1-(6,7-dimethyl)naphthyl]-10-dodecenylamine and (*S*)-2-phenylpropanoic acid. Of the two diastereomeric CSPs, the (*S,S*) and the (*R,S*), the former is found to be better than the latter in separating the enantiomers of the racemic thiazide diuretics and their analogues with complete separation being observed on the (*S,S*)-CSP.

Another newly developed Pirkle-type straight chiral stationary phase, based on the 3,5-dinitrobenzoyl derivative of 1,2 diphenylethylene-diamine and known as ULMO, has been successfully applied to the direct resolution of the enantiomers of several diuretics (althiazide, butizide and chlortiazide). A mobile phase consisting of hexane and propan-2-ol appears the most appropriate for the chiral separation of the tested diuretics on the ULMO-column [151]. Enantioseparation of chlortalidone and indapamide was performed on macrocyclic antibiotic-based CSP. Chirobiotic V (vancomycin), Chirobiotic T (teicoplanin), Chirobiotic TAG (teicoplanin aglycone) a Chirobiotic R (ristocetin A) using three possible separation modes: reversed phase with methanol/buffer mobile phases, normal phase with hexane/ ethanol mobile phases and polar ionic mode (PIM) with 100% methanol mobile phase with trace amounts of acid and/or base. All separation were studied in a 5-45 °C temperature range. In the majority, the enantioresolution decreased or even vanished when temperature increased [152-3].

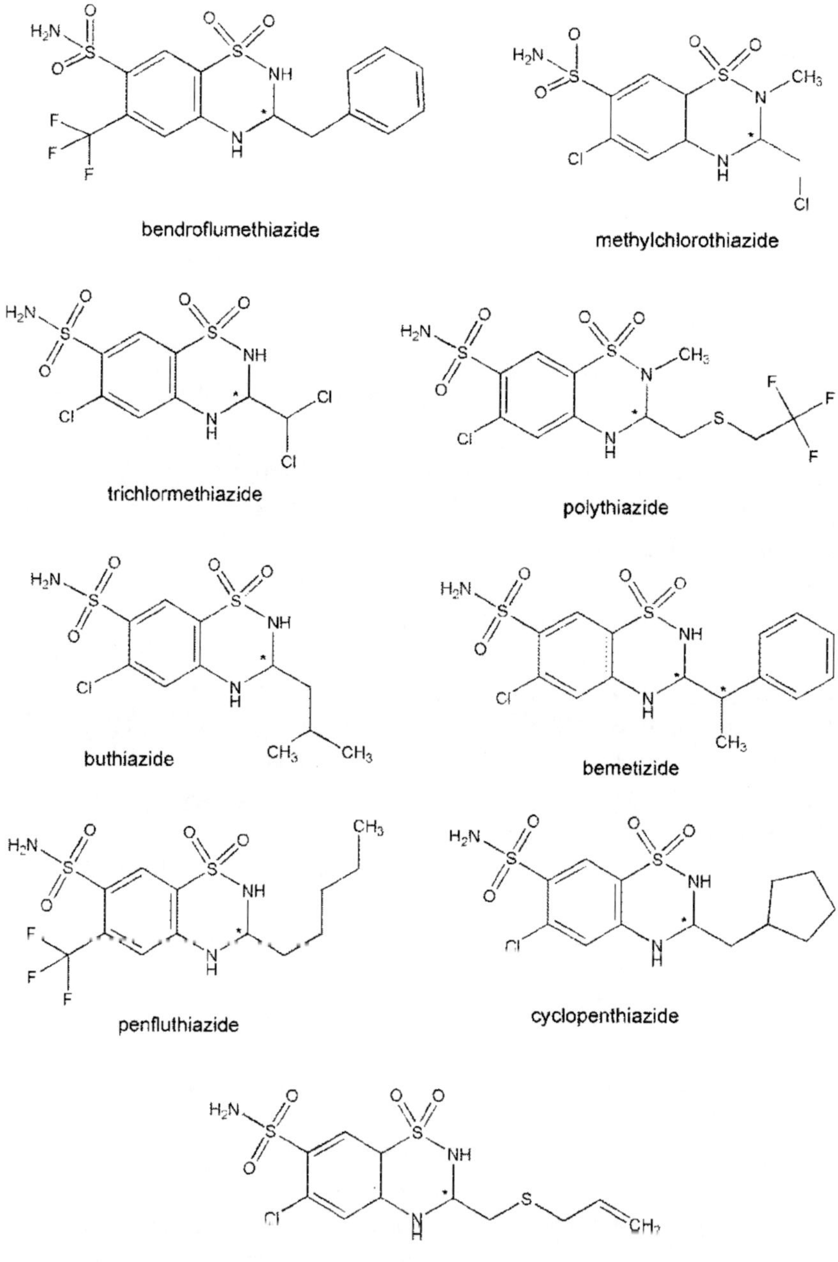

The asterisk denotes the stereogenic centre.

Figure 3. Chemical structure of major thiazide diuretics.

Protein based CSPs containing cellobiohydrolase (CBG-58) from *Phanerochaete chrysosporium* and cellobiohydrolase (CBH 58) from *Trichoderma reesei* were used for enantioseparation of chlortalidone. Resolution of enantiomers was similar on both chiral phases column, but retention was higher on CBH 58 phase [154].

For diuretics, in addition to enantioseparation by HPLC, successful use was made of other methods such as supercritical fluid chromatography, capillary electrochromatography, and capillary electrophoresis.

Barnhart et al. [155] compared enantioseparation of different drugs, including diuretics - bendroflumethiazide, indapamide, chlortalidone, althiazide on poly(trans-1,2-cyclohexanediyl-bis acrylamide) (P-CAP) with polysaccharide-based CSPs (Chiralpak AD-H and AS-H, Chiralcel OD-H and OJ-H columns) using supercritical fluid chromatography. Overall, the synthetic polymer-based P-CAP showed less chiral discrimination power compared to the derivatized polysaccharide-based CSPs.

Rapid enantioseparation with high resolution of chlortalidone enantiomers was achieved on 3,5-dimethylphenyl carbamate cyclofructan 7 chiral stationary phase in supercritical fluid chromatography. The mobile phase consisted from carbon dioxide: propan-2-ol: trifluoroacetic acid (80:20:0.1) [156]. Mangelings, et al. [157] used the miniaturised techniques, capillary electrochromatography (CEC) and capillary liquid chromatography (CLC), for the chiral separation of chlortalidone. In both cases, HP-β-CDn was used as a chiral selector in the mobile phase, while an achiral stationary phase was used.

Fillet et al. [158] accomplished enantioseparation of acidic drugs including chlortalidone by capillary electrophoresis (CE) using polyanionic sulfobutyl-β-cyclodextrin in combination with a neutral cyclodextrin derivative such as trimethyl-β-cyclodextrin (TMCD) or dimethyl-β-cyclodextrin (DMCD) as the chiral selector, at pH=3 with the phosphoric acid – triethanolamine buffer. CE method for enantioseparation of indapamide was developed by Tero-Vescan et al. [159]. Sulfobuthyl ether-β-CD was proved as a optimal chiral selector for the enantioseparation. Using a buffer solution (25 mM Na_2HPO_4, 25 mM NaH_2PO_4, and 5 mM sulfobuthyl ether-β-CD at pH=7, (a voltage of + 25 kV, 15°C), the separation of the two enantiomers was succeeded in 6 minutes, with a resolution of 4.30.

3.2. Stereoselective Synthesis of Diuretics

There are several papers describing stereoselective syntheses of diuretics or their intermediates. An efficient method for (*S*)-(+)-indacrinone was developed involving a *cinchona* alkaloid using catalyzed asymmetric methylation for preparation of intermediate that was converted in three additional steps to final chiral compounds [160].

Both enantiomers of indacrinone were prepared in high yield and enantiomeric purity by efficient catalytic asymmetric alkylations [161]. Zhu et al. [162] performed Nazarov-type cyclization for preparation of polysubstituted indanones as intermediates for chiral indacrinone. Starting materials were 1,4-enediones and $AlCl_3$ was highlighted as the most efficient promoter for this reaction. Allin et al. [163] reported stereoselective approach to the indolino[8,7-b]indole used also in the preparation of diuretic compounds. Spironolactone is an aldosterone antagonist, and has been used for more than thirty years as one of the preferred diuretics in the treatment of hypertension without symptomes.

7α-Methylthio-3β-hydroxy-17α-pregn-4-ene-21,17-carbolactone and 7α-methylthio-3β-hydroxy-17α-pregn-4-ene-21,17-carbolactone, the two major metabolites of spironolactone, were prepared stereoselectively by exploring different types of reduction reagents. For the 3β-hydroxyl isomer, the application of $NaBH_4/CeCl_3 \cdot 7H_2O$ gave the best result while for the 3α-hydroxyl isomer, K-selectride seemed to provide the highest stereoselectivity [164].

4. α_2-Adrenergic Agonists

Indirect acting antihypertensives that have a stereogenic centre in their structure include methyldopa - (*S*)-(-)-2-amino-3-(3,4-dihydroxyphenyl)-2-methylpropanoic acid (Figure 6). It is a prodrug that exerts its antihypertensive action via an active metabolite by several mechanisms:

Stimulation of central inhibitory α_2-receptors reducing sympathetic tone;

- Substitution of endogenous dopamine on dopaminergic nerve terminals as a false neurotransmitter;
- Reduction in plasma renin activity and peripheral vascular resistance

Although used frequently as antihypertensive agent in the past, metyldopa´s significant advere effects limit its current use largely to treatment of hypertension in pregnancy, where it has a record for safety [165].

The (*R*)- and (*S*)- enantiomers of α-methyldopa (mDOPA) were prepared from chiral hydantoins, obtained in a good yield from phenyl isocyanates and *N*-[(*S*)-α-phenylethyl] glycinate. Dialkyl hydantoins (*S*,*S*)-7 and (*S*,*R*)-7, after flash chromatography separation followed by hydrolysis, provide (*S*) and (*R*)-α-methyldopa in good yield [166].

Capillary electrophoresis method was employed for enantiomeric separation of methyldopa and structurally related compounds – DOPA (3,4-dihydroxyphenylalanine) and carbidopa (2-hydrazino-2-methyl-3-(3,4-dihydroxyphenyl)propanoic acid) using several sulfobutylated beta-cyclodextrin as a chiral additive and uncoated fused-silica capillaries. Resolution was strongly influenced by the concentration of the chiral selector added to the background electrolyte. In fact, 2-5 mM of SBE-CD enabled the resolution of DOPA and mDOPA enantiomers, while CDOPA optical isomers were resolved by using either 0.5 mM or 6-20 mM of SBE-CD. The latter separation conditions (reversed polarity mode) made it possible to obtain inversion of migration order [167].

Chiral HPLC methods were also used successfully for the determination of the enantiomeric purity of levodopa, methyldopa, carbidopa and tryptophan. The investigated method uses phenylalanine and copper sulfate in the mobile phase and a C18 column [168]. The determination of enantiomeric purity of methyldopa and levodopa was accomplished using a chiral ligand-exchange chromatography with an ordinary C18 column and a chiral mobile phase containing *N*,*N*-dimethyl-L-phenylalanine and Cu(II) acetate. Beside this method, chiral teicoplanin column in polar organic mode with methanol-acetic acid-triethylamine (1.00:0.05:0.05, v/v/v) mobile phase was used for determination of D enantiomers. In comparison with pharmacopoeial polarimetric methods (according to the European

Pharmacopoeia), the LC methods proved to be much more sensitive giving detection limits of 0.04% for D-DOPA and 0.3% for D-methyldopa [169].

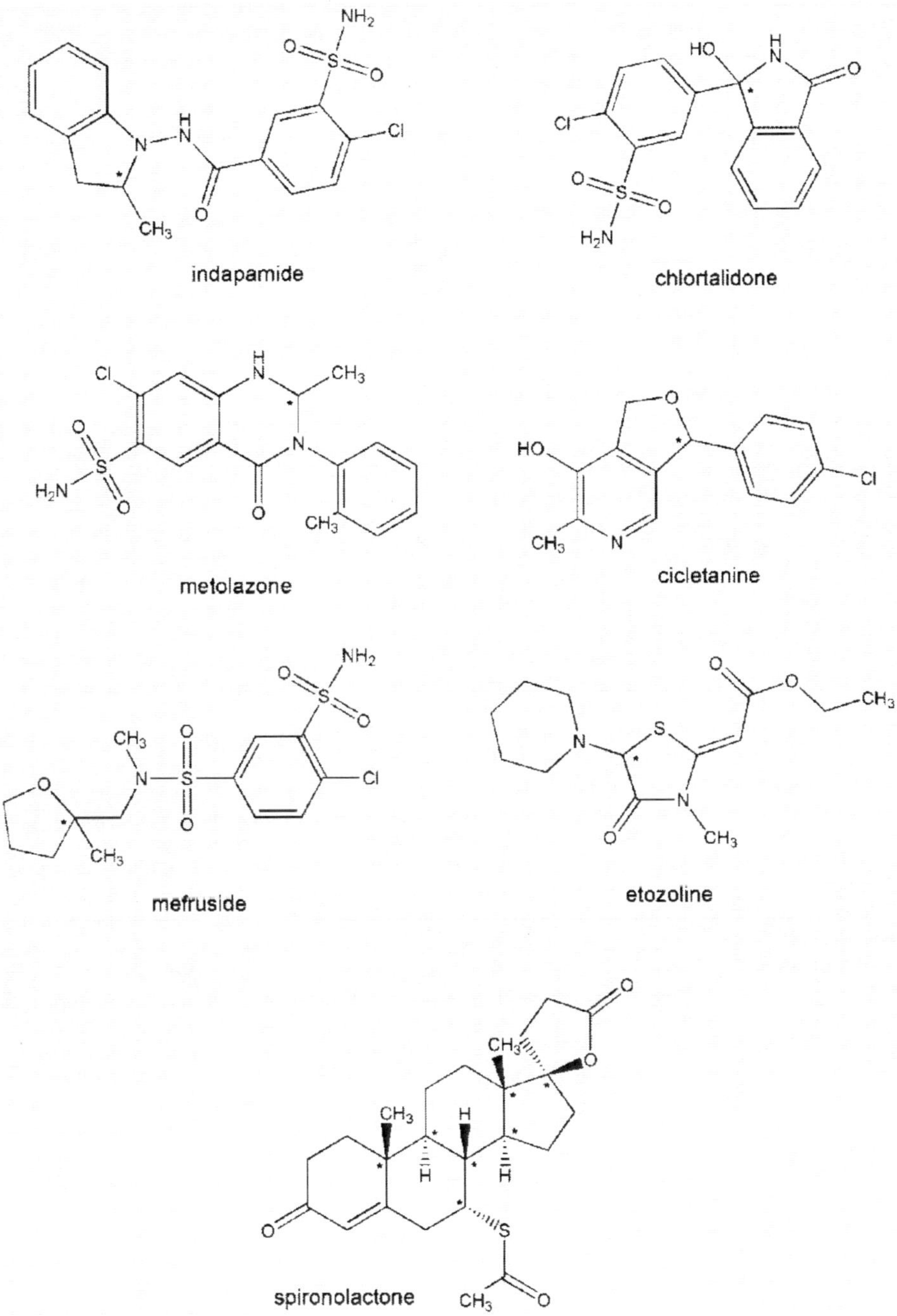

The asterisk denotes the stereogenic centre.

Figure 4. Chemical structure of various diuretics.

5. Ace Inhibitors

ACE inhibitors represent drugs that, in addition to the antihypertensive effect, also have cardioprotective, vasodilatory, and renal protective effects; captopril was found to also possess antioxidant activity.

Combination with diuretics or other antihypertensive agents leads to an increase in their antihypertensive effect [170]. The effect of ACE inhibitors is based on influencing the renin-angiotensin-aldosterone system. The key role is played by renin and the angiotensin converting enzyme (ACE), which is a metalloprotease having Zn^{2+} in its active site.

Renin itself functions as an enzyme that cleaves angiotensinogen (alpha$_1$-globulin) into an inactive decapeptide angiotensin I. Angiotensin I is converted by the action of angioconvertase into an octapeptide – angiotensin II with a significant vasoconstrictive effect. Blocking the production of angiotensin II by means of ACE inhibitors leads to a decrease of blood pressure and subsequently aldosterone level is reduced. ACE inhibitors inactivate the active site of angioconvertase by forming coordination bonds with the Zn^{2+} cations [171].

Possible mechanisms of action of these drugs include inhibition of hydrolysis of *N*-acetyl -seryl-aspartyl-lysyl-proline (Ac-SDKP) [172].

According to the nature of the functional group (ligand), ACE inhibitors can be classified as [173]:

- sulfanyl ACE inhibitors (captopril, alacepril, zofenopril, and others)
- carboxylic ACE inhibitors (enalapril, perindopril, ramipril, cilazapril, lisinopril and others)
- phosphinyl ACE inhibitors (fosenopril, ceranapril and others) (Figures 5, 5a)

ACE inhibitors have at least two chiral centres and can form several optically active isomers. Only one of the stereoisomers is capable of interacting with the active site of the receptor. For virtually all isomers, only one enantiomer is used in clinical practice – an eutomer having all of the stereogenic centres in the (*S*)-configuration [174]. One of the first drugs of this class is captopril bearing a sulfanyl group. It is used in arterial hypertension and heart failure. A recent study confirmed that as a result of the presence of the sulfanyl groups, it also acts as a free radical quencher [175]. Captopril has the absolute configuration of (2*S*,2*S*) and of the three other diastereomers, only (2*R*,2*S*) is considered an undesirable product.

5.1. Stereoselective Analysis of ACE Inhibitors

Captopril has been analysed mainly by chromatographic methods: TLC, GC-MS, HPLC with UV, fluorescence, electrochemical detection [176] and LC-MS/MS method [177]. The GC method developed for the stereoisomeric purity determination of captopril was based on the combined information derived from the analyses of the captopril sample on two GC systems, one with a chiral and the other with an achiral column [178].

Owens et al. [179] developed a method to separate the diastereomers and rotamers of captopril by reversed-phase LC using teicoplanin as the chiral selector. Captopril is relatively unstable, which does not permit its detection by UV absorbance in clinical studies. The detection of captopril in HPLC analyses is improved using derivatization agents such as Ellmans reagent or 2,4'-dibromoacetophenone [180]. Other methods used for the analysis of captopril include capillary electrophoresis and capillary isotachophoresis [181, 182]. An alternative to the preceding captopril detection methods is the electrochemical detection using graphite or selective membrane electrodes [183, 184]. The advantages include simplicity, speed, and low cost. The sensitivity and reproducibility of these electrodes was not high and contamination of the surface often occurred. These undesirable effects were successfully eliminated with a thin-film electrode consisting of boron and diamond [185]. Most other ACE inhibitors are used in practice in the form of prodrugs (e.g. enalapril, lisinopril). These drugs in the form of carboxylic or phosphinic esters are metabolised in the body to the active substance. Kocijan et al. [186] monitored the chromatographic behaviour of lisinopril, enalapril and its two degradation products – enalaprilat (a hydrolytic degradation product) and diketopiperazine (cyclisation degradation product) depending on the temperature of the column and the pH of the mobile phase.

It was found that the rate of isomerisation increased with temperature. At 80 °C and pH = 2, all the studied compounds appear as narrow chromatographic peaks. Reducing the temperature causes the peaks to spread or split. At 6 °C, enalapril appears in two peaks which belong to its *cis*- and *trans*- rotation isomers.

The ACE inhibitor, enalapril and its metabolite enalaprilat can exist in solution as *cis* and *trans* conformers which interconvert around the amide bond at room temperature. Both of conformers were resolved using HPLC or capillary electrophoresis method [187]. In addition nuclear overhauser enhancement difference was used for the identification of the conformers of enalaprilat. The *trans* isomer was the major form [188].

Bouabdallah [189] investigated the separation of *cis* and *trans*- isomers of lisinopril by HPLC. It was demonstrated that complete separation of the two isomers can be achieved at low temperature at either neutral or low pH together with appropriate type and concentration of organic solvent. The classical analytical methods for ACE inhibitors are being replaced with biosensors making enantioseparation of a sample a simple process. ACE inhibitors (*S*)-cilazapril, (*S*)-trandolapril, and (*S*)-pentopril were enantioselectively determined using an amperometric biosensor based on L-amino oxidase using a chemically modified carbon paste. The low limits of detection obtained were 5 pmol/l (I), 15 mumol/l (II), and 5 mumol/l (III), respectively [190]. This type of amperometric biosensor has been developed also for the enantiolysis from raw material as well as from dosage forms for the (*S*)-enantiomers of enalapril, ramipril, and pentopril [191].

(*S*)- and (*R*)-perindopril were also simultaneously detected using an amperometric biosensor based on L-amino oxidase as a detector in a flow system. The method was developed to enable the separation of the inactive (*R*)-enantiomer from the (*S*)-enantiomer [192].

5.2. Stereoselective Syntheses of ACE Inhibitors

Stereoselective synthesis is an alternative method for obtaining of pure isomers of ACE inhibitors. Ciabatti et al. [193] described the synthesis of 1-[(2-mercaptocyclopentyl) carbonyl]-L-prolines, 1-[(2-mercaptocyclobutyl) carbonyl]-L-prolines and related benzoyl derivatives as pure isomers.

The abilities of all of the compounds to inhibit angiotensin converting enzyme (ACE) in vitro and in vivo and to lower the systolic blood pressure in renal hypertensive dogs were determined.

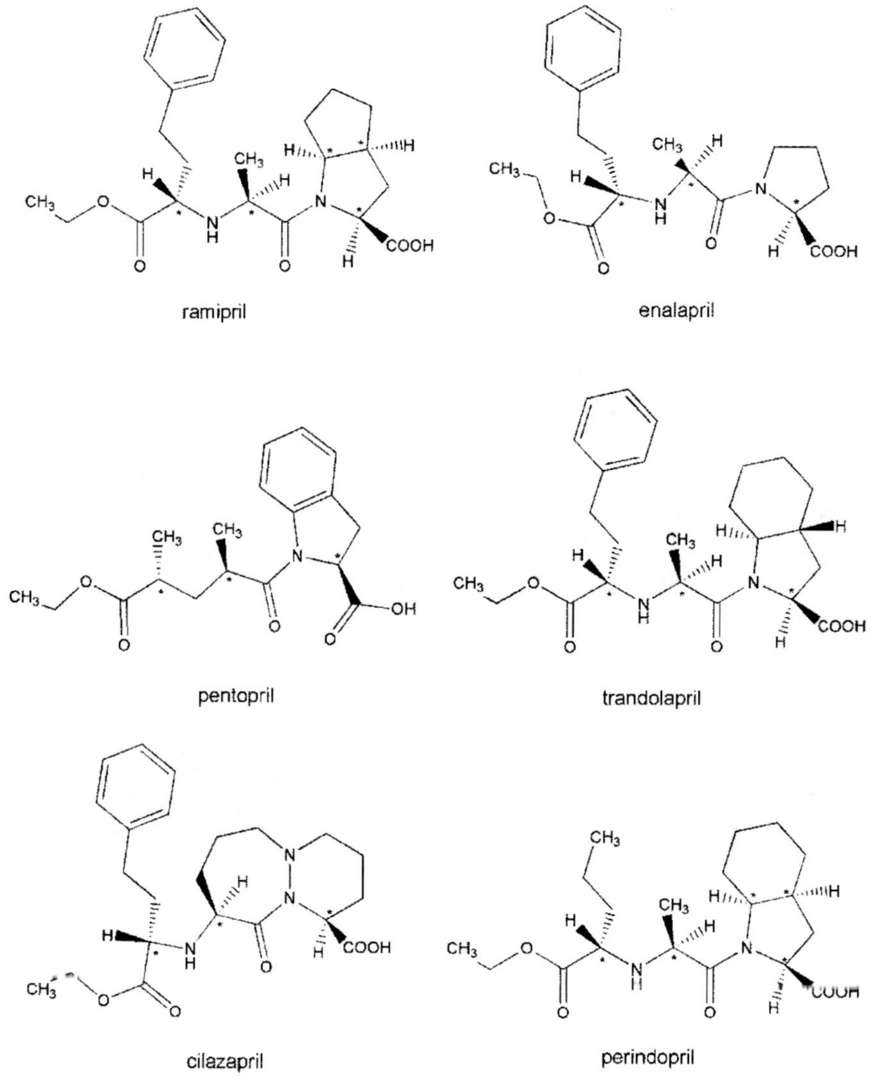

The asterisk denotes the stereogenic centre.

Figure 5. Chemical structure of major ACE inhibitors.

Three of them, namely 1-[[2-(benzoylthio)cyclopentyl]carbonyl]-L-proline (10f(*R,S*], 1-[(2-mercaptocyclopentyl)carbonyl]-L-proline (10g(*R,S*], and 1-[[2-(benzoylthio)cyclobutyl] carbonyl]-L-proline (16f(*R,S*], were found to be as potent as captopril in reducing blood pressure. The influence of chirality and ring size on the ACE inhibition is described.

The work of Oritz et al. [194] described the synthesis of two new diastereomers of captopril derivatives. These epimers were achieved by conjugate addition of thioacetic acid and α-toluenethiol to α,β-unsaturated system. Their isolation of epimers was possible because of the high crystallinity showed by one epimer compared to the other one.

An enantioselective synthesis of the ACE inhibitor benazepril was achieved through an asymmetric reduction of 4-(2-nitrophenyl)-2,4-dioxobutyric acid ethyl ester employing baker's yeast as the reductive catalyst.

The enantiomeridc purity of prepared intermediate was checked using chiral analysis on Chiralcel OC column with mobile phase hexane: propan-2-ol (97:3, v/v) [195].

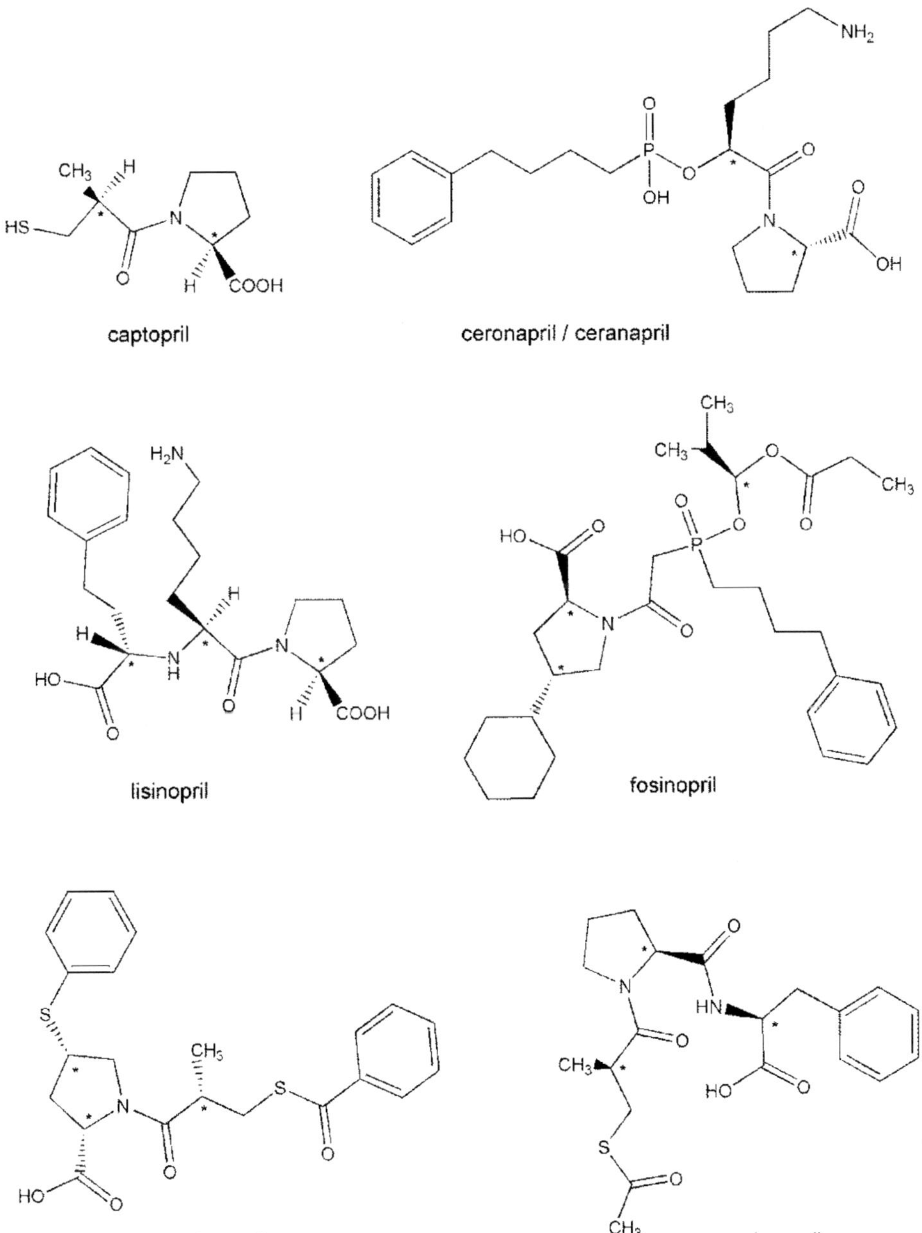

The asterisk denotes the stereogenic centre.

Figure 5a. Chemical structure of major ACE inhibitors.

Mistra et al. [196] prepared an important intermediate of benazepril ethyl 3-phthalimido-2,3,4,5-tetrahydro-1H-[1]benzazepin-2-one-1-acetate under the influence of microwave irradiation. An formal enantioselective synthesis of benazepril·HCl, an antihypertensive drug, was reported by Yu et al. [197]. The desribed synthesis employed an asymmetric aza-Michael addition of L-homophenylalanine ethyl ester to 4-(2-nitrophenyl)-4-oxo- but-2-enoic acid methyl ester as the key step to prepare (2*S*,3'*S*)-2-(2-oxo-2,3,4,5- tetrahydro-1*H*-benzo[b] azepin-3-ylamino)-4-phenylbutyric acid ethyl ester, which is the key intermediate leading to benazepril.

Over the past decade, L-homophenylalanine is extensively used in the pharmaceutical industry as a precursor for production of ACE inhibitors. A number of chemical methods have been reported thus far for the synthesis of L-homophenylalanine. However, chemical methods generally suffer from process complexity, high cost and environmental pollution. On the other hand, enantiomerically pure L-homophenylalanine can be obtained efficiently by employing biocatalytic methods. [198].

Other types of syntheses of ACE inhibitors were reviewed by Lima et al. [199].

6. Renin Inhibitors

Some of the currently used antihypertensive drugs intervene at different point of the renin-angiotensin system. Aliskiren became the first clinicaly used drug from this group [200]. It selectively inhibits human renin, the enzyme responsible for the conversion of angiotensiogen to angiotensin I, therefore, the final production of the vasoconstrictor angiotensin II is inhibited [201, 202]. Aliskiren has four chiral centers, but is obtained as a single diastereomer, all (*S*)-configured (Figure 6). Validated HPLC method for enantioseparation of aliskiren was described by Ashok et al. [203]. Separation of aliskiren enantiomers was achieved on an immobilized type Chiralpak IC chiral stationary phase (cellulose tris(3,5-dichlorophenycarbamate) using a mixture of acetonitrile: *n*-butyl amine (100:0.1 v/v) as a mobile phase. Resolution between the two enantiomers was greater than 3.0. The method is recommended for the routine determination of (*R*)-aliskiren in aliskiren bulk drug sample.

7. Angiotensin II Receptor Antagonists

Angiotensin II receptor antagonists, also known as angiotensin receptor blockers (ARBs), or sartans, are a group of pharmaceuticals that modulate the renin–angiotensin–aldosterone system by inhibition of angiotensin II receptor type and are widely employed for treatment of all grades hypertension [204]. They encompass the group of tetrazole derivative and imidazole derivatives. The chiral structure appears in valsartan, which belongs to the nonpeptide terazole derivative. Pure (*S*)-enantiomer is essentially used in the therapy of hypertension (Figure 6). Several techniques were reported for the determination of valsartan individually in pharmaceutical dosage forms or human serum samples such as HPLC [205] LC-MS/MS [206] or high performance capillary electrophoresis [207-8]. However, for determination of enantiomeric purity of valsartan the enantioselective analytical methods are necessary.

A few HPLC method have been reported for separation of valsartan and its enantiomers in bulk drug and tablet. The enantioseparation of valsartan was achieved on α_1-glycoprotein (Chiral AGP) with a phosphate buffer, pH=7, containing 2% (v/v) propan-2-ol as a mobile phase [209]. Rane et al. [210] achieved enantioseparation of valsartan on Chiralpak AD-H (amylose based stationary phase) column using a mobile phase consisting of hexane: propan-2-ol:trifluoroacetic acid (85:15:0.2, v/v/v).

Recently, capillary zone electrophoresis method for enantioseparation of valsartan has been developed. Acetyl-β-cyclodextrin was used as chiral selector. The assay was validated for (*R*)-enantiomer of valsartan in the range 0.04-3 % and was applied to the determination of the chiral purity of valsartan tablets [211].

8. Calcium Channel Blocking Agents

Calcium channel blocking agents inhibit the movement of calcium ion across the cell membrane by blocking the L-type (slow) calcium channel. Calcium channel blocking agents are used for treatment of hypertension, angina pectoris and supraventricular arrhythmias.

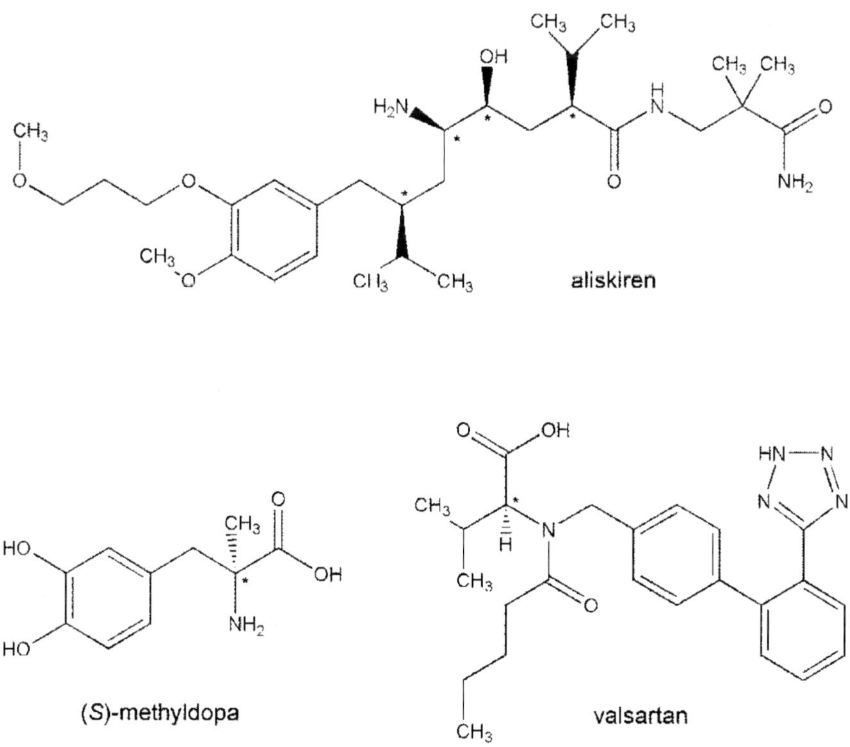

The asterisk denotes the stereogenic centre.

Figure 6. Chemical structure of (*S*)-methyldopa, aliskiren, valsartan.

In this chapter calcium channel blocking agents are classified into three groups according to their chemical structure:

- dihydropyridines (nitrendipine, nimodipine, nicardipine, nilvadipine, isradipine, felodipine, lercanidipine, benidipine and amlodipine)
- phenylalkylamines (verapamil, gallopamil, prenylamine, fendiline)
- benzothiazepines (diltiazem); [212-214] (Figures 7, 8)

8.1. Dihydropyridines

4-Aryl-substituted 1,4-dihydropyridines belong to the most potent cardioactive compounds. Structural modification at various positions of the phenyl ring in dihydropyridines affect the activity profile of this class of calcium channel blockers [215].

Nifedipine is a chiral compound, a prototype of this class of compounds (first generation), has been used in general medical practice wordwide for the treatment of hypertension and vasospastic angina for over two decades. Different substituents in compounds of the second – generation such as amlodipine, nitrendipine and nicardipine lead to chiral derivatives whose enantiomers differ in their pharmacological effects. In the case of the calcium antagonist, the differences are quantitative.

However, the introduction of certain substituent in position 3 or 5 can lead to calcium agonists. The pharmacological efficiency as calcium agonist or antagonist depends on the configuration at the stereogenic C4-atom. In the case of felodipine, nitrendipine and niguldipine, the (*S*)-enantiomers are more potent than (*R*)-enantiomers. There are also well-known examples, within this series of agents whose individual enantiomers have opposite effect on channel function. Thus (*S*)-enantiomers are calcium channel activators, whereas the (*R*)-enantiomers are antagonists [216, 139]. Stereoselectivity of differing degrees has been reported in the pharmacokinetics of this class of drugs (amlodipine, felodipine, gallopamil, nicardipine, nivaldipine, prenylamine). For all the drugs in this class, it appears that plasma concentrations of more active enantiomers are equal to or higher than those of the less active enantiomer. When these drugs have been given intravenously, stereoselectivity is considerably less than given orally, suggesting enantioselective presystemic metabolism [11].

Jabor et al. [217] evaluated stereoselectivity of pharmacokinetic of lercanidipine. The results showed that plasma levels after an oral dose of rac lercanidipine administered to a healthy volunteers were found to be higher for the more active (*S*)-enantiomer. Enantioselective pharmacokinetics the enantiomers of clevidipine an ultrashort-acting dihydropyridine antagonist was described by Ericsson et al. [218]. Both enantiomers were high-clearance compounds with similar blood clearance values. The volume of distribution for the enantiomers was slightly different, presumably due to differences in the protein binding. From a pharmacokinetic point of view, the use of a single enantiomer as an alternative to the racemic clevidipine will not offer any clinical advantages.

8.1.1. Stereoselective Analysis of Dihydropyridines

Many of analytical methods have been used for the separation of enantiomers of the dihydropyridines. HPLC seems to be the most widely used technique for the enantioseparation and quantification of enantiomers as well as in preceding chiral compounds (β-blockers, diuretic, ACE-inbitors). Many chiral stationary phases such as polysaccharides (cellulose or amylose derivatives) or proteins were used for the direct enantioseparation of different compounds such a isradipine, nimodipine, benidipine, nitrendipine, nicardipine etc. Isradipine (second generation of dihydropyridines) is commercially available as a racemic mixture of its (+)-(*S*) and (-)-(*R*)-enantiomers. In therapeutic concentrations, the calcium entry blocking effect is primarily due to (+)-enantiomer. Isradipine was separated by HPLC on a Chiral AGP column and an analytical CN column. Using mobile phase containing 10 mM phosphate butter (pH=7) and acetonitrile (88:12) with 25 mM tetrapropylammonium bromide, the enantiomers were baseline separated [219].

Chiral-AGP as the chiral stationary phase was also used in enantioseparation of a pharmacological active dihydropyridines including felodipine. In this study was found, that mobile phase pH, organic modifier(s) and column temperature influenced the chiral recognition [220].

Japanese authors examined the optical resolution of six dihydropyridines, nimodipine, nilvadipine, benidipine, nitrendipine, isradipine and nicardipine, on six HPLC columns with chiral selectors xylan bis(3,5-dichlorophenyl carbamate), xylan bis(3,5-dimethylphenyl carbamate), cellulose tris (4- *tert-* butylphenyl carbamate), cellulose tris(3,5-dimethylphenyl carbamate), amylose tris (3,5-dimethylphenyl carbamate) and amylose tris(4-*tert*-butylphenyl carbamate).

Semi-preparative separation was studied in 0.5 mg of nitrendipine with cellulose tris(4-tert-butylphenyl carbamate) using hexane:propan-2-ol:chloroform 85:10:5 v/v/v as mobile phase. Nitrendipine was completely separated with a resolution of $R_s = 0.97$ [221].

Cellulose tris(3,5-dimethyl carbamate) as chiral selector was also performed for enantioseparation of other dihydropyridine derivatives. It was a long lasting analysis with very broad peaks [222]. For this reason previous authors have used nine modified Pirkle type chiral stationary phases. Nine urea type chiral phases were derived from (*R*)-1-(α-naphthyl) ethylamine with (*S*)-proline or from (*S*)-1-(α-naphthyl) ethylamine with (*S*)-*tert*-leucine chemically bonded to the 3- aminopropylsilanized silica stationary phase (Sumichiral OA-4500 and Suchimiral OA-4600) [223].

Isradipine, and structurally related compounds derived from 1,4 and 1,2-dihydropyridines were separated by HPLC on a Chiralpak OT-chiral selector based on poly (triphenylmetacrylate) using the mobile phase hexane: propan-2-ol (90:10, 95:5 v/v). The best chiral resolution were recognized in the compound in which the nitrogen is attached to the dihydropyridine methyl group [224].

Separation of six 1,4-dihydropyridines (isradipine, nimodipine, nisoldipine, felodipine, lercanidipine and amlodipine) were examined on the macrocyclic antibiotic vancomycin as chiral selector (Chirobiotic V). Chromatographic data obtained on the vancomycin CSP phase were compared with those on an α_1-acid glycoprotein (Chiral AGP) CSP [225].

HPLC technique was used also in the determination of dihydropyridines in biological fluids during the pharmacokinetic study.

The stereoselective pharmacokinetics of dihydropyridine calcium antagonists were reviewed in detail in 1995. Pharmacokinetics of nilvadipine, nitrendipine, felodipine, nimodipine, manidipine, benidipine and nisoldipine were reviewed in animals, healthy subjects and patients with hepatic disease. Enantiomer-enantiomer interaction, enantiomeric inversion and the stereochemical aspects of pharmacokinetic drug interaction in these drugs were also described [226].

The present review article updates the methods for the stereoselective determination of dihydropyridines using chromatographic techniques and summarizes the pharmacokinetics of the dihydropyridines, including the newest drugs under development [227].

Antihypertensive activity of (*S*)-(+)-enantiomer of manidipine (another example of 1,4-dihydropyridines) was studied in rats showing to be 30-fold more potent than the (*R*)-(-)-isomer. It acts as calcium antagonists with long–lasting activity. Yamaguchi et al. [228] described a stereoselective and highly sensitive method using chiral chromatography and successive column-switching liquid chromatography for the determination of manidipine enantiomers in human serum. The enantiomers in the extract from serum were separated on a chiral stationary phase column Chiralcel OJ based on cellulose tris (4-methylbenzoate). The favorable result for enantioseparation was achieved with the mobile phase of hexane: ethanol: methanol 80: 15: 4 (v/v/v). at elevated temperature (α =1.3, RS = 1.2). This method might be appropriate for the pharmacokinetic study of manidipine.

From the other chiral columns, ovomucoid based and cyclodextrin columns have been used for enantioseparation in this group of compounds [229, 230].

A sensitive and simple method was developed for determination of the enantiomers of azelnidipine: (*R*)-(-)-azelnidipine and (*S*)-(+)-azelnidipine, in human plasma using chiral liquid chromatography with positive ion atmospheric pressure chemical ionization tandem mass spectrometry. Plasma samples were spiked with stable isotope-labeled azelnidipine. Azelnidipine enantiomers were separated on α_1-acid glycoprotein CSP (Chiral AGP) under isocratic mobile phase conditions [231].

Enantiomeric determination of amplodipine in human plasma was performed by LC-MS/MS method. The chiral stationary phase used for this determination was a Chiral-AGP column. Other chiral selectors tested in this study were celullose tris-(3,5-dimethylphenyl carbamate), celullose tris-4-methylbenzoate and amylose tris-(3,5-dimethylphenyl carbamate) [232].

Margues et al. [233] used HPLC method combined with GC-MS for the analysis of nisoldipine in human plasma. The enantiomers were resolved on a Chiralcel OD-H column and the (+)- and (-)-fractions were collected separately. For the quantification of the nisoldipine enantiomers a GC-MS with an Ultra 1 column was used with the detector operated in the single-ion monitoring mode with electron-impact ionization. The method proved to be suitable for pharmacokinetic studies.

Felodipine enantiomers were determined in plasma using LC-MS method with enantioseparation on Chiralcel OJ-R column [234].

Another Separation Techniques

Besides HPLC enantioseparation, separation by thin layer chromatography is another fast method for the optical resolution. Nimodipine and other chiral compounds were separated by TLC technique using β-cyclodextrin as chiral stationary phase. Enantioseparation mechanism is mainly based on the formation of inclusion complexes [235].

The simultaneous enantiomeric separation of three neutral 1,4-dihydropyridine derivatives (nimodipine, nisoldipine and nitrendipine) was studied using electrokinetic chromatography. Bile salts allowed the non-chiral separation of these DHP derivatives.

Enantiomeric separation of nimodipine and nisoldipine was observed using taurine-conjugated bile salts. Achiral micelles of sodium dodecyl sulphate mixed with neutral cyclodextrins did not allow enantioseparation. Baseline chiral separation of nisoldipine and nimodipine was obtained with carboxymethyl-CD at pH 5.0. The buffer type affected the chiral separation, especially in the case of nisoldipine. The addition of organic solvent decreased the enantioresolution of nimodipine.

However, the resolution between the nisoldipine enantiomers was increased when methanol or ethanol were added to the background electrolyte. Varying the temperature had almost no effect on the enantioresolution of nisoldipine, whereas a clear improvement at lower temperatures was observed in case of nimodipine.

Using the optimised method, the selectivity of this method was investigated for three possible impurities of nisoldipine [236].

Nimodipine was developed for the treatment of high blood pressure. It is not frequently used for this indication, it has shown good results in preventing a major complication of subarachnoid hemorrhage (a form of cerebral hemorrhage) termed vasospasm; this is now the main use of nimodipine. The aim of study [237] was to investigate the concentration time profiles of the nimodipine enantiomers in patiens with subarachnoid bleeding after i.v. oral administration of nimodipine. The plasma concentration of nimodipine was analyzed by HPLC with UV detection using isradipine and N-desmethyl-diazepam as internal standards. The results indicate, that (*S*)-(-)-nimodipine is metabolized at a much faster rate compared to (+)-(*R*)-enantiomer.

Long-acting calcium channel blocker amlodipine is considered among the third generation of dihydropyridines. Amlodipine in clinical practice is mostly used as a racemate. (*S*)-amlodipine is 1000 times more effective, but only the (*R*)-enantiomer has the capacity to cause the release of nitric oxide from the vascular endothelium [238].

The use of highly sulfated cyclodextrins (HS-CDs) as chiral selectors in CE was examined for rapid and reproducible enantioseparation of amlodipine [239].

In the other work, hydroxypropyl-β-CD (HP-βCD) and an ionic liquid (1-ethyl-3-methylimidazolium-l-lactate) were used as additives in CE for the enantioseparation of 10 analytes, including amlodipine. The effects of ionic liquid concentrations, salt effect, cations, and anions of ionic liquids on enantioseparation were investigated and the results proved that there was a synergistic effect between hydroxypropyl-β-CD and the ionic liquid, and the cationic part of the ionic liquid played an important role in the increased resolution [240].

In the paper Tabani et al. [241], for the first time, sulfated maltodextrin (SMD) was synthesized as a new anionic chiral selector and then it was successfully applied for the enantioseparation of five basic drugs (amlodipine, hydroxyzine, fluoxetine, tolterodine, and tramadol) as model chiral compounds using CE. Under the optimized condition (buffer solution: 50 mM phosphate (pH 3.0) and 2% w/v SMD (voltage: 18 kV; 20°C), the baseline enantioseparation was observed for all mentioned chiral drugs.

In the study [242] four chondroitin sulfate-based chiral dual systems, namely chondroitin sulfate C/glycogen, chondroitin sulfate C/chondroitin sulfate A, chondroitin sulfate C/hydroxypropyl-β-cyclodextrin, as well as chondroitin sulfate C/β-cyclodextrin, were evaluated for separation of amlodipine and chlorphenamine enantiomers by CE method.

The work [243] describes a capillary zone electrophoresis separation technique coupled with on-capillary diode array detector for highly reliable enantioselective determination of amlodipine in commercial tablets. For the separation of amplodipine enantiomers, HP-β-CD was an appropriate chiral selector providing complete enantioresolution [244].

8.2. Phenylalkylamines

Verapamil, the first calcium channel blocker, is used for treatment of hypertension, angina pectoris and supraventricular arrhythmias. Verapamil is available as a racemate (rac-verapamil). Two enantiomers differ in their pharmacokinetic and pharmacodynamic properties. (*S*)-(-)verapamil is pharmacodynamically more potent than (*R*)-(+)-verapamil. It is preferentially metabolised during the first-pass and has a greater volume of distribution than (*R*)-verapamil [245]. Serum concentrations of the (*S*)-(-) enantiomer are lower than those of the (*R*)-(+)-enantiomer after both oral and intravenous administration of rac-verapamil. (*S*)-(-)-verapamil was about 20 times more potent than (*R*)-(+)- verapamil with regard to negative dromotropic effects on AV node conduction [246].

8.2.1. Stereoselective Analysis of Phenylalkylamines

Enantioseparation of racemic verapamil was performed by chromatographic techniques, mainly by HPLC similarly to dihydropyridines. Enantioselective separation of verapamil and its metabolite norverapamil in serum and urine was achieved using ChiralcelChiralcel OD [24] and Chiralpak AD chiral stationary phase [247-249].

Chiralpak-AD column based on amylose tris (3,5-dimethylphenyl carbamate) CSP was the most suitable compared to other chiral polysaccharide columns used without derivatization [250]. Verapamil and its methoxy derivative gallopamil were separated on an AGP-column, eluting with ammonium acetate, pH 6.8: acetonitrile 89:11 v/v using UV and MS detection [251]. Verapamil and its desmethyl metabolite norverapamil were studied on the same chiral AGP column in conjunction with achiral. Results from the separation using AGP column were compared with results for another glycoprotein column - ovomucoid [252].

In addition to HPLC, capillary electrophoresis method was utilised for enantioseparation of verapamil and its metabolite using carboxymethyl-β-CD as a chiral selector. Capillary electrophoresis results were compared with the results obtained by HPLC [253].

Prenylamine and its analog fendiline is calcium channel blocker using as a vasodilatans in the treatment of angina pectoris. Enantioseparation of prenylamine and other racemic compounds by HPLC was performed using urea bonded cyclodextrin derivatives on silica [254]. Fendiline and its sixteen analogues were resolved on a chiral stationary phase based on (+)-(18-crown-6)-2,3,11,12-tetracarboxylic acid. Chromatographic behaviour of its analogues indicated that 3,3-diphenylpropyl group bonded to the secondary amino group is important in the chiral recognition [255]. In an attempt to separate the enantiomers of these drugs β-cyclodextrins are the most studied in capillary electrophoresis as chiral selectors, mainly HP-β-CD [256]. Enantiomers of fendiline and verapamil were separated by capillary electrophoresis using a raw cyclodextrin compared to heptakis (2,3-di-*O*-acetyl) -substituted cyclodextrin and randomly acetylated cyclodextrin. The best distribution was achieved by randomly substituted cyclodextrin [257].

Gotti et al. studied the applicability of linear polysaccharide Dextran 20 and Dextran 70 for enantioseparation of various chiral drugs including fendiline by CE. Using Dextran 20 very good separation of enantiomers was achieved. In contrast, Dextran 70 exhibited poorer enantioresolution but had wider applicability [258]. Six cyclodextrins as chiral selectors were used to separate the enantiomers of different linear and cyclic bis(phenethyl)amines including prenylamine by capillary electrophoresis. The best separation of prenylamine was achieved using heptakis (2,3-*O*-diacetyl-6-sulfato) β-cyclodextrin. The successful resolution of other enantiomers, but with a longer migration time and the worse separation was performed with the use of cyclodextrins with negatively charged groups at high pH [259]. In an extended screening program enantioseparations of 50 racemic compounds including fendiline was tested by using a reverse mode of CE with chiral selector based on a sulfated β-cyclodextrin. At this study 37 compounds were resolved but enantioseparation fendiline was unsuccessful [260]. Micellar electrokinetic capillary chromatography (MECC) using surfactant solutions containing sodium deoxycholate (NaDC), polyoxyethylene ethers, and methanol produced simultaneous baseline separation of the enantiomers of verapamil, norverapamil and gallopamil [261]. The authors Bhushan and Guta [262] separated verapamil enantiomers by thin layer chromatography using macrocyclic antibiotics as chiral selectors. In the study, the mobile phase of acetonitrile: methanol:water (15: 2.5: 2.5 v/v/v) was used.

8.3. Benzothiazepines

Diltiazem belongs to the benzothiazepines and contains two chiral centers in its structure. Diltiazem exists in the form of four stereoisomers from which only (+)-(*cis*)-(2*S*,3*S*)-diltiazem is the clinically used in the treatment of angina pectoris, hypertension and supraventricular tachyarrhythmias. The enantiomer (2*R*, 3*R*) and the two diastereoisomers of (2*R*, 3*S*) and (2*S*, 3*R*) are ineffective [263].

8.3.1. Stereoselective Analysis of Benzothiazepines

The direct resolution of four isomers of diltiazem hydrochloride was studied on both normal- and reversed-phase chiral HPLC columns. Four optical isomers of diltiazem·HCl were completely resolved on a Chiralcel OF column (cellulose-tris(4-chlorophenyl) carbamate) within 30 min [264]. Yaku et al. studied chiral resolution of four optical isomers of diltiazem by packed-column sub- and/or supercritical fluid chromatography (p-SubFC and/or p-SFC) on a column of modified cellulose coated onto silica, using a mixture of carbon dioxide with a polar modifier and additive [265].

Cellulose tris(4-chlorophenylcarbamate) coated on silica was used as a chiral stationary phase for the separation of optical isomers of diltiazem in packed-column supercritical fluid chromatography. The effect of temperature on the separation of the *cis*- and *trans*-enantiomers was studied in detail. The thermodynamic parameters revealed that the separation of *trans*-enantiomers was entropy-controlled in the range of temperatures examined, whereas enthalpy-controlled separation was observed for *cis*-enantiomers [266].

The separation and determination of enantiomers of diltiazem in dog plasma by a two-column HPLC technique was studied. Diltiazem and its metabolites were extracted from dog plasma and analyzed on a conventional column (Nucleosil 5C_{18}) with a volatile buffer system with 0.1% TFA and acetonitrile in a ratio of 7: 3 v / v.

The enantiomeric ratio of the collected diltiazem was determined on a chiral column (Chiralcel OC) using ethanol: diethyl amine in a ratio of 100:1 v/v as mobile phase [267].

8.4. Stereoselective Syntheses of Calcium Channel Blocking Agents

Various synthetic method have been developed for preparation of enantiomers of 1,4-dihydropyridines. Hantzsch reaction is one of the earliest synthesis for preparation of dihydropyridine derivatives.

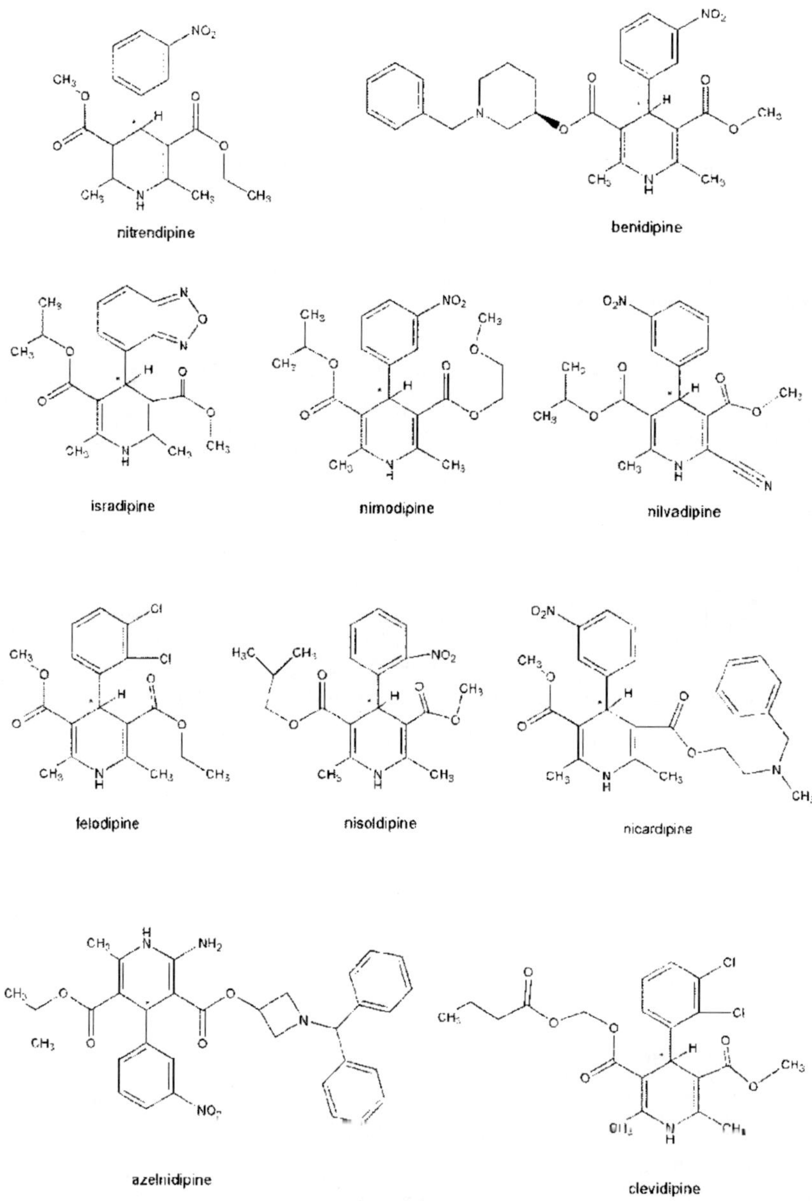

The asterisk denotes the stereogenic centre.

Figure 7. Chemical structure of major dihydropyridine calcium channel blockers.

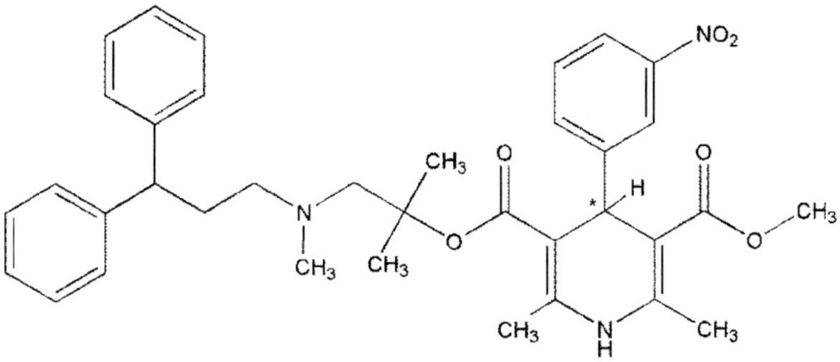

lercanidipine

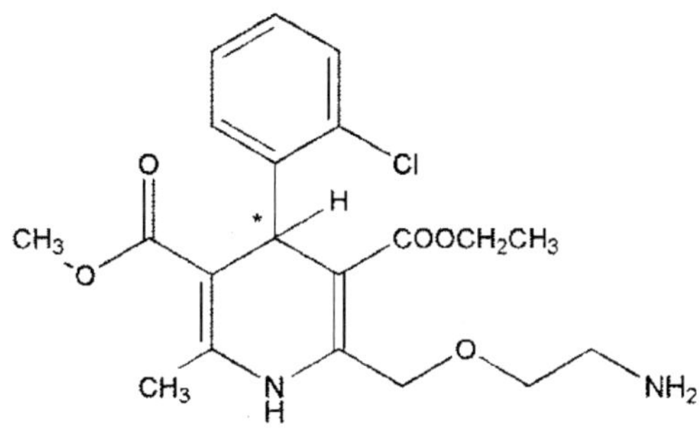

amlodipine

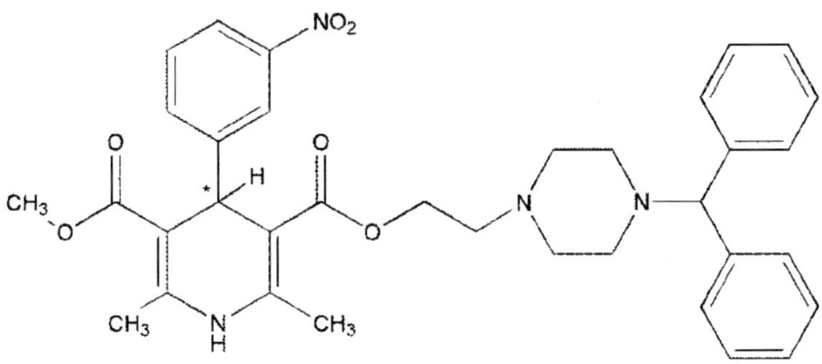

manidipine

The asterisk denotes the stereogenic centre.

Figure 7a. Chemical structure of major dihydropyridine calcium channel blockers.

This reaction is based on condensation of an aldehyde with two equivalents of a β-ketoester in the presence of ammonia [268]. First intermediate of this reaction is Knoevenagel condensation product. A second key intermediate is an ester enamine, which is produced by condensation of the second equivalent of the β-ketoester with ammonia: condensation between these two fragments gives the dihydropyridine derivatives [269]. Saini et al. [270] presented synthesis called Hantzsch-Bayer reaction as major reaction for the preparation of

1,4-dihydropyridines. The other paper [271] described a Brönsted acid-bifunctional thiourea co-catalyzed asymmetric cycloaddition of β-enamino esters and α, β-unsaturated aldehydes to afford trisubstituted and tetrasubstituted 1,4-dihydropyridines, which used novel thiourea catalyst as a source of chirality. Using this methods both enantiomers of 4-substituted 1,4-dihydropyridine can be synthesized from the same starting compounds.

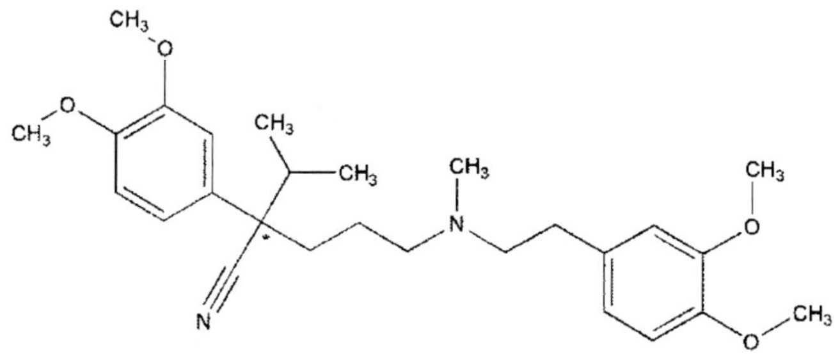

verapamil

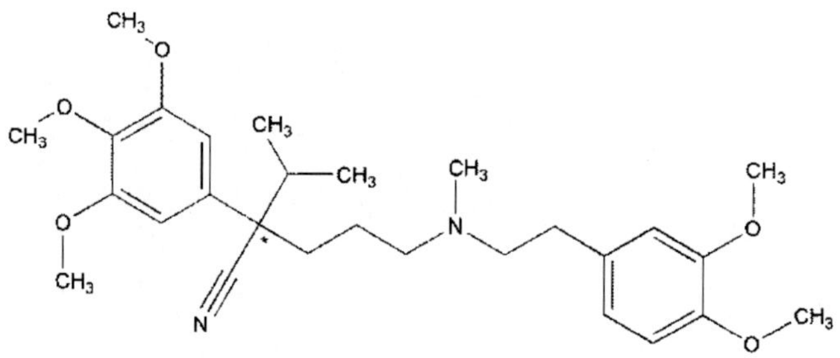

gallopamil

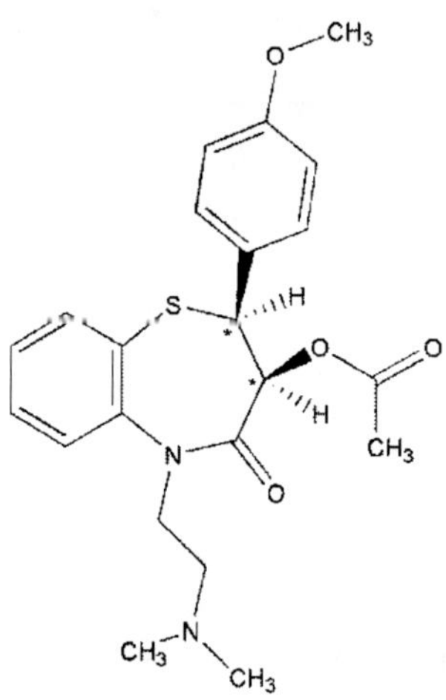

diltiazem

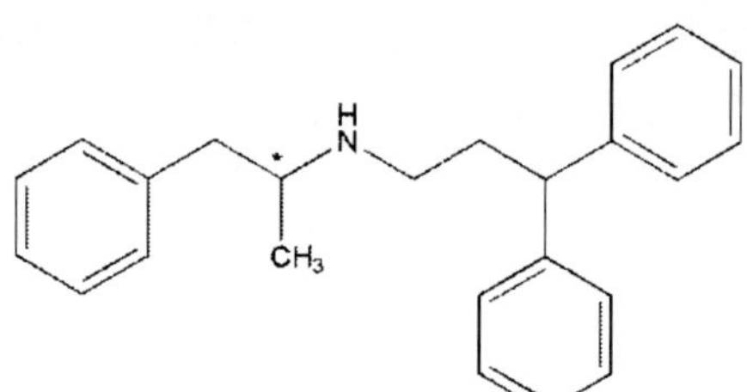

prenylamine

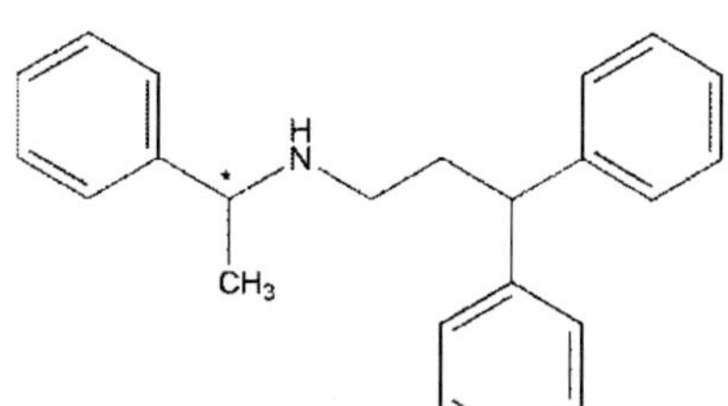

fendiline

The asterisk denotes the stereogenic centre.

Figure 8. Chemical structure of various calcium channel blockers.

An enantioselective synthesis of verapamil based on nucleophile-catalyzed asymmetric acylation of a silyl ketene imine was performed [272]. In the next paper [273] 4-cyano-4-(3,4-dimethoxyphenyl)-5-methylhexanoic acid resolved with α-methylbenzylamine was used as the key intermediate for synthesis of verapamil enantiomers.

Pharmacologically active stereoisomeric (2S, 3S) form of diltiazem was obtained by enantioselective synthesis from optically active glycidester as the starting material by means of an enantioselective enzymatic hydrolysis [274].

Levai [275] described synthesis of optically active 1,5-benzothiazepines. During reaction of 2-nitrophenol with phenylglycidester, the corresponding nitrocarboxylic acids which form a diastereoisomeric mixture of 2-aryl-2,3-dihydro-3-hydroxy-1,5-benzothiazepine-4 (5H)-ones were obtained.

Stereoisomers of diltiazem were also prepared by stereoselective synthesis of oxazolidinone [276] or by addition of 2-aminothiophenol to α-alkoxycinnamic acid derivatives [277]. A suitable way to prepare chiral intermediates methyl trans -3- (4-methoxyphenyl) glycidate and methyl threo-2-hydroxy-3- (4-methoxyphenyl) -3- (2-nitrophenylthio) propionate for the synthesis of diltiazem is enzymatically catalyzed kinetic resolution using lipase [278].

Another efficient synthesis of diltiazem has been developed using dynamic kinetic resolution as a key step. The methyl (2*S*,3*S*)-2-chloro-3-hydroxy-3-(4-methoxyphenyl) propionate was synthesized from a racemic mixture of α-chloro-β-keto ester, with high *anti* diastereoselectivity (92%) and enantioselectivity (95%), based on an asymmetric hydrogenation reaction with a chiral ruthenium (II) catalyst.

By treatment of this α-chloro-β-hydroxy ester with a base, the corresponding *trans* methyl glycidate, a key intermediate of diltiazem, was easily obtained [279]. Hashiyama, T. et al. [280] described reaction of 2-nitrotiophenol with trans-3-phenylglycidic ester carrying various substituent on the aromatic ring as part of stereoselective synthesis of diltiazem. A catalytic effect of various Lewis acids in the performed reaction was investigated.

The efficient catalytic activity in this synthesis was shown using $SnCl_4$. Process of preparing optically active benzothiazepine compounds by asymmetric reduction is described in patent [281] and the preparation of optically active intermediates methyl trans-3-(4-methoxyphenyl)glycidates by microbial asymmetric reduction is published by Nishida et al. [282].

Conclusion

To conclude, a large number of antihypertensive drugs are chiral and marketed as racemates. Most of racemates exhibit stereoselectivity in both, pharmacodynamic as well as pharmacokinetic properties. Resolution and enantioseparation of chiral antihypertensive drugs using optimal stereoselective methods is a potentially promising research area in this group of drugs. Development of analytical methods for the quantitative determination of stereoisomers of chiral drugs is an important and challenging task in drug synthesis and drugs formulation in pharmaceutical industry. Current methods for identification and determination of enantiomers in biological fluids are necessary for pharmacological, pharmacokinetic, and toxicological studies as well as for therapeutic drug monitoring.

Acknowledgments

This work was supported by the project implementation: The Centre of Excellence of Security Research code ITMS: 26240120034 supported by the Research and Development Operational Programme funded by the ERDF.

References

[1] Kearney, P., Whelton, M., Reynolds, K., Muntner, P., Whelton, P., He, J.: Global burden of hypertension: analysis of worldwide data. *Lancet* 2005, 365, 217-223.

[2] Tobe, S. W.: β-adrenergic receptor blockers in hypertension. *Can. J. Cardiol.* 2014, 30, 1-2.

[3] Baker, J. G., Hill, S. J., Summers, R. J.: Evolution of β-blockers: from anti-anginal drugs to ligand-directed signalling. *Trends Pharmacol. Sci.* 2011, 32, 227-234.

[4] Migliazzo, C. V., Hagan, J. C.: Beta blocker eye drops for treatment of acute migraine. *Mo. Med.* 2014, 111, 283-288.

[5] Larochelle, P., Tobe, S. W., Lacourcière, Y.: β-blockers in hypertension: studies and meta-analyses over the years. *Can. J. Cardiol.* 2014, 30, 16-22.

[6] Cizmarikova, R.: β-adrenergic receptor blockers – the group of chiral drugs: Different effects of individual enantiomers. *Ces. Slov. Farm.* 2002, 51, 121-128 (in slovak).

[7] Tenero, D., Boike, S., Boyle, D., Ilson, B., Fesniak, H. F., Brozena, S., Jorkasky, D.: Steady-state pharmacokinetics of carvedilol and its enantiomers in patients with congestive heart failure. *J. Clin. Pharmacol.* 2000, 40, 844-853.

[8] Riva, E., Mennini, T., Latini, R.: The alpha- and beta-adrenoceptor blocking activities of labetalol and its *RR-SR* (50:50) stereoisomers. *Br. J. Pharmacol.* 1991, 104, 823-828.

[9] Srinivas, N. R., Barr, W. H., Shyu, W. C., Mohandoss, E., Chow, S., Staggers, J., Balan, G., Belas, F. J., Blair, I. A., Barbhaiya, R. H.: Bioequivalence of two tablet formulations of nadolol using single and multiple dose data: assessment using stereospecific and nonstereospecific assays. *J. Pharm. Sci.* 1996, 85, 299-303.

[10] Siebert, C. D., Hänsicke, A., Nagel, T.: Stereochemical comparison of nebivolol with other beta-blockers. *Chirality* 2008, 20, 103-109.

[11] Mehvar, R., Brocks, D. R.: Stereospecific pharmacokinetics and pharmacodynamics: cardiovascular drugs. In: Reddy, I. K., Mehvar, R., ed.: *Chirality in drug design and development.* New York, Marcel Dekker 2004, 281-350.

[12] Walle, T., Webb, J. G., Walle, U. K., Bagwell, E. E.: Stereoselective accumulation of the beta-receptor blocking drug atenolol by human platelets. *Chirality* 1991, 3, 451-453.

[13] Walle, T., Webb, J. G., Bagwell, E. E., Walle, U. K., Daniell, H. B., Gaffney, T. E.: Stereoselective delivery and actions of beta receptor antagonists. *Biochem. Pharmacol.* 1988, 37, 115-124.

[14] Narimatsu, S., Nakata, T., Shimizudani, T., Nagaoka, K., Nakura, H., Masuda, K., Katsu, T., Koeda, A., Naito, S., Yamano, S., Miyata, A., Hanioka, N.: Regio- and stereoselective oxidation of propranolol enantiomers by human CYP2D6, cynomolgus monkey CYP2D17 and marmoset CYP2D19. *Chem. Biol. Interact.* 2011, 189, 146-52.

[15] Yu, L., Qian, M., Liu, Y., Yao, T., Zeng, S.: Stereoselective metabolism of propranolol glucuronidation by human UDP-glucuronosyltransferases 2B7 and 1A9. *Chirality* 2010, 22, 456-461.

[16] Hanioka, N., Tanaka, S., Moriguchi, Y., Narimatsu, S.: Stereoselective glucuronidation of carvedilol in human liver and intestinal microsomes. *Pharmacology* 2012, 90, 117-124.

[17] Seeringer, A., Brockmöller, J., Bauer, S., Kirchheiner, J.: Enantiospecific pharmacokinetics of metoprolol in CYP2D6 ultra-rapid metabolizers and correlation with exercise-induced heart rate. *Eur. J. Clin. Pharmacol.* 2008, 64, 883-888.

[18] Gübitz, G., Schmid, M. G.: Chiral separation principles. In: Gübitz, G., Schmid, M. G., eds. *Chiral separations*, Totowa, New Jersey, Humana Press, 2004, 1-28.

[19] Singh, A. K., Kedor-Hackmann, Erika R. M., Santoro, Maria Inês R. M.: Enantiomeric separation and quantitative determination of propranolol enantiomers in pharmaceutical preparations by chiral liquid chromatography. *Rev. Bras. Cienc. Farm.* 2004, 40, 301-304.

[20] Petersen, P. V., Ekelund, J., Olsen, L., Ovesen, S. V.: Chiral separations of β-blocking drug substances using the Pirkle-type alpha-Burke 1 chiral stationary phase. *J. Chromatogr. A.* 1997, 757, 65-71.

[21] Younes, A. A., Mangelings, D., Vander Heyden, Y.: Chiral separations in normal phase liquid chromatography: enantioselectivity of recently commercialized polysaccharide-based selectors. Part I: enantioselectivity under generic screening conditions. *J. Pharm. Biomed. Anal.* 2011, 55, 414-423.

[22] Cizmarikova, R., Nemethy, A., Valentova, J., Hrobonova, K., Bruchata, K.: Synthesis and HPLC enantioseparation of derivatives of the 3-hydroxyphenylethanone. *Acta Fac. Pharm. Univ. Comen.* 2012, 59, 5-13.

[23] Enquist, M., Hermansson, J.: Separation of the enantiomers of beta-receptor blocking agents and other cationic drugs using a CHIRAL-AGP column. Binding properties and characterization of immobilized alpha 1-acid glycoprotein. *J. Chromatogr.* 1990, 519, 285-298.

[24] Matsunaga, H., Haginaka, J.: Separation of enantiomers on chiral stationary phase based on chicken α_1-acid glycoprotein: effect of silica particle diameters on column performance. *J. Chromatogr. A.* 2014, 1363, 96-100.

[25] Matchett, M. W., Branch, S. K., Jefferies, T. M.: Polar organic chiral separation of propranolol and analogues using a β-cyclodextrin bonded stationary phase. *Chirality.* 1996, 8, 126-130.

[26] Pham-Huy, C., Radenen, B., Sahui-Gnassi, A., Claude, J. R.: High-performance liquid chromatographic determination of (*S*)- and (*R*)-propranolol in human plasma and urine with a chiral beta-cyclodextrin bonded phase. *J. Chromatogr. B Biomed. Appl.* 1995, 665, 125-132.

[27] Kafkova, B., Bosakova, Z., Tesarova, E., Coufal, P.: Chiral separation of beta-adrenergic antagonists, profen non-steroidal anti-inflammatory drugs and chlorophenoxypropionic acid herbicides using teicoplanin as the chiral selector in capillary liquid chromatography. *J. Chromatogr. A.* 2005, 1088, 82-93.

[28] Cizmarikova, R., Racanska, E., Hrobonova, K., Lehotay, J., Aghova, Z., Halesova, D.: Synthesis, pharmacological activity and chromatographic separation of some novel

potential β-blockers of the aryloxy aminopropanol type. *Pharmazie* 2003, 58, p. 237-241.

[29] Ansell, R. J.: Molecularly imprinted polymers for the enantioseparation of chiral drugs. *Adv. Drug Deliv. Rev.* 2005, 57, 1809-1835.

[30] Nie, Y., Liu, X., Yang, X., Zhao, Z.: Recent application of chiral liquid chromatography-tandem mass spectrometric methods for enantiomeric pharmaceutical and biomedical determinations. *J. Chromatogr. Sci.* 2013, 51, 753-763.

[31] Wang, D., Li, F., Jiang, Z., Yu, L., Guo, X.: Chiral Recognition Mechanisms of four β-Blockers by HPLC with Amylose Chiral Stationary Phase. *Iran. J. Pharm. Res.* 2014, 13, 449-457.

[32] Ilisz, I., Berkecz, R., Peter, A.: Retention mechanism of high-performance liquid chromatographic enantioseparation on macrocyclic glycopeptide-based chiral stationary phases. *J. Chromatogr. A.* 2009, 1216, 1845-1860.

[33] Pirkle, W. H., Burke, J. A.: Chiral stationary phase designed for beta-blockers. *J. Chromatogr.* 1991, 557, 173-185.

[34] Welch, CH. J.: Evolution of chiral stationary phase design in the Pirkle laboratories. *J. Chromatogr.* 1994, 666, 3-26.

[35] Zhang, X., Ouyang, J., Baeyens, W. R., Zhai, S., Yang, Y., Huang, G.: Enantiomeric separation of beta-blockers by HPLC using (*R*)-1-naphthylglycine and 3,5-dinitrobenzoic acid as chiral stationary phase. *J. Pharm. Biomed. Anal.* 2003, 31, 1047-1057.

[36] Dyas, A. M.: The chiral chromatographic separation of beta-adrenoceptor blocking drugs. *J. Pharm. Biomed. Anal.* 1992, 10, 383-404.

[37] Torul, H., Tamer, U.: Determination of enantiomers of atenolol and propranolol in pharmaceutical formulations by HPLC. *J. AOAC Int.* 2011, 94, 833-888.

[38] Küsters, E., Giron, D.: Enantiomeric separation of the β-blocking drugs pindolol and bopindolol using a chiral-immobilized protein stationary phase *J. High Resolut. Chromatogr.* 1986, 9, 531-533.

[39] Barbato, F., Carpentiero, C., Grumetto, L., La Rotonda, M. I.: Enantioselective retention of beta-blocking agents on human serum albumin and alpha1-acid glycoprotein HPLC columns: relationships with different scales of lipophilicity. *Eur. J. Pharm. Sci.* 2009, 38, 472-478.

[40] Tamai, G., Edani, M., Imai, H.: Chiral separation and determination of propranolol enantiomers in rat or mouse blood and tissue by column switching high performance liquid chromatography with ovomucoid bonded stationary phase. *Biomed. Chromatogr.* 1990, 4, 157-160.

[41] Ståhlberg, J., Henriksson, H., Divne, C., Isaksson, R., Pettersson, G., Johansson, G., Jones, T. A.: Structural basis for enantiomer binding and separation of a common beta-blocker: crystal structure of cellobiohydrolase Cel7A with bound (*S*)-propranolol at 1.9 A resolution. *J. Mol. Biol.* 2001, 305, 79-93.

[42] Bojarski, J.: Stereoselective chromatography of cardiovascular drugs: an update. *J. Biochem. Biophys. Methods*. 2002, 54, 197-220.

[43] Lehotay, J., Hrobonova, K., Cizmarik, J., Celkova, H.: Separation of enantiomers of some 1,4-piperazine derivatives of aryloxyaminopropanols on a vancomycin chiral stationary phase, *Pharmazie* 1999, 54, 743-745.

[44] Hrobonova, K., Lehotay, J., Cizmarikova, R., Armstrong, D. W.: Study of mechanism of enantioseparation. Part I. Chiral analysis of alkylaminoderivatives of aryloxypropanols by HPLC using macrocyclic antibiotics as chiral selectors. *J. Liq. Chromatogr. Rel. Technol.* 2001, 24, 2225-2237.

[45] Cizmarikova, R., Nemethy, A., Valentova, J., Hrobonova, K., Adamcova, K.: Synthesis of new compounds of the aryloxyaminopropanol type and their HPLC enantioseparation. *Acta Facult. Pharm. Univ. Comenianae* 2013, 60, 37-42.

[46] Hrobonova, K., Lehotay, J., Bruchata, K., Cizmarikova, R.: Enantioselective HPLC analysis and in vitro- kinetic study decomposition of potential β-blocker drug in guinea pig serum. *J. Liq. Chromatogr. Rel. Technol.* 2009, 32, 80-94.

[47] Lamprecht, G., Kraushofer, T., Stoschitzky, K., Lindner, W.: Enantioselective analysis of (*R*)- and (*S*)-atenolol in urine samples by a high-performance liquid chromatography column-switching setup. *J. Chromatogr. B Biomed. Sci. Appl.* 2000, 740, 219-226.

[48] Xia, Y. Q., Bakhtiar, R., Franklin, R. B.: Automated online dual-column extraction coupled with teicoplanin stationary phase for simultaneous determination of (*R*)- and (*S*)-propranolol in rat plasma using liquid chromatography-tandem mass spectrometry. *J. Chromatogr. B. Analyt. Technol. Biomed. Life Sci.* 2003, 788, 317-329.

[49] D'Orazio, G., Fanali, S.: Enantiomeric separation by using nano-liquid chromatography with on-column focusing. *J. Sep. Sci.* 2008, 31, 2567-2571.

[50] MacLeod, S. L., Sudhir, P., Wong, C. S.: Stereoisomer analysis of wastewater-derived beta-blockers, selective serotonin re-uptake inhibitors, and salbutamol by high-performance liquid chromatography-tandem mass spectrometry. *J. Chromatogr. A.* 2007, 1170, p. 23-33.

[51] Ribeiro, A. R., Santos, L. H., Maia, A. S., Delerue-Matos, C., Castro, P. M., Tiritan, M. E.: Enantiomeric fraction evaluation of pharmaceuticals in environmental matrices by liquid chromatography-tandem mass spectrometry. *J. Chromatogr. A.* 2014, 1363, p. 226-235.

[52] Bagnall, J. P., Evans, S. E., Wort, M. T., Lubben, A. T., Kasprzyk-Hordern, B.: Using chiral liquid chromatography quadrupole time-of-flight mass spectrometry for the analysis of pharmaceuticals and illicit drugs in surface and wastewater at the enantiomeric level. *J. Chromatogr. A.* 2012, 1249, 115-129.

[53] Hefnawy, M. M., Al-Shehri, M. M., Abounassif, M. A., Mostafa, G. A.: Enantioselective quantification of atenolol in mouse plasma by high performance liquid chromatography using a chiral stationary phase: application to a pharmacokinetic study. *J. AOAC Int.* 2013, 96, 976-980.

[54] Poggi, J. C., Da Silva, F. G., Coelho, E. B., Marques, M. P., Bertucci, C., Lanchote, V. L.: Analysis of carvedilol enantiomers in human plasma using chiral stationary phase column and liquid chromatography with tandem mass spectrometry. *Chirality* 2012, 24, 209-214.

[55] Szymura-Oleksiak, J., Bojarski, J., Aboul-Enein, H. Y.: Recent applications of stereoselective chromatography. *Chirality* 2002, 14, 417-435.

[56] Sharma, S. C., Evans, M. B., Evans, S. J.: The enantiomeric separation of metipranolol and desacetylmetipranolol on a cellulose tris-3,5-dimethylphenyl-carbamate chiral stationary phase. *J. Pharm. Biomed. Anal.* 1995, 13, 129-137.

[57] Agustian, J., Kamaruddin, A. H., Aboul-Enein, H. Y.: Chromatographic comparison of atenolol separation in reaction media on cellulose tris-(3,5-dimethylphenylcarbamate)

chiral stationary phase using ultra fast liquid chromatography. *Chirality* 2012, 24, 356-367.

[58] Antunes Nde, J., Cavalli, R. C., Marques, M. P., Lanchote, V. L.: Stereoselective determination of metoprolol and its metabolite α-hydroxymetoprolol in plasma by LC-MS/MS: application to pharmacokinetics during pregnancy. *Chirality* 2013, 25, 1-7.

[59] Aboul-Enein, H. Y., Ali, I.: HPLC enantiomeric resolution of nebivolol on normal and reversed amylose based chiral phases. *Pharmazie* 2001, 56, 214-216.

[60] Valentova, J., Cizmarikova, R., Bui, T. T. T., Drake, A. F., Hutt, A. J.: Enantiomeric resolution of novel aryloxyaminopropanol derivatives with β-adrenoceptor antagonist activity on a derivatised amylose chiral stationary phase. *Chromatographia* 2003, 58, 733-740.

[61] Al-Othman, Z. A., Ali, I.: Rapid and economic chiral-HPLC method of nebivolol enantiomers resolution in dosage formulation. *Biomed. Chromatogr.* 2012, 26, 775-780.

[62] Ribeiro, A. E., Rodrigues, A. E., Pais, L. S.: Separation of nadolol stereoisomers by chiral liquid chromatography at analytical and preparative scales. *Chirality* 2013, 25, 197-205.

[63] Heberer, T.: Occurrence, fate, and removal of pharmaceutical residues in the aquatic environment: a review of recent research data. *Toxicol. Lett.* 2002, 131, 5-17.

[64] Maurer, M., Escher, B. I., Richle, P., Schaffner, C., Alder, A. C.: Elimination of beta-blockers in sewage treatment plants. *Water Res.* 2007, 41, 1614-1622.

[65] Morante-Zarcero, S., Sierra. I.: Simultaneous enantiomeric determination of propranolol, metoprolol, pindolol, and atenolol in natural waters by HPLC on new polysaccharide-based stationary phase using a highly selective molecularly imprinted polymer extraction. *Chirality* 2012, 24, 860-866.

[66] Morante-Zarcero, S., Sierra, I.: Comparative HPLC methods for β-blockers separation using different types of chiral stationary phases in normal phase and polar organic phase elution modes. Analysis of propranolol enantiomers in natural waters. *J. Pharm. Biomed. Anal.* 2012, 62, 33-41.

[67] Ghanem, A., Hoenen, H., Aboul-Enein, H. Y.: Application and comparison of immobilized and coated amylose tris-(3,5-dimethylphenyl carbamate) chiral stationary phases for the enantioselective separation of beta-blockers enantiomers by liquid chromatography. *Talanta.* 2006, 6, 602-609.

[68] Ahmed, M., Gwairgi, M., Ghanem, A.: Conventional Chiralpak ID vs. capillary Chiralpak ID-3 amylose tris (3 chlorophenylcarbamate)-based chiral stationary phase columns for the enantioselective HPLC separation of pharmaceutical racemates. *Chirality* 2014, 26, 677-682.

[69] Subert, J.: Progress in the separation of enantiomers of chiral drugs by HPLC without their prior derivatization, *Pharmazie* 1994, 49, 3-13.

[70] Chang, S. C., Reid, G. L., Chen, S., Chang, C. D., Armstrong, D. W.: Evaluation of a new polar—organic high-performance liquid chromatographic mobile phase for cyclodextrin-bonded chiral stationary phases. *Trends Anal. Chem.* 1993, 12, 144-153.

[71] Armstrong, D. W., Chen, S., Chang, C., Chang, S.: A New Approach for the Direct Resolution of Racemic Beta Adrenergic Blocking Agents by HPLC. *J. Liq. Chromatogr.* 1992, 15, 545-556.

[72] Guillarme, D., Bonvin, G., Badoud, F., Schappler, J., Rudaz, S., Veuthey, J. L.: Fast chiral separation of drugs using columns packed with sub-2 microm particles and ultra-high pressure. *Chirality* 2010, 22, 320-330.
[73] Ghanem, A., Ahmed, M., Ishii, H., Ikegami, T.: Immobilized β-cyclodextrin-based silica vs polymer monoliths for chiral nano liquid chromatographic separation of racemates. *Talanta* 2015, 132, 301-14.
[74] Cizmarikova, R., Valentova, J., Hutt, A. J.: Beta-adrenergic receptor blockers – a group of chiral drugs: Enantioseparation in the group of β-blockers. *Ces. Slov. Farm.* 2004, 7-17.
[75] Bhushan, R., Tanwar, S.: Reversed-phase high-performance liquid chromatographic enantioresolution of six beta-blockers using dinitrophenyl-L-Pro-*N*-hydroxysuccinimide ester, *N*-succinimidyl-(*S*)-2-(6-methoxynaphth-2-yl) propionate and twelve variants of Sanger's reagent as chiral derivatizing reagents. *Biomed. Chromatogr.* 2009, 23, 1291-1299.
[76] Bhushan, R., Dixit, S.: Enantioresolution of five β-blockers by reversed-phase high-performance liquid chromatography using fifteen chiral derivatizing reagents having amino acids or their amides as chiral auxiliaries on a cyanuric chloride platform. *Biomed. Chromatogr.* 2012, 26, 239-246.
[77] Tivert, A. M., Backman, A.: Separation of the enantiomers of β-blocking drugs with a chiral mobile phase additive. *J. Planar Chromatogr.* 1993, 6, 216-219.
[78] Suedee, R., Heard, CH. M.: Direct resolution of propranolol and bupranolol by thin-layer chromatography using cellulose derivatives as stationary phase. *Chirality* 1997, 9, 139-144.
[79] Cizmarikova, R., Hrobonova, R., Lehotay, J., Racanska, E., Bruchata, K.: Preparation, pharmacological activity and enantioseparation of [3-(cyclopentyloxymethyl)-4-(hydroxy-3-isopropylaminopropoxy)phenyl] ethanone as potential β-blocker. *Acta Facult. Pharm. Univ. Comenianae.* 2005, 52, 79-88.
[80] Bhushan, R., Thiongo, G. T.: Direct enantioseparation of some beta-adrenergic blocking agents using impregnated thin-layer chromatography. *J. Chromatogr. B Biomed. Sci. Appl.* 1998, 708, 330-334.
[81] Bhushan, R., Arora, M.: Direct enantiomeric resolution of (+/-)-atenolol, (+/-)-metoprolol, and (+/-)-propranolol by impregnated TLC using L-aspartic acid as chiral selector. *Biomed. Chromatogr.* 2003, 17, 226-230.
[82] Bhushan, R., Dixit, S.: Aminoacids as chiral selector in enantioresolution by liquid chromatography. *Biomed. Chromatogr.* 2012, 26, 962-971.
[83] Cizmarikova, R., Bruchatá, K., Pastirová, Z., Lehotay, J., Hrobonova, K.: HPLC and TLC enantioseparation of the nitro-positioned aryloxysubstituted aminopropranols. *Pharmazie* 2010, 65, 387-388.
[84] Bhushan, R., Tanwar, S.: Direct TLC resolution of atenolol and propranolol into their enantiomers using three different chiral selectors as impregnating reagents. *Biomed. Chromatogr.* 2008, 22, 1028-1034.
[85] Suedee, R., Srichana, T., Saelim, J., Thavonpibulbut, T.: Thin-layer chromatographic separation of chiral drugs on molecularly imprinted chiral stationary phases. *J. Planar Chromatogr. Modern TLC.* 2001, 4, 194-198.

[86] Suedee, R., Srichana, T., Saelim, J., Thavornpibulbut, T.: Chiral determination of various adrenergic drugs by thin-layer chromatography using molecularly imprinted chiral stationary phases prepared with α-agonists. *Analyst* 1999, 124, 1003-1009.

[87] Gübitz, G., Schmid, M. G.: Chiral separation by capillary electrochromatography. *Enantiomer* 2000, 5, 5-11.

[88] Gübitz, G., Schmid, M. G.: Advances in chiral separation using capillary electromigration techniques. *Electrophoresis* 2007, 28, 114-126.

[89] Aturki, Z., D'Orazio, G., Rocco, A., Fanali, S.: Advances in the enantioseparation of β-blocker drugs by capillary electromigration techniques. *Electrophoresis* 2011, 3, 2602-2628.

[90] Scriba, G. K.: Cyclodextrins in capillary electrophoresis enantioseparations-recent developments and applications. *J. Sep. Sci.* 2008, 31, 1991-2011.

[91] Tsioupi, D. A., Stefan-Vanstaden, R. I.: Kapnissi-Christodoulou, C. P.: Chiral selectors in CE: recent developments and applications. *Electrophoresis* 2013, 34, 178-204.

[92] Chankvetadze, B., Blaschke, G.: Enantioseparations using capillary electromigration techniques in nonaqueous buffers. *Electrophoresis* 2000, 21, 4159-4178.

[93] Hashem, H., Kinzig, M., Jira, T.: The effect of achiral calixarenes on chiral separation of propranolol-HCl and brompheniramine maleate in capillary electrophoresis using cyclodextrin as chiral selector. *Pharmazie* 2008, 63, 256-262.

[94] Juvancz, Z., Kendrovics, R. B, Iványi, R., Szente, L.: The role of cyclodextrins in chiral capillary electrophoresis. *Electrophoresis* 2008, 29, 1701-1712.

[95] Servais, A. C., Rousseau, A., Fillet, M., Lomsadze, K., Salgado, A., Crommen, J., Chankvetadze, B.: Capillary electrophoretic and nuclear magnetic resonance studies on the opposite affinity pattern of propranolol enantiomers towards various cyclodextrins. *J. Sep. Sci.* 2010, 33, 1617-1624.

[96] Peterson, T. E.: Separation of drug stereoisomers by capillary electrophoresis with cyclodextrins. *J. Chromatogr.* 1993, 630, 353-363.

[97] Bechet, I., Paques, P., Fillet, M., Hubert, P., Crommen, J.: Chiral separation of basic drugs by capillary zone electrophoresis with cyclodextrin additives. *Electrophoresis* 1994, 15, 818-823.

[98] Proksa, B.: Capillary zone electrophoretic separation of (*R,S*)-metipranolol and related substances. *Pharmazie* 1999;54:431-434.

[99] Proksa, B., Cizmarikova, R.: Separation of β-adrenolytics derived from 4-hydroxyacetophenone by capillary zone electrophoretic in the presence of cyclodextrins. *Anal. Chim. Acta* 2001, 434, 15-79.

[100] Matthijs, N., Vander Heyden, Y.: Enantiomeric impurity determination in capillary electrophoresis using a highly-sulfated cyclodextrins-based method. *Biomed. Chromatogr.* 2006, 26, p. 4116-4126.

[101] Chankvetadze, L., Servais, A. C., Fillet, M., Salgado, A., Crommen, J., Chankvetadze, B.: Comparative enantioseparation of talinolol in aqueous and non-aqueous capillary electrophoresis and study of related selector-selectand interactions by nuclear magnetic resonance spectroscopy. *J. Chromatogr. A.* 2012, 1267, 206-216.

[102] Lomsadze, K., Salgado, A., Calvo, E., López, J. A., Chankvetadze, B.> Comparative NMR and MS studies on the mechanism of enantioseparation of propranolol with heptakis(2,3-diacetyl-6-sulfo)-β-cyclodextrin in capillary electrophoresis with aqueous and non-aqueous electrolytes. *Electrophoresis* 2011, 32, 1156-1163.

[103] Xu, H., Yu, X., Chen, H.: Enantiomeric separation of basic drugs with partially filled serum albumin as chiral selector in capillary electrophoresis. *Anal. Sci.* 2004, 20, 1409-1413.
[104] Yu, T., Du, Y., Chen, B.: Evaluation of clarithromycin lactobionate as a novel chiral selector for enantiomeric separation of basic drugs in capillary electrophoresis. *Electrophoresis* 2011, 32, 1898-1905.
[105] Beck, G. M., Neau, S. H.: Optimization of lambda-carrageenan as a chiral selector in capillary electrophoresis separations. *Chirality* 2000, 12, 614-620.
[106] Stavrou, I. J., Moore, L. J., Fernand, V. E., Kapnissi-Christodoulou, C. P., Warner, I. M.: Facile preparation of polysaccharide-coated capillaries using a room temperature ionic liquid for chiral separations. *Electrophoresis* 2013, 34, 1334-1338.
[107] Dixit, S., Park, J. H.: Penicillin G as a novel chiral selector in capillary electrophoresis. *J. Chromatogr. A.* 2014, 1326, 134-138.
[108] Hsieh, M. L., Chau, L. K., Hon, Y. S.: Single-step approach for fabrication of vancomycin-bonded silica monolith as chiral stationary phase. *J. Chromatogr. A.* 2014, 1358, 208-216.
[109] Chen, Z., Zeng, S., Yao, T.: Separation of beta-receptor blockers and analogs by capillary liquid chromatography (CLC) and pressurized capillary electrochromatography(pCEC) using a vancomycin chiral stationary phase column. *Pharmazie* 2007, 62, 585-592.
[110] D'Orazio, G., Fanali, S.: Coupling capillary electrochromatography with mass spectrometry by using a liquid-junction nano-spray interface. *J. Chromatogr. A.* 2010, 1217, 4079-4086.
[111] Karlsson, C., Wikström, H., Armstrong, D. W., Owens, P. K.: Enantioselective reversed-phase and non-aqueous capillary electrochromatography using a teicoplanin chiral stationary phase. *J. Chromatogr. A.* 2000, 897, 349-363.
[112] Chen, X., Qin, F., Liu, Y., Kong, L., Zou, H.: Preparation of a positively charged cellulose derivative chiral stationary phase with copolymerization reaction for capillary electrochromatographic separation of enantiomers. *Electrophoresis* 2004, 25, 2817-2824.
[113] Aturki, Z., Vichi, F., Messina, A., Sinibaldi, M.: Indirect resolution of beta-blocker agents by reversed-phase capillary electrochromatography. *Electrophoresis* 2004, 25, 607-614.
[114] Guo, W. P., Rong, Z. B., Li, Y. H., Fung, Y. S., Gao, G. Q., Cai, Z. M.: Microfluidic chip capillary electrophoresis coupled with electrochemiluminescence for enantioseparation of racemic drugs using central composite design optimization. *Electrophoresis.* 2013, 34, 2962-2969.
[115] Belin, G. K., Seeger, S.: Rapid analysis of serotonin and propranolol using miniaturized CE with deep-UV fluorescence detector. *Electrophoresis* 2009, 30, 2565-2571.
[116] Agustian, J., Kamarrudin, A. H., Bhatia, S.: Single enantiomeric β-blockers - The existing technologies. *Process Biochem.* 2010, 45, 1587-1604.
[117] Cho, B. T., Kang, S. K., Yang, K. Y.: Convenient synthesis of enantiopure β-adrenergic blockers: (*R*)-nifenalol, (*R*)-denopamine, (*R*)-dichloroisoproterenol and (*R*)-pronethalol. *Bull. Korean Chem. Soc.* 2002, 2, 1328-1330.

[118] Klunder, M. K., Ko, S. Y., Sharpless, K. B.: Asymmetric epoxidation od allyl alcohol: efficient routes to homochiral β-adrenergic blocking agents. *J. Org. Chem.* 1986, 51, 3710-3712.

[119] Sayyed, I. A., Thakur, V. V., Nikalje, M. D., Dewkar, G. K., Kotkar, S. P., Sudalai, A.: Asymmetric synthesis of aryloxypropanolamines via OsO_4-catalyzed asymmetric dihydroxylation. *Tetrahedron* 2005, 61, 2831-2838.

[120] Jacobsen, E. N.: Asymmetric catalysis of epoxide ring-opening reactions. *Acc. Chem. Res.* 2000, 33, 421-431.

[121] Joshi, R. A., Garud, D. R., Muthukrishnan, M., Joshi, R. R., Gurjar, M. K.: A convenient. synthesis of the enantiomerically pure β-blocker (*S*)-betaxolol using hydrolytic kinetic resolution. *Tetrahedron: Asymmetry* 2005, 16, 3802-3806.

[122] Schaus, S. E., Brandes, B. D., Larrow, J. F., Tokunaga, M., Hansen, K. B., Gould, A. E., Furrow, M. E., Jacobsen, E. N.: Highly selective hydrolytic kinetic resolution of terminal epoxides catalyzed by chiral (salen)CoIII complexes. Practical synthesis of enantioenriched terminal epoxides and 1,2-diols. *J. Am. Chem. Soc.* 2002, 124, 1307-1315.

[123] Muthukrishnan, M., Garud, D. R., Joshi, R. R., Joshi, R. A.: Concise synthesis of β-blockers (*S*)-metoprolol and (*S*)-betaxolol using hydrolytic kinetic resolution. *Tetrahedron* 2007, 63, 1872-1876.

[124] Bose, D. S., Narsaiah, A. V.: An efficient asymmetric synthesis of (*S*)-atenolol: using hydrolytic kinetic resolution. *Bioorg. Med. Chem.* 2004, 13, 627-630.

[125] Eshghi, H., Porkar Yazdi, H.: A facile synthesis of (*S*)-(-)-propranolol. *J. Sci. I. R. Iran* 2003, 14, 17-19.

[126] Singh, N., Kumar, A., Singh, R.: Concise synthesis of (*S*)-(-)-propranolol: Using acid catalysed kinetic resolution. *J. Chem. Pharm. Res.* 2012, 12, 5111-5113.

[127] Inkum, R., Teerawutgulrag, A., Puangsombat, P., Rakariyatham, N.: Stereoselective reduction of amino ketone with sodium borohydride in the presence of metal chloride. A Simple pathway to (*S*)-Propranolol. *World Academy of Science, Engineering and Technology* 2012, 67, 960-963.

[128] Panchgalle, S. P., Gore, R. G., Chavan, S. P., Kalkote, U. R.: Organocatalytic enantioselective synthesis of β-blockers: (*S*)-propranolol and (*S*)-naftopidil. *Tetrahedron: Asymmetry* 2009, 20, 1767-1770.

[129] Zhang, J. Y., Liu, H. M., Wang, X. J., Wang, P., Zheng, J. X.: Application of kinetic resolution using HCS as chiral auxilliary: novel synthesis of β-blockers (*S*)-betaxolol and (*S*)-metoprolol. *Chirality* 2009, 21, 745-750.

[130] Wunsche, K., Schwaneberg, U., Bornscheuer, U. T., Meyer, H. H.: Chemoenzymatic route to β-blockers via 3-hydroxy esters. *Tetrahedron: Asymmetry* 1996, 7, 2017-2022.

[131] Banoth, L., Narayan, T. K., Banerjee, U. C.: New chemical and chemo-enzymatic routes for the synthesis of (*RS*)- and (*S*)-enciprazine. *Tetrahedron: Asymmetry* 2012, 23, 1272-1278.

[132] Kamal, A., Khanna, G. B. R., Krishnaji, T., Tekumalla, V., Ramu, R.: New chemoenzymatic pathway for β-adrenergic blocking agents. *Tetrahedron: Asymmetry* 2005, 16, 1485-1494.

[133] El Gihani, M. T., Williams, M. J.: Dynamic kinetic resolution. *Curr. Opin. Chem. Biol.* 1999, 3, 11-15.

[134] Pamies, O., Backvall, J. E.: Dynamic kinetic resolution of β-azido alcohols. An efficient route to chiral aziridines and β-amino alcohols. *J. Org. Chem.* 2001, 66, 4022-4025.

[135] Yang, W., Xu, J. H., Xie, Y., Xu, Y., Zhao, G., Lin, G. Q.: Asymmetric reduction of ketones by employing Rhodotorula sp. AS2.2241 and synthesis of the β-blocker (*R*)-nifenalol. *Tetrahedron: Asymmetry* 2006, 17, 1769-1774.

[136] Cizmarikova, R., Valentova, J., Hutt, A. J., Sedlakova, S.: Blockers of β-adrenergic receptors – group of chiral agents. Stereoselective synthesis of β-blockers. *Čes. Slov. Farm.* 2005, 5, 201-206 (in slovak).

[137] Jung, M. E., Shaw, T. J.: Total synthesis of (*R*)-glycerolacetonide and the antiepileptic and hypotensive drug (-)-γ-amino-β-hydroxybutyric acid (GABOOB): use of vitamin C as a chiral starting material. *J. Am. Chem. Soc.* 1980, 102, 6304-6311.

[138] Dorsch, M. P., Gillespie, B. W., Erickson, S. R., Bleske, B. E., Weder, A. B.: Chlorthalidone reduces cardiovascular events compared with hydrochlorothiazide: a retrospective cohort analysis. *Hypertension* 2011, 57, 689-694.

[139] Patel, B. H., Hutt, A. J.: Stereoselectivity in drug action and disposition. In: Reddy, I. K., Mehvar, R., ed.: *Chirality in drug design and development.* New York, Marcel Dekker 2004, 281-350.

[140] Visegrády, B., Konecsni, T., Grobuschek, N., Schmid, G., Kilár, F., Aboul-Enein, H. Y.: Chiral separation of thiazide diuretic by HPLC on Chiral OD-RH®, Chiralcel OJ-R® and Chirobiotic T™® phases. *J. Biochem. Biophysic. Methods* 2002, 53, 15-24.

[141] Chankvetadze, B., Chankvetadze, L., Sidamonidze, S. H., Yashima, E., Okamoto, Z.: High performance liquid chromatography enantioseparation of chiral pharmaceutical using tris (chloromethylphenylcarbamate)s of cellulose. *J. Pharm. Biomed. Anal.* 1996, 14, 1295-1303.

[142] Chankvetadze, B., Kartozia, I., Yamamoto, C., Okamoto, Y.: Comparative enantioseparation of selected chiral drugs on four different polysaccharide-type chiral stationary phases using polar organic mobile phases. *J. Pharm. Biomed. Anal.* 2002, 27, 467-478.

[143] Du, B., Pang, L., Li, H., Ma, S., Li, Y., Jia, X., Zhang, Z.: Chiral liquid chromatography resolution and stereoselective pharmacokinetic study of indapamide enantiomers in rats. *J. Chromatogr. B Analyt. Technol. Biomed. Life Sci.* 2013, 932, 88-91.

[144] Ates, H., Mangelings, D., Heyden, Y. V.: Chiral separations in polar organic solvent containing polysacharide-based stationary phases. *J. Chromatogr. B* 2008, 875, 57-64.

[145] Herraez-Hernandez, R., Campins-Falco, P.: Chromatographic separation of chlorthalidone enantiomers using beta-cyclodextrins as chiral additives. *J. Chromatogr. B* 2000, 740, 169-177.

[146] Cabrera, K., Jung, M., Fluck, M., Schurig, V.: Determination of enantiomerization barriers by computer simulation of experimental elution profiles obtained by high-performance liquid chromatography on a chiral stationary phase. *J. Chromatogr. A* 1996, 731, 315-321.

[147] Wang, Y., Young, D. J., Tan, T. T., Ng, S. C.: "Click" immobilized perphenylcarbamated and permethylated cyclodextrin stationary phases for chiral high-performance liquid chromatography application. *J. Chromatogr. A.* 2010, 1217, 5103-5108.

[148] Zhong, Q., He, L., Beesley, T. E., Trahanovsky, W. S., Sun, P., Wang, C., Armstrong, D. W.: Development of dinitrophenylated cyclodextrin derivatives for enhanced

enantiomeric separations by high-performance liquid chromatography. *J. Chromatogr. A*. 2006, 1115, 19-45.

[149] Welch, CH. J., Szczerba, T., Perrin, S. R.: Some recent high-performance liquid chromatography separations of enantiomers of pharmaceuticals and other compounds using the Whelk-O I chiral stationary phase. *J. Chromatogr. A* 1997, 758, 93-98.

[150] Hyun, M. H., Pirkle, W. H.: Liquid chromatographic separation of the stereoisomers of thiazide diuretics. *J. Chromatogr A*. 2000, 876, 221-227.

[151] Vercauteren, A., Van der Weken, G., Vankeirsbilck, T., Aboul-Enein, H. Y., Baeyens, W. R.: Enantiomeric separation of diuretics on a novel Pirkle-type chiral stationary phase. *Biomed. Chromatogr*. 2002, 16, 437-440.

[152] Berthod, A., Nair, U. B., Bagwill, C., Armstrong, D. W.: Derivatized vancomycin stationary phases for LC chiral separation. *Talanta* 1996, 43, 1767-1782.

[153] Berthod, A., He, L. F., Beesley, T. E.: Temperature and enantioseparation by macrocyclic glykopeptide chiral stationary phase. *J. Chromatogr. A*. 2004, 1060, 205-21.

[154] Henriksson, H., Muñoz, I. G., Isaksson, R., Pettersson, G., Johansson, G.: Cellobiohydrolase 58 (P.c. Cel 7D) is complementary to the homologous CBH I (T.r. Cel 7A) in enantioseparations. *J. Chromatogr. A*. 2000, 898, 63-74.

[155] Barnhart, W. W., Gahm, K. H., Hua, Z., Goetzinger, W.: Supercritical fluid chromatography comparison of the poly(*trans*-1,2-cyclohexanediyl-bis acrylamide) (P-CAP) column with several derivatized polysaccharide-based stationary phases. *J. Chromatogr. B Analyt. Technol. Biomed. Life Sci.* 2008, 875, 217-229.

[156] Vozka, J., Kalikova, K., Roussel, C., Armstrong, D. W., Tesarova, E.: An insight into the use of dimethylphenyl carbamate cyclofructan 7 chiral stationary phase in supercritical fluid chromatography: the basic comparison with HPLC. *J. Sep. Sci.* 2013, 36, 1711-1719.

[157] Mangelings, D., Maftouh, M., Massart, D. L., Vander Heyden, Y.: Comparison of the miniaturised techniques capillary electrochromatography and capillary liquid chromatography for the chiral separation of chlorthalidone. *J. Pharm. and Biomed. Anal.* 2004, 35, 789-799.

[158] Fillet, M., Fotsing, L., Crommen, J.: Enantioseparation of uncharget compounds by capillary electrophoresis using mixture of anionic and neutral β-cyclodextrin derivatives. *J. Chromatogr. A* 1998, 817, 113-119.

[159] Tero-Vescan, A., Ilancu, G., Oroian, M., Cârje, A.: Chiral separation of indapamide enantiomers by capillary electrophoresis. *Adv. Pharm. Bull.* 2014, 4, 267-272.

[160] Dolling, U. H., Davis, P., Grabowski, E. J. J.: Efficient catalytic asymmetric alkylations. 1. Enantioselective synthesis of (+)-indacrinone via chiral phase-transfer catalysis. *J. Am. Chem. Soc.* 1984, 106, 446-447.

[161] Hughes, D. L., Dolling, U. H., Ryan, K. M., Schoenewaldt, E. F., Grabowski, E. J. J.: Efficient catalytic asymmetric alkylations. 3. A kinetic and mechanistic study of the enantioselective phase-transfer methylation of 6,7-dichloro-5-methoxy-2-phenyl-1-indanone. *J. Org. Chem.* 1987, 52, 4745-4752.

[162] Zhu, Y.-P., Cai, Q., Jia, F.-Ch., Liu, M.-C., Gao, Q.-H., Meng, X.-G., Wu, A.-X: Electronic tuning cyclization of aryl-1,4-enediones: $AlCl_3$-mediated Nazarov-type cyclization to synthesize polysubstituted-1-indanones. *Tetrahedron* 2014, 70, 9536-9544.

[163] Allin, S. M., Thomas, Ch. I., Allard, J. E., Duncton, M., Mark, R. J., Elsegood, M. R. J., Edgar, M.: Stereoselective synthesis of the indolizinoindole ring system. *Tetrahedron Letters* 2003, 44, 2335-2337.

[164] Li, G., Zhang, Y.: Stereoselective synthesis of the two major metabolites of spironolactone, 3- and 3-hydroxy-7-methylthio-17-pregn-4-ene-21, 17-carbolactone. *Steroids* 2007, 72, 569-572.

[165] Brunton, L. L., Chabner, B. A., Knollmann, B. C. (eds.): *Goodman nad Gilmanś The pharmacological basic of therapeutics*, 12th ed. McGraw-Hill Companies 2011.

[166] Leon-Romo, J. L., Virues, C. I., Avina, J., Regla, I., Juaristi, E.: Preparation of (*R*) and (*S*)-alpha methyldopa from a chiral hydantoin containing the alpha phenylethyl group. *Chirality* 2002, 14, 144-50.

[167] Dolezalova, M., Fanali, S.: Enantiomeric separation dihydroxyphenylalanine (DOPA), methyldihydroxyphenylalanine (MDOPA) and hydrazinomethyldihydroxy phenylalanine (CDOPA) by using capillary electrophoresis with sulfobutyl ether-beta-cyclodextrin as a chiral selector. *Electrophoresis* 2000, 3264-3269.

[168] Gelber, L. R., Neumeyer, J. L.: Determination of the enantiomeric purity of levodopa, methyldopa, carbidopa and tryptophan by use of chiral mobile phase high-performance liquid chromatography. *J. Chromatogr.* 1983, 257, 317-326.

[169] Dolezalova, M., Tkaczykova, M.: Direct high-performance liquid chromatographic determination of the enantiomeric purity of levodopa and methyldopa: comparison with pharmacopoeial polarimetric methods. *J. Pharm. Biomed. Anal.* 1999, 19, 555-567.

[170] Waeber, B.: Combination therapy with ACE inhibitors/angiotensin II receptor antagonists and diuretics in hypertension. *Expert Rev. Cardiovasc. Ther.* 2003, 1, 9-16.

[171] Brown, N. J., Vaughan, D. E.: Angiotensin-converting enzyme inhibitors. *Circulation* 1998, 97, 1411-1420.

[172] Peng, H., Carreters, O. A., Vuljaj, N., Liao, T. D., Motivala, A., Peterson, E. L., Rhaleb, N. E.: Angiotensin-converting enzyme inhibitors: a new mechanism of action. *Circulation* 2005, 112, 2436-2445.

[173] Sramko, M., Remko, M.: Angiotensin converting enzyme inhibitors. *Ceska Slov. Farm.* 2006, 55, 160-167 (in slovak).

[174] Nemec, K., Schubert-Zsilavecz, M.: Vom Teoprotid zum Captopril. Rationales design von ACE-hemmern. *Pharm. Unserer Zeit.* 2003, 32, 11-15.

[175] Chopra, M., Beswick, H., Clapperton, M., Dargie, H. J., Smith, W. E., McMurray, J.: Antioxidant effects of angiotensin-converting enzyme (ACE) inhibitors: free radical and oxidant scavenging are sulphydryl dependent, but lipid peroxidation is inhibited by both sulphydryl- and nonsulphydryl-containing ACE inhibitors. *J. Cardiovasc. Pharmacol.*, 1992, 19, 330-340.

[176] Mansour, F. R., Danielson, N. D.: Separation methods for captopril in pharmaceuticals and biological fluids. *J. Sep. Sci.* 2012, 35, 1213-1226.

[177] Rudzki, P. J., Buś, K., Ksycinska, H., Kobylinska, K.: An overview of chromatographic methods coupled with mass spectrometric detection for determination of angiotensin-converting enzyme inhibitors in biological material. *J. Pharm. Biomed. Anal.* 2007, 44, 356-367.

[178] Both, D. A., Jemal, M.: Stereoisomeric purity determination of captopril by capillary gas chromatography. *J. Chromatogr.* 1991, 558, 257-263.

[179] Owens, P. K., Svensson, L. A., Vessman, J.: Direct separation of captopril diastereoisomers including their rotational isomers by RP-LC using a teicoplanin column. *J. Pharm. Biomed. Anal.* 2001, 25, 453-464.

[180] Russell, J., McKeown, J. A., Hensman, C., Smith, W. E., Reglinski, J.: HPLC determination of biologically active thiols using pre-column derivatization with 5,´5-dithio-(bis-2-nitrobenzoic acid). *J. Pharm. Biomed. Anal.* 1997, 15, 1757-1763.

[181] Hillaert, S., Van Den Bossche, W.: Determination of captopril on a coated capillary by capillary electrophoresis. *J. Pharm. Belg.* 1999, 54, 83-84.

[182] Wronski, M.: Separation of urinary thiols as tributyltinmercaptides and determination using capillary isotachophoresis *J. Chromatogr. B Biomed. Appl.* 1996, 676, 29-34.

[183] Stefan, R. I., Van Staden, J. K., Aboul-Enein, H. Y.: Simultaneous detection of *S*- and *R*-captopril using sequetial injection analysis. *Talanta,* 2000, 51, 969-975.

[184] Stefan, R. I., Van Staden, J. K., Aboul-Enein, H. Y.: Amperometric biosensor/sequetial injection analysis system for simultaneous determination of *S*- and *R*-captopril. *Biosens. Bioelectron.* 2000, 15, 1-5.

[185] Siangproh, W., Ngamukot, P., Chailapakul, O.: Electrochemical determination of captopril at boron-doped diamond thin film electrode applied to a flow injection system. *Sensors and Actuators B,* 2005, 91, 60-66.

[186] Kocijan, A., Grahek, R., Kocjan, D., Zupancic-Kralj, L.: Effect of column temperature on the behaviour of some angiotensin converting enzyme inhibitors during high-performance liquid chromatographic analysis. *J. Chromatogr. B Biomed. Sci.* 2001, 755, 229-35.

[187] Trabelsi, H., Bouabdallah, S., Sabbah, S., Raouafi, F., Bouzouita, K.: Study of the *cis*-trans isomerization of enalapril by reversed-phase liquid chromatography. *J. Chromatogr. A.* 2000, 871,189-199.

[188] Bouabdallah, S., Trabelsi, H., Ben Dhia, T., Sabbah, S., Bouzouita, K., Khaddar, R.: RP-HPLC and NMR study of *cis-trans* isomerization of enalaprilat. *J. Pharm. Biomed. Anal.* 2003, 31, 731-41.

[189] Bouabdallah, S., Trabelsi, H., Bouzouita, K., Sabbah, S.: Reversed-phase liquid chromatography of lisinopril conformers. *J. Biochem. Biophys. Methods* 2002, 54, 391-405.

[190] Aboul-Enein, H. Y., Stefan, R. I., Radu, G. L.: Biosensor for enantioselective analysis of *S*-cilazapril, *S*-trandolapril, and *S*-pentopril. *Pharm. Dev. Technol.* 1999, 4, 251-5.

[191] Stefan, R. I., Staden, J. F., Bala, C., Aboul-Enein, H. Y.: On-line assay of the *S*-enantiomers of enalapril, ramipril and pentopril using a sequential injection analysis/amperometric biosensor system. *J. Pharm. Biomed. Anal.* 2004, 36, 889-892.

[192] Stefan, R. I., Staden, J. F., Mulaudzi, L. V., Aboul-Enein, H. Y.: On line simultaneous determination of *S*- and *R*-perindopril using amperometric biosensor as detector in flow system. *Analyt. Chim. Acta* 2002, 467, 189-195.

[193] Ciabatti, R., Padova, G., Bellasio, E., Tarzia, G., Depaoli, A., Battaglia, F., Cellentani, M., Barone, D., Baldoli, E.: Angiotensin converting enzyme inhibitors as antihypertensive agents. 1-[(2-mercaptocycloalkyl)carbonyl] L prolines. *J. Med. Chem* 1986, 29, 411-417.

[194] Oritz, A., Arellano, O., Sansinenea, E., Bernes, S.: Stereoselective crystallization as a key step for the synthesis of new epimers of captopril derivatives. *J. Mex. Chem. Soc.* 2007, 5, 245-248.

[195] Chang, Ch. Y., Yang, T. K.: Asymmetric synthesis of ACE inhibitor-Benazepril HCl via a bioreductive reaction. *Tetrahedron: Asymmetry* 2003, 14, 2239-2245.
[196] Mistra, B., Medhane, D., Mohanraj, K., Ghonr, S. A.: Microwave-assisted synthesis of an important intermediate of benazepril. *Ind. J. Pharm. Science* 2010, 72, 378-380.
[197] Yu, T. L., Huang, J. L., Chang, Ch. Y., Yang, T. K.: Formal synthesis of the ACE inhibitor benazepril.HCl via an asymmetric aza-Michael reaction. *Molecules* 2006, 11, 641-648.
[198] Ahmad, Al.L., Oh, P.C., Abd Shukor, S.R.: Sustainable biocatalytic synthesis of L-homophenylalanine as pharmaceutical drug precursor. *Biotechnol. Adv.* 2009, 27, 286-296.
[199] De Lima, D. P.: Synthesis of angiotensin-converting enzyme (ACE) inhibitors as important class of antihypertensive drug. *Quimica Nova* 1999, 22, 375-381.
[200] Jensen, C., Herold, P., Brunner, H. R.: Aliskiren: the first renin inhibitor for clinical treatment. *Nat. Rev. Drug Discov.* 2008, 7, 399-410.
[201] Friedrich, S., Schmieder, R. E.: Review of direct renin inhibition by aliskiren. *J. Renin Angiotensin Aldosterone Syst.* 2013, 14, 193-196.
[202] Zaporowska-Stachowiak, I., Hoffmann, K., Bryl, W., Minczykowski, A.: Aliskiren - an alternative to angiotensin-converting enzyme inhibitors or angiotensin receptor blockers in the therapy of arterial hypertension. *Arch. Med. Sci.* 2014, 10, 830-836.
[203] Ashok, S., Varma, M. S., Swaminathan, S.: A validated LC method for the determination of the enantiomeric purity of aliskiren hemifumarate in bulk drug samples. *J. Chromatogr. Sci.* 2012, 50, 799-802.
[204] Flesch, G., Muller, P., Lloyd, P.: Absolute bioavailability and pharmacokinetics of valsartan, an angiotenin II receptor antagonist, in man. *Eur. J. Clin. Pharmacol.* 1997, 52, 115-120.
[205] Raju, V. B., Rao, A. L.: 2011. Reversed phase HPLC analysis of valsartan in pharmaceutical dosage forms. *IjCEPr*, 2011, 2, 56-60.
[206] Gonzalez, O., Iriarte, G., Rico, E., Ferreirós, N., Maguregui, M. I., Alonso, R. M., Jiménez, R. M.: LC–MS/MS method for the determination of several drugs used in combined cardiovascular therapy in human plasma. *J. Chromatogr. B*, 2010, 878, 2685-2692.
[207] Hillaert, S., Bossche, W.: Simultaneous determination of hydrochlorothiazide and several angiotensin-II-receptor antagonists by capillary electrophoresis. *J. Pharm. Biomed. Anal.* 2003, 31, 329-339.
[208] Alnajjar, A. O.: Validation of a capillary electrophoresis method for the simultaneous determination of amlodipine besylate and valsartan in pharmaceuticals and human plasma. *J. AOAC Inter.* 2011, 94, 498-502.
[209] Francotte, E., Davatz, A., Richert, P.: Development and validation of chiral high-performance liquid chromatographic methods for the quantitation of valsartan and of the tosylate of valinebenzyl ester. *J. Chromatogr. B* 1996, 686, 77-83.
[210] Rane, V., Patil, K., Shinde, D.: Enantiomeric LC separation of valsartan on amylose based stationary phase. *Pharmazie* 2009, 64, 495-498.
[211] Lee, K. R., Nguyen, N. T., Lee, Y. J., Choi, S., Kang, J. S., Mar, W., Kim, K. H.: Determination of the *R*-enantiomer of valsartan in pharmaceutical formulation by capillary electrophoresis. *Arch. Pharm. Res.* 2014, DOI 10.1007/s12272-014-0449-7 [Epub. ahead of print].

[212] Romero, M., Sánchez, I., Pujol, M. D.: New advances in the field of calcium channel antagonists: cardiovascular effects and structure-activity relationships. *Curr. Med. Chem. – Cardiovasc. Hematol. Agents*. 2003, 1, 113-141.

[213] Bkaily, G., Jacques, D.: L-Type Calcium Channel Antagonists and Suppression of Expression of Plasminogen Receptors Is the Missing Link the L-Type Calcium Channel. *Circ. Res.* 2009, 105, 112-113.

[214] Cizmarikova, R., Nemethy, A., Bruchata, K.: Chiral aspects in the group of antihypertensive drugs III. Calcium channel blockers. *Farm. Obzor* 2014, 83, 167-175 (in slovak).

[215] Kendall, H. E., Luscombe, D. K.: Calcium channel blocking drugs. In: Ellis, G. P., West, G. B. ed: *Progress in medicinal chemistry*. Elsevier, 24, 1987, 249-299.

[216] Moshtaghi, Z. A., Raisossadat, O. M., Sadeghi, Sh. Q.: Synthesis of novel unsymmetrically substituted 1,4-dihydropyridines and separation of the enantiomers of racemic 1,4-dihydropyridine containing isothioureido group. *ARKIVOC*, 2006, 14, 15-21.

[217] Jabor, V. A. P., Coelho, E. B., Ifa, D. R., Bonato, P. S., Santos, N. A. G., Lanchote, V. L.: Enantioselective determination of lercanidipine in human plasma for pharmacokinetic studies by normal-phase liquid chromatography-tandem mass spectrometry. *J. Chromatogr. B.* 2003, 796, 429-437.

[218] Ericsson, H., Schwieler, J., Lindmark, B., Löfdahl, P., Thulin, T., Regardh, C. G.: Enantioselective pharmacokinetics of the enantiomers of clevidipine following intravenous infusion of the racemáte in essentials hypertensive patiens. *Chirality* 2001, 13, 130-134.

[219] Rask, H. S., Angelo, H. R., Christensen, H. R.: Enantioselective determination of isradipine in human serum using chiral stationary phase liquid chromatography and gas chromatography with nitrogen selective detection. *Chirality* 1998, 10, 808-812.

[220] Gottfries, J., Johanson, P., Karlson, A.: Influence of chromatographic descriptors on enantioresolution of a dihydropyridine and structurally related compounds. *J. Chromatogr. A.* 1997, 763, 115-123.

[221] Okamoto, Y., Aburatani, R., Hatala, K., Honda, M., Inotusme, N., Nakano, M.: Optical resolution of dihydropyridine enantiomers by high-performance liquid chromatography using phenylcarbamates of polysaccharides as a chiral stationary phase. *J. Chromatogr. A.* 1990, 513, 375-378.

[222] Okamoto, T., Uno, T., Sugawara, K.: Enantiomer separation of dihydropyridine derivatives by liquid chromatography with chiral stationary phase. *Chromatographia*, 33, 1992, 287-288.

[223] Ohkubo, T., Uno, T., Sugawara, K.: Enantiomer separation of dihydropyridine derivative by high-performance liquid chromatography with chiral stationary phase. *J. Chromatogr. A.* 1994, 659, 467-471.

[224] Küsters, E., Dosenbach, C., Gerber, G.: Enantiomeric separation of isradipine and related compounds by liquid chromatography with a chiral stationary phase. *J. High Resolut. Chromatogr.* 1991, 14, p. 769-770.

[225] Boato, G., Neiddu, M., Faedda, M. V., De Caprariis, P.: Enantiometric separation by HPLC of 1,4-dihydropyridines with vancomycin as chiral selector. *Chirality* 2003, 15, 494-497.

[226] Tokuma Y., Noguchi, H.: Stereoselective pharmacokinetic of dihydropyridine calcium antagonists. *J. Chromatogr. A.* 1995, 694, 181-193.

[227] Inotsume, N., Nakano, M.: Stereoselective determination and pharmacokinetics of dihydropyridines : an updated review. *J. Biochem. Biophys. Methods*. 2002, 54, 255-274.

[228] Yamaguchi, M., Yamashita, K., Aoki, I., Tabata, T., Hirai, S. I., Yashiki, T.: Determination of manidipine enantiomers in human serum using chiral chromatography and column switching liquid chromatography. *J. Chromatogr.* 1992, 575, 123-129.

[229] Berthod, A., Jin, H. L., Beesley, T. E., Duncan, J. D., Armstrong, D. W.: Cyclodextrin chiral stationary phases for liquid chromatographic separation of drug stereoisomers. *J. Pharm. Biomed. Anal.*, 1990, 8, 123-130.

[230] Qiang, F. U., Matsunaga, H., Haginaka, J.: Resolution of dihydropyridine calcium antagonist enantiomers using HPLC with ovoglycoprotein as a chiral stationary phase. *Anal. Sci.* 2001, 17, 897-900.

[231] Kawabata, K., Samata, N., Urasaki, Y., Fukazawa, I., Uchida, N., Uchida, E., Yasuhara, H.: Enantioselective determination of azelnidipine in human plasma using liquid chromatography-tandem mass spectrometry. *J. Chromatogr. B Analyt. Technol. Biomed. Life Sci.* 2007, 852, 389-397.

[232] Streel, B., Lainé, C., Zimmer, C., Sibenaler, R., Ceccato, A.: Enantiomeric determination of amlodipine in human plasma by liquid chromatogramy coupled to tandem mass spectrometry. *J. Biochem. Biophys. Methods* 2002, 54, 357-368.

[233] Marques, M. P., Santos, N. A. G., Coelho, E. B., Bonato, P. S., Lanchote, V. L., Enantioselective assay of nisoldipine in human plasma by chiral high-performance liquid chromatogramy combined with gas chromatographic-mass spectrometry: applications to pharmacokinetics. *J. Chromatogr. B* 2001, 762, 87-95.

[234] Lindmark, B., Ahnoff, M., Persson, B. A.: Enantioselective determination of felodipine in human plasma by chiral normal-phase liquid chromatography and electrospray ionisation mass spectrometry. *J. Pharm. Biomed. Anal.* 2002, 27, 489-495.

[235] Zhu, Q., Yu, P., Deng, O., Zeng, L.: β-Cyclodextrin-bonded chiral stationary phase for thin-layer chromatographic separation of enantiomers. *J. Planar Chromatogr.* 2001, 14, 137-139.

[236] Van Eeckhaut, A., Detaevernier, M. R., Michotte, Y.: Separation of neutral dihydropiridines and their enantiomers using electrokinetic chromatography. *J. Pharm. Anal.* 2004, 36, 799-805.

[237] Wanner-Olsen, H., Gaarskaer, F. B., Mikkelsen, E. O., Jacobsen, O., Voldby, B.: Studies on concentration-time profiles of nimodipine enantiomers following intravenous and oral administration of nimodipine in patients with subarachnoid hemorrhage. *Chirality* 2000, 12, 660-664.

[238] Zhang, X. P., Loke, K., Mital, S., Chahwala, S., Hintze, S. H.: Paradoxical release of nitric oxide by an L-type calcium channel antagonist, the *R*-enantiomer of amlodipine. *J. Cardiovasc. Pharmacol.* 2002, 39, 208-214.

[239] Zandkarimi, M., Shafaati, A., Foroutan, S. M., Charles, A. Lucy.: Rapid enantioseparation of amlodipine by highly sulfated cyclodextrins using short-end injection capillary electrophoresis. *DARU J. Pharm. Sci.* 2009, 17, 269-276.

[240] Cui, Y., Ma, X., Zhao, M., Jiang, Z., Xu, S., Guo, X.: Combined use of ionic liquid and hydroxypropyl-β-cyclodextrin for the enantioseparation of ten drugs by capillary electrophoresis. *Chirality* 2013, 25, 409-414.

[241] Tabani, H., Mahyari, M., Sahragard, A., Fakhari, A. R., Shaabani, A.: Evaluation of sulfated maltodextrin as a novel anionic chiral selector for the enantioseparation of basic chiral drugs by capillary electrophoresis. *Electrophoresis* 2015, 36, 305-311.

[242] Chen, J., Du, Y., Zhu, F., Chen, B., Zhang, Q., Du, S., Li, P.: Study of the enantioseparation capability of chiral dual system based on chondroitin sulfate C in capillary electrophoresis. *Electrophoresis* 2015, 36, 607-614.

[243] Mikus, P., Marakova, K., Valaskova, I., Havranek, E.: Determination of amlodipine enantiomers in pharmaceuticals using capillary electrophoresis separation and diode array detection. *Pharmazie* 2009, 64, 76-79.

[244] Mikus, P., Marakova, K., Marak, J., Nemec, I., Valaskova, I., Havranek, E.: Direct quantitative determination of amlodipine enantiomers in urine samples for pharmacokinetic study using on line coupled isotachophoresis-capillary zone electrophoresis separation method with diode array detection. *J. Chromatogr. B. Analyt. Technol. Biomed. Life Sci.* 2008, 875, 266-272.

[245] Laethem, M. E., Belpaire, F. M., Wijnant, P., Bogaert, M. G.: Stereoselective pharmacokinetics of oxprenolol, propranolol, and verapamil. Species differences and influence of endotoxin. *Chirality* 1995, 7, 616-622.

[246] Sasaki, M., Taheishi, T., Ebihara, A.: The effects of age and gender on the stereoselective pharmacokinetics of verapamil. *Clin. Pharmacol. Ther.* 1993, 54, 278-285.

[247] Chu, Y. Q., Wainer, I. W.: Determination of the enantiomers of verapamil and norverapamil in serum using coupled achiral-chiral high-performance liquid chromatography. *J. Chromatogr.* 1989, 497, 191-200.

[248] Brandsteterová, E., Wainer, I. W.: Achiral and chiral high-performance liquid chromatography of verapamil and its metabolites in serum samples. *J. Chromatogr. B* 1999, 732, 395-404.

[249] Shibukawa, A., Wainer, I. W.: Simultaneous direct determination of the enantiomers of verapamil and norverapamil in plasma using a derivatized amylose high-performance liquid chromatographic chiral stationary phase. *J. Chromatogr.* 1992, 574, 85-92.

[250] Perrin, C., Vu, V. A., Matthijs, N., Maftouh, M., Massart, D. L., Van Der Heyden, Y.: Screening approach for chiral separation of pharmaceuticals Part I. Normal-phase liquid chromatography. *J. Chromatogr. A.* 2002, 947, 69-83.

[251] Rustichelli, C., Ferioli, V., Gamberini, G.: Resolution of the enantiomers of verapamil and galopamil by chiral liquid chromatography-mass spectrometry. *Chromatographia.* 1997, 44, 477-483.

[252] Sandström, R., Lennernäs, H., Öhlér, K., Karlsson, A.: Enantiomeric separation of verapamil and norverapamil using Chiral-AGP as the stationary phase. *J. Pharm. Biomed. Anal.* 1999, 21, 43-49.

[253] Brandsteterova, E., Endresz, G., Blaschke, G.: Chiral separation of verapamil and some of its metabolites by HPLC and CE. *Pharmazie* 2001, 56, 536-541.

[254] Muderawan, I. W., Ong, T. T., Ng, S. C.: Urea bonded cyclodextrin derivatives onto silica for chiral HPLC. *J. Sep. Sci.* 2006, 29, 1849-1871.

[255] Lee, G. R., Hyun, M. H.: Liquid chromatographic resolution of fendiline and its analogues on a chiral stationary phase based on (+)-(18-crown-6)-2,3,11,12-tetracarboxylic acid. *Molecules* 2014, 19(12), 21386-97.
[256] Lin, B., Zhu, X., Wuerthner, S., Epperlein, U., Koppenhoefer, B.: Separation of enantiomers of drugs by capillary electrophoresis part 8. beta-cyclodextrin as chiral solvating agent. *Talanta* 1998, 46, 743-749.
[257] Chankvetadze, B., Lomsadze, K., Burjanadze, N., Breitkreutz, J., Pintore, G., Chessa, M., Bergander, K., Blaschke, G.: Comparative enantioseparations with native beta-cyclodextrin, randomly acetylated beta-cyclodextrin and heptakis-(2,3-di-o-acetyl)-beta-cyclodextrin in capillary electrophoresis. *Electrophoresis* 2003, 24, 1083-1091.
[258] Gotti, R., Pomponio, R., Cavrini, V.: Linear, neutral polysaccharides as chiral selectors in enantioresolution of basic drug racemates by capillary electrophoresis. *Chromatographia* 2000, 52, 273-277.
[259] Wedig, M., Thunhorst, M., Laug, S., Decker, M., Lehmann, J., Holzgrabe, U.: Enantioseparation of linear and cyclic chiral bis (phenethyl)amines by means of cyclodextrin-modified capillary electrophoresis. *Fresenius J. Anal. Chem.* 2001, 371, 212-217.
[260] Yang, G. S., Chen, D. M., Yang, Y., Tang, B., Gao, J. J., Aboul-Enein, H. Y., Koppenhoefer, B.: Enantioseparation of some clinically used drugs by capillary electrophoresis using sulfated β-cyclodextrin as a chiral selector. *Chromatographia* 2005, 62, 441-445.
[261] Clothier, Jr, J. G., Tomellini, S. A.: Chiral separation of verapamil and related compounds using micellar electrokinetic capillary chromatography with mixed micelles of bile salts and polyoxyethylene ethers. *J. Chromatogr. A.* 1996, 723, 179-187.
[262] Bhushan, R., Gupta, D.: Thin-layer chromatography separation of enantiomers of verapamil using macrocyclic antibiotic as a chiral selector. *Biomed. Chromatogr.* 2005, 19, 474-478.
[263] Tanaka, T., Inoue, H., Date, T., Aoe, K., Takeda, M., Kugita, H., Murata, S., Yamaguchi, T., Kikkawa, K., et al.: Synthesis of the optically active *trans*-isomers of diltiazem and their cardiovascular effects and Ca-antagonist activity. *Chem. Pharm. Bull.* 1992, 40, 1476 -1480.
[264] Ishii, K., Minato, K., Nishimura, N., Miyamoto, T., Sato, T.: Direct chromatographic resolution of four optical isomers of diltiazem hydrochloride on Chiralcel OF column. *J. Chromatogr.* 1994, 686, 93-100.
[265] Yoku, K., Aoe, K., Nishimura, N., Sato, T., Morishita, F.: Chiral resolution of four optical isomers of diltiazem hydrochloride on chiral columns by packed-column supercritical fluid chromatography. *J. Chromatogr. A.* 1997, 785, 185-193.
[266] Yoku, K., Aoe, K., Nishimura, N., Morishita, F.: Thermodynamic study and separation mechanism of diltiazem optical isomers in packed-column supercritical fluid chromatography. *J. Chromatogr.* 1999, 848, 337-345.
[267] Ishii, K., Banno, K., Miyamoto, T., Kakimoto, T.: Determination of diltiazem hydrochloride enantiomers in dog plasma using stationary-phase liquid chromatography. *J. Chromatogr.* 1991, 564, 338-345.
[268] Jain, P., Narang, G., Jindal, D. P., Bansal, R., Calle, C., Carron, R., Pemperton, K., Harvey, A. L.: Synthesis of a new series of 4-aryl-1,4-dihydropyridines with calcium channel blocking and vasodilatory activity. *Pharmazie* 61, 2006, 400-405.

[269] http://www.organic-chemistry.org/namedreactions/hantzsch-dihydropyridine-synthesis.shtm.

[270] Saini, A., Kumar, S., Sandhu, J. S.: Hantzch reaction: recent advances in Hantzch 1,4-dihydropyridines. *J. Sci. Ind. Res.* 67, 2008, 95-111.

[271] Yoshida, K., Inokuma, T., Takasu, K., Takemoto, Y.: Catalytic asymmetric synthesis oif both enantiomers of 4-substituted 1,4-dihydropyridines with use of bifunctional thiourea-ammonium salts bearing different counterions. *Molecules* 15, 2010, 8305-8326.

[272] Mermerian, A. H., Fu, G. C.: Nucleophile-catalyzed asymmetric acylations of silyl ketene imines: application to the enantioselective synthesis of verapamil. *Angew. Chem. Int. Ed.* 2005, 44, 949-952.

[273] Banister, R. M., Brookes, M. H., Evans, G. R., Katz, R. B., Tyrrell, N. D.: A scaleable route to the pure enantiomers of verapamil. *Org. Process Res. Dev.* 2000, 4, 467-472.

[274] Knabe, J.: Synthetische Enantiomere als Arzneistoffe. *Pharmazie in unserer Zeit* 1995, 24, 324-330.

[275] Lévai, A.: Optically active 1,5-benzothiazepines. *Pharmazie*, 54, 1999, 719-726.

[276] Mannhold, R., Kubinyi, H., Timmerman, H.: *New trends in synthetic medicinal chemistry.* Wiley – VCH Vol. 7, 2000, 118-120.

[277] Miyata, O., Shinada, T., Naito, T., Ninomiya, I., Date, T., Okamura, T.: Stereoselective addition of 2-aminothiophenol to α-alkoxycinnamic acid derivatives—alternative synthesis of (±)-diltiazem. *Tetrahedron* 1993, 49, 8119-8128.

[278] Liisa, T., Kanerva, L., Sundholm, O.: Lipase catalysis in the resolution of racemic intermediates of diltiazem synthesis in organic solvents. *J. Chem. Soc. Perkin Trans.* 1993, 1, 1385-1389.

[279] Mordant, C., Caño de Andrade, C., Touati, R., Ratovelomanana-Vidal, V., Hassine, B. B.: Stereoselective Synthesis of Diltiazem via Dynamic Kinetic Resolution. *Synthesis* 2003, 15, 2405-2409.

[280] Hashiyama, T.: Applications of Lewis acids for the efficient syntheses of diltiazem, cephems, and taxoids. *Med. Res. Rev.* 2000, 20, 485-501.

[281] Ozaki, Y., Yamada, S., Seko, H.: Process for preparing optically active benzothiazepine compounds by asymmetric reduction. *Patent:* US5310904 A, 1994, http://www.google.com.br/patents/US5310904.

[282] Nishida, T., Matsumae, H., Machida, I., Shibatani, T.: Microbial asymmetric reduction. Preparation of optically active methyl *trans*-3-(4-methoxyphenyl)glycidates. *Bioanal. Biotransform.* 1995, 12, 205-214.

In: Antihypertensive Drugs
Editor: Scott Caldwell

ISBN: 978-1-63463-829-6

Chapter II

Evaluation of Genotoxic Effects of Antihypertensive Drugs: Angiotensin II Receptor Blockers

Iratxe Huerta[1,2], Maitane Barasoain[1], Mercedes Télez[1,2], Eduardo Ortiz-Lastra[3], Javier González[3], Mikel Longa[2], Javier Muga[2], Gorka Barrenetxea[3], Begoña Criado[4] and Isabel Arrieta*[*1]

[1]Department of Genetics,Physical Anthropology and Animal physiology, Faculty of Science and Technology, University of the Basque Country, Bilbao, Spain
[2]Virgen de Begoña Clinical Analysis Laboratory (Medikosta), Erandio, Spain
[3]Department of Medical-Surgical Specialities, Faculty of Medicine, University of the Basque Country, Bilbao, Spain
[4]Cooperativa de Ensino Superior Politecnico e Universitario (CESPU), Porto, Portugal

Abstract

Arterial Hypertension is one of the most important preventable contributors to disease and death, and is commonly treated with antihypertensive drugs combined with appropriate changes in life-style. The large majority of hypertensive patients need long-term therapy and because of the long duration of the pharmacological treatment, documentation of safety and efficiency is required, including sensitive indices of genotoxic damage.

In this study, the potential genotoxic effect of five Angiotensin II receptor blockers (ARBs: Candesartan, Telmisartan, Eprosartan, Valsartan, Olmesartan) was analyzed *in*

[*]Corresponding author at: Department of Genetics, Physical Anthropology and Animal Physiology, Faculty of Science and Technology, University of the Basque Country, Apdo. 644-48080, Bilbao, Spain. Tel.: +34 946012605; fax: +34 946013145.E-mail address: mariaisabel.arrieta@ehu.es (I. Arrieta).

vivo and *in vitro* in human peripheral blood lymphocytes (PBLs) by means of the cytokinesis-block micronucleus (CBMN) assay in combination with fluorescence *in situ* hybridization (FISH) with a centromeric probe, and by the analysis of structural chromosomal aberrations (sCA) and expression of fragile sites (FS). The *in vivo* study was carried out in 55 hypertensive patients while the *in vitro* study was performed in 10 control individuals by adding the drugs to the culture medium at a final concentration similar to the levels found in plasma in patients. In relation to the CBMN assay, our results showed a significant increase in the frequencies of MN and binucleated cells with MN (BNMN) *in vivo* and especially *in vitro*. FISH analysis revealed no significant differences between patients and control individuals in the frequency of centromeric signals. Regarding the incidence of sCA, the data revealed again a significantly higher rate of sCA *in vivo*, and mostly *in vitro*. Chromosomal location analysis pointed at chromosomes 16 and 17 as preferential targets for the clastogenic effect of ARBs drugs. Several FS emerged as specific; among them, the *locus* 17q21, recently proposed as a new FS, was only expressed in ARBs-treated patients, supporting the findings for a linkage between hypertension and a telomeric *locus* on chromosome 17.

Therefore, these results are consistent with our previous studies of beta-blockers genotoxicity and provide evidence for an association among the antihypertensive therapy, arterial hypertension and DNA damage in human lymphocytes.

1. Introduction

Arterial Hypertension (AHT) is the most prevalent treatable risk factor for diseases of the heart, brain and kidneys, being therefore associated with increased cardiovascular morbidity and mortality [Kearney et al., 2005; Mancia et al., 2013]. Nowadays, the condition affects to more than 1 billon adults worldwide, although because of the increasing longevity and prevalence of contributing factors such as obesity, AHT is project to increase to 1.56 billion people affected by the year 2020 [Chobanian et al., 2003; Messerly et al., 2007]. In Spain, according to the Spanish Society of Hypertension, the disorder affects to the 40% of the general adult population, increasing up to the 85% of the population above 65 years [Banegas et al., 1998; Banegas et al., 2002; Banegas et al., 2009].

Apart from appropriate lifestyle changes which are mandatory to control AHT, the condition should be usually treated with antihypertensive drugs [Chobanian et al., 2003; Mancia et al., 2007; Mancia et al., 2013; James et al., 2014]. Angiotensin-receptor blockers (ARBs) are a class of antihypertensive agents that are growing in popularity due to their excellent blood control pressure and tolerability. These pharmaceutical agents modulate the rennin-angiotensin-aldosterone system which is responsible for blood pressure regulation and fluid and electrolyte homeostasis [Streeten et al., 1976; De Gasparo et al., 2000; Taylor et al., 2011].

The first ARB, Losartan, was approved for clinical use in 1995, followed by six other drugs including Valsartan, Candesartan, Irbesartan, Telmisartan, Olmesartan and Eprosartan [Schaefer et al., 1996]. Despite belonging to the same drug class, ARBs vary in several aspects of their chemical structure, feature that leads to important differences in pharmacokinetic and pharmacodynamic characteristics [Song et al., 2000; Tamargo et al., 2006; Miura et al., 2011]. These differences may translate into differences in the antihypertensive effects, and thus they should be taken into account.

The antihypertensive therapy for the large majority of hypertensive patients need to be long-term administration and, therefore, patients are usually exposed to prolonged contact with these drugs. Thus, the long-term treatment requires documentation of safety and efficacy, including sensitive indices of genotoxic and carcinogenic damage [Kikland et al., 2005; Pfuhler et al., 2007; De Miguel et al., 2012]. In fact, genotoxicity testing of pharmaceuticals prior to commercialization is mandated by regulatory agencies worldwide. From a drug development standpoint, it is important to have a thorough understanding of the mechanism of any positive genetic toxicology findings so that informed decisions may be made with respect to risk [Snyder and Green, 2001]. Specifically, related to antihypertensive drugs, epidemiological genotoxicity and carcinogenicity studies show conflicting results, making it difficult to establish whether antihypertensive therapy while preventing cardiovascular complications, may be associated with an increase in genotoxic-carcinogenic risk [Bambrilla and Martelli, 2006; Bambrilla and Martelli, 2009; Bambrilla and Martelli, 2010].

However, as for almost every antihypertensive drug class which carcinogenic potential has been debated for decades, recent concerns have surfaced about possible links between ARBs and an increased cancer risk [Weinmann et al., 1994; Sipahi et al., 2010; Wuerzner et al., 2011; Olin et al., 2011; Wang et al., 2013; Coogan et al., 2013; Chiang et al., 2014]. Concerning genotoxicity assays, a few positive responses were obtained although results were not published in peer-reviewed journals. A review of genotoxicity and carcinogenicity testing of marketed pharmaceuticals indicates that only three ARBs, specifically Eprosartan, Irbesartan and Telmisartan have been tested for genotoxicity in human cells. Genotoxic results for Telmisartan were unclear while for Eprosartan resulted negative, and surprisingly Irbesartan showed genotoxic positive effects [Muller andKasper, 2000; Bambrilla andMartelli, 2006; Bambrilla andMartelli, 2009; Bambrilla andMartelli, 2010]. Based on the evidences, a thorough evaluation of the genotoxic and subsequently carcinogenic effects of ARBs in humans is greatly needed.

The cytokinesis-block micronucleus test (CBMNT) is a well-established method for measuring micronuclei (MN), which are cytogenetic markers extensively used for the detection of early biological effects of DNA-damaging agents [Fenech et al., 1985; Fenech et al., 1997; Fenech et al., 2007; Au et al., 2007; Kirsch-Volders et al., 2014]. Combination of fluorescence *in situ* hybridization (FISH) using pancentromeric regions with the CBNM assay allows for discrimination between clastogenic (inducing MN containing chromosome fragments) and aneugenic agents (inducing MN containing whole chromosomes) [Lindberg et al., 2008; Decodier et al., 2011]. In studies of human genotoxic effects, discriminating between these two phenomena is highly recommended [Norppa and Falck, 2003].

Structural chromosomal aberrations (sCA) represent the most validated biomarker in populations exposed to genotoxic agents and it is extensively accepted that a high frequency of sCA is predictive of an increased risk of cancer [Obe et al., 2002; Bonassi et al., 2008]. Previous studies have found a non-random distribution in the observed number of structural sCA [Bender et al., 1990; Télez et al., 2010].

Chromosomal fragile sites (FS) are specific loci that preferentially exhibit gaps and breaks on metaphase chromosome, involved in chromosomal instability [Sutherland et al., 2007]. A connection between FS and the cellular DNA-damage response was demonstrated. FS has also been proposed to be preferential targets for mutagens and carcinogens, being considered as regions of the genome particularly sensitive to genotoxic stress [Guler et al., 2007; Durkin and Glover, 2007].

Previous works reported by our group have revealed a possible genotoxicity of two antihypertensive drugs, the beta blocker Atenolol and the calcium antagonist Nimodipine [Télez et al., 2000; Télez et al., 2001]. In the present study, we evaluated the genotoxic potential *in vivo* and *in vitro* of five ARBs: Candesartan, Eprosartan, Olmesartan, Telmisartan and Valsartan. These drugs were cytogenetically tested for their ability to induce MN and sCA in cultured peripheral lymphocytes of patient under ARBs therapy and *in vitro* exposed control individuals. The origin of MN was determinate by FISH with a probe detecting all human centromeres. The information on FS indicates that non-random processes underlie the expression of FS, and thus the analysis of the FS significantly expressed in our samples has allowed the identification of possible specific and exclusive FS in hypertensive patients treated with ARBs.

2. Materials and Methods

Study Sample

The sample was made up of two different groups: 55 hypertensive patients (treated by Dr. Ortiz-Lastra) and 10 control individuals, matched with respect to sex, age and smoking habit (in the present study all individuals were non-smokers). Patients (29 females and 26 males) ranged in age from 49 and 77 years, with an average age of 61.6 years (Table I). The mean duration of the treatment was 2.8 years (5 months - 10 years). None of them was undergoing other medical treatments.

Table I. Descriptive characteristic of the different groups of patients according to the ARB treatment and the mean concentration used in culture mediums *in vitro*

	Candesartan	Eprosartan	Olmesartan	Telmisartan	Valsartan	Total
All patients	10	13	10	9	13	55
Males	5	6	5	5	5	26
Females	5	7	5	4	8	29
Age (years)						
Mean±SD	68.20±11.01	73.85±6.70	69.80±11.14	68.44±9.08	69.77±8.50	70.24±9.14
Duration of treatment (months)						
Range	5-60	12-120	8-120	12-96	2-108	2-120
Mean±SD	25.20±18.93	36.46±28.27	32.10±34.05	40.00±27.50	33.92±32.22	33.60±28.20
Dose (mg/day)						
Range	8-32	300-600	20-40	80	80-160	8-600
Dose in culture medium (mg/ml)	0.0016	0.12	0.004	0.016	0.016	

They did not have a previous history of known exposure to genotoxic compounds or a recent X-ray examination. The control group (5 females and 5 males) had an average age of 57.8 years, ranged from 50 to 62 years. All of them were healthy individuals not undergoing any pharmaceutical compound intake, without recent alcohol and/or drug consumption in the recent past.

All protocols were approved by the Ethical Committee of the University of the Basque Country and all subjects gave their informed consent. All participants in the patient and control groups provided a venous blood sample for cytogenetic analysis.

Blood Collection and Cell Cultures

Peripheral blood was collected by venipuncture into sterile vials containing sodium heparin (BD Vacutainer®) and vials were transferred to the laboratory where duplicate whole blood cultures were established within 24 h. For patients, the cultures were numbered with a code P1-P55 according to the sequence of blood collection. For control individuals, two different cultures were performed: one set number C1/T-1-C10/T-1 (control/T-1) and another set where the drug was added to the culture medium at the start of the culture. Drugs, kindly provided by Dr. Ortiz-Lastra, had previously been dissolved in distilled water, to give a final concentration in the culture medium that matched the average found in patients after oral intake (these analyses were performed by capillary zone electrophoresis in the Department of Analytical Chemistry, University of the Basque Country, Spain). Data are presented in Table 1. These cultures were numbered C1/medium-C10/medium (control/medium).

This methodology was based on the study by Kirkland [Kirkland et al., 1992].

Cytogenetic Tests

Lymphocytes cultures were set up by adding 0.5 ml of heparinised whole blood to 4.5 ml of RPMI 1640 medium (Gibco®), supplemented with 10% foetal bovine serum (Gibco®), 1% antibiotics (penicillin and streptomycin) (Gibco®) and HEPES buffer solution (Gibco®). Lymphocytes were stimulated by adding 4% phytohaemagglutinin (Gibco®).

For the MN assay, the cultures were incubated for 72 h at 37ºC. Binucleated (BN) cells were accumulated by adding cytochalasin B (Sigma Aldrich®) at 48 h following initiation of culture. At the end of the incubation time, the cells were collected by centrifugation. The cells were washed once in RPMI 1640 medium and then a mild hypotonic treatment (2–3 min in 0.075M KCl at room temperature) was carried out. The cells were then centrifuged and a methanol:acetic acid (5:1) solution was added. This fixation step was repeated twice. Air-dried preparations were made and the slides were stained with 10% Giemsa in phosphate buffer for 20 min [Fenech et al., 2007].

For the sCA analysis, the cultures were incubated for 72 h at 37ºC. One hour prior to harvest, 0.4 μg/ml of colcemid (Gibco®) was added to arrest the cells at metaphase. After recollecting the cells by centrifugation, the cells were resuspended in a pre-warmed hypotonic solution (0.075 M KCl) for 10 min and fixed three times in methanol:acetic acid (3:1). Chromosomal preparations were uniformly stained with Giemsa to detect chromosomal damage, expressed mainly as chromosomal lesions (gaps and breaks) [Moorhead et al., 1960].

Lately, for the FS analysis, a G banding technique was applied in order to re-examinate the preparations for an accurate identification of the breakpoints involved in the chromosomal damage [Seabright et al., 1971]. Criteria for cytogenetic evaluations were determined according to the International System for Human Cytogenetic Nomenclature [Shaffer et al., 2013].

Fluorescence *In Situ* Hybridization (FISH)

For the identification of centromeres in MN, FISH was performed with a probe for all human centromeres (QBIOgene®) following the protocol recommended by the manufacturer. Slides were incubated for 30 min at 37° C in 2× SSC/0.5% NP-40, pH 7.0 and then dehydrated in a series of ice-cold ethanol washes and dried at room temperature. The probe was applied to slides and cover slipped. Slides were denatured at 75° C on a hot plate for 5 min and incubated overnight at 37° C in a humidified chamber. After hybridization, slides were washed in 1× Wash Buffer (0.5× SSC/0.1% SDS) for 5 min at 65° C and 1× PBD (phosphate-buffered saline) at room temperature for 5 min. Slides were counterstained with propidium iodide (Q-BIOgene®). To evaluate probe-hybridization efficiency, metaphase spreads were also examined [Eastmont and Tucker, 1989; Migliore et al., 1996].

Slide Scoring and Statistical Methods

For the MN assay, 1,000 BN cells with well-preserved cytoplasm were examined for each individual and type of culture on coded slides in a blind study. The identification of MN was according to the criteria described by Fenech [Fenech et al., 1993]. A nuclear division index (NDI) was calculated according to the formula NDI = (M1+ 2M2+ 3M3+ 4M4)/n, where M1–M4 represent the number of cells with one to four nuclei, respectively, and n is the number of cells scored. In addition, a minimum of 500 lymphocytes were also scored to determine the percentage of cells with 1, 2, 3, 4 or >4 nuclei [Eastmond et al., 1989].

For the sCA analysis, a total of 100 well-spread metaphases were examined for each individual on coded slides. The metaphases were scored for the chromosomal number and for the type of structural chromosomal aberrations. The mitotic index (MI) was expressed as the number of cells in mitotic division stage per 1000 cells [Parry and Parry, 2012].

All data was expressed as mean ± standard deviation (SD). Parametric tests (the Student's *t*-test for the *in vivo* study and for the analysis *in vitro*) were used after logarithmic transformation because MN were not normally distributed. Non parametric test were also used when the size of the compared groups was small (U- Mann Whitney, Kruskall Wallis, Wilcoxon and Friedman test). The level of significance considered was 0.05. Statistics Package for the Social Sciences (SPSS) v20.0 software was utilized for analysis.

For the FISH analysis, to identify centromeres, a total of 50 MN for each individual and type of culture on coded slides in a blind study were analyzed for the presence of a fluorescent signal. MN were classified as centromere-negative (CN^-) or centromere-positive (CN^+) by considering the presence of a hybridization signal in a MN as a direct indication of the presence of a centromere. Among CN^+MN, signals of different intensities were found due to variable amounts of alpha-satellite DNA on different human chromosomes [Tusell et al.,

1996; Migliore et al., 1996]. However, hybridization on metaphase chromosome preparations confirmed the extremely precise location of the signals only at the centromere, varying only in intensity. Statistical evaluation of the results was performed using the Student's *t*-test and the Kruskall Wallis test. In order to identify which chromosomes and chromosomal bands were involved in chromosomal damage using standard cultures, two statistical methods were used. Firstly, a chi-square test was performed to test the hypothesis of a non uniform distribution of the breakpoints among chromosomes based on their length and estimated using the diagram of standardized human karyotype [Shaffer et al., 2013]. Secondly, the Fragile Site Multinomial method, FSM version 995, was used to distinguish novel FS from random breakage events by estimating the minimal number of events that must be present at a given band to be considered as a significantly expressed FS in the sample [Bohm et al., 1995; Greenbaum et al., 1995; Greenbaum et al., 1997].

3. Results

Micronucleus Analysis

The results of the MN study are shown in Table II. The means of total MN and BMNM obtained in patients (13.40±7.01 and 10.71±5.38, respectively) were higher than those observed in controls/T-1 (8.46±2.62 and 7.27±2.09, respectively); these differences were statistically significant ($p<0.05$ in both cases).

Table II. Distribution of micronuclei (MN) in the binucleated (BN) cells scored, total number of MN, total number of micronucleated BN cells (BNMN) and nuclear division index (NDI) after different treatments. Mean ± SD

Group	Distribution of MN in BN cells			Total MN	Total BNMN	NDI
	1	2	>2			
Patients						
Candesartan	96	18	3	14.10±4.36	11.70±3.09	1.82±0.16
Eprosartan	102	18	3	11.31±4.68	9.48±3.69	1.86±0.09
Olmesartan	75	15	2	11.10±4.41	9.20±3.16	1.91±0.08
Telmisartan	67	17	4	12.56±3.84	9.78±2.64	1.85±0.16
Valsartan	125	35	9	17.31±11.57	13.00±9.31	1.75±0.12
Mean in patients	8.50±4.36	1.90±1.41	0.40±0.56	13.40±7.01[a]	10.71±5.38[a]	1.83±0.13
Controls						
Mean in controls/T-1	6.10±1.91	1.20±0.76	0	8.46±2.62	7.27±2.09	1.83±0.21
Controls/medium						
C/Candesartan	118	23	4	17.54±9.24	14.36±6.60	1.65±0.19
C/Eprosartan	88	23	3	14.40±5.62	11.40±4.01	1.69±0.15
C/Olmesartan	131	21	11	21.10±6.82[b]	16.40±5.15[b]	1.51±0.12[c]
C/Telmisartan	104	21	8	16.76±6.65	13.27±5.04	1.64±0.13
C/Valsartan	107	24	9	18.30±6.86	14.00±4.52	1.66±0.16
Mean in controls/medium	10.96±4.10	2.24±1.50	0.70±0.50	17.62±7.12	13.89±5.12	1.63±0.16

[a] Patients vs. controls/T-1 ($p<0.05$, Student´s *t-test*).

[b] Controls/T-1 vs. controls/medium ($p<0.01$, Student´s *t-test*).

[c] Controls/T-1 vs. controls/medium ($p<0.01$, Student´s *t-test*).

On the other hand, when the means of total MN and BNMN obtained in controls/T-1 were compared with those obtained in controls/medium (17.62±7.12 and 13.89±5.12, respectively), the high increased observed in the last group showed statistical significance ($p<0.01$ in both cases).

Variability in the mean frequencies of total MN and BNMN among the five different types of ARBs analyzed could be observed in patients and in controls/medium. By one hand, although the two variables studied were found to be increased among patients treated with the five ARBs with respect to controls/T-1, the differences were statistically significant just for Candesartan (14.10±4.36 and 11.70±3.09, respectively), Telmisartan (12.56±3.84 and 9.78±2.64, respectively) and Valsartan (17.31±11.57 and 13.00±9.31, respectively) ($p<0.05$ in all cases). By the other hand, the mean frequencies of MN and BNMN in controls/medium respect to controls/T-1 were increased and the differences were statistically significant for all the ARBs analyzed (Candesartan 17.54±9.24 and 14.36±6.60, respectively; Telmisartan 16.76±6.65 and 13.27±5.04, respectively; Valsartan 18.30±6.86 and 14.00±4.52, respectively; Eprosartan 14.40±5.62 and 11.40±4.01, respectively and Olmesartan (21.10±6.82 and 16.40±5.15, respectively) ($p<0.05$ in all cases).

The NDI value reflecting the average number of nuclei per cell, did not show statistically significant differences when the mean value were compared between patients (1.82±0.16) with controls/T-1 (1.83±0.21) ($p>0.05$). Although, by other hand, statistical differences were found when the mean of NDI values was compared between controls/T-1 and the data obtained in controls/medium (1.63±0.16) ($p<0.05$).

Variability among the five ARBs studied in the NDI measure could be observed in patients under treatment as well as in controls/medium. When the mean of each group of patients treated with the five drugs was compared to controls/T-1, the NDI parameter showed a not statistically significant difference ($p>0.05$). But, when each group of controls/medium was compared with controls/T-1, in all cases the NDI values were decreased and these differences were statistically significant for the five analyzed ARBs (Candesartan 1.65±0.19, Telmisartan 1.64±0.13, Valsartan 1.66±1.60, Eprosartan 1.69±0.15 and Olmesartan 1.51±0.12, $p<0.05$ in all cases).

FISH Analysis

The application of FISH with a centromeric probe to determine the nature of analyzed ARA II-induced MN is presented in Table III.

In the sample of patients, 38.72% of the MN was CN+ whereas 61.05% did not present hybridization signal. In controls/T-1 the percentage of CN+MN and CN-MN were approximately the same than in patients (61.21% CN+MN and 38.78% CN-MN). When the percentage of CN+MN in patients was compared with the same percentage in controls no statistical differences were found ($p>0.05$).

Slight variability among the five antihypertensive analyzed was observed. The patients treated with Candesartan and Valsartan presented the highest percentage of CN+ (40.88% and 40.04%, respectively) and the patients treated with Eprosartan presented the lowest percentage (35.64%) but no statistical differences were found between patients/medium and controls/T-1 ($p>0.05$), suggesting that in patients and controls/T-1 there were a higher number of MN that contain only acentric chromosome fragments than MN with at least a whole chromosome or centric fragments.

Table III. Total number and mean frequency of centromere-negative (CN^-) and centromere-positive (CN^+) micronuclei (MN)

Group	Total CN^-MN	CN^- MN %	Total CN^+MN	CN^+ MN %
Patients				
Candesartan	29	59.11±7.66	21	40.88±7.66
Eprosartan	32	64.35±6.52	18	35.64±6.52
Olmesartan	30	60.57±9.31	20	39.43±9.31
Telmisartan	31	61,92±8.21	19	38.08±8.21
Valsartan	30	59.03±8.63	20	40.04±7.45
Mean in patients	30.40±1.14	61.05±8.04	19.60±1.14	38.72±7.73
Controls				
Mean in controls/T-1	30.50±0.58	61.21±9.53	19.50±0.58	38.78±9.53

Structural Chromosomal Aberrations (sCA)

The effect of the ARBs drugs on the induction of sCA independent of chromosomal location is summarized in Table IV. The most frequently sCA observed corresponded to chromatid breaks in the three groups studied (65.50%, 62.96% and 57.17% of the total sCA in patients, controls/T-1 and controls/medium, respectively), followed by chromosome type breaks (34.33%, 35.19% and 42.65% of the total sCA in patients, controls/T-1 and controls/medium, respectively).

When the percentage of aberrant cells and the mean frequency of CA/aberrant cell between patients (9.85±4.56 and 0.11±0.06, respectively) and controls/T-1 (5.40±5.00 and 0.06±0.03, respectively) were compared, a statistically significant increase was found in patients ($p<0.05$).

Also, when the means of the two variables were analyzed between those obtained in controls/medium (10.30±2.56 and 0.11±0.03, respectively) and in controls/T-1 a statistical significant increase was observed in the first group ($p<0.05$).

Taking into account the percentage of aberrant cell and the mean frequency of CA/aberrant cell among the five different ARBs, a wide variability could be noted among groups in patients and also in controls/medium. Although it could be observed in patients that the two analyzed variables were increased in all the groups treated with the five ARBs respect to controls/T-1, the differences were statistically significant only for Valsartan (8.62±4.40 and 0.10±0.06, respectively), Olmesartan (10.50±3.78 and 0.12±0.05, respectively) and Eprosartan (11.85±4.70 and 0.14±0.07, respectively) ($p<0.05$ for Valsartan and for Olmesartan and $p<0.001$ Eprosartan) whereas for Candesartan (8.80±5.37 and 0.10±0.07, respectively) and Telmisartan (9.22±4.49 and 0.11±0.06, respectively), there were no significant differences observed ($p>0.05$).

On the other hand, the variable percentage of aberrant cell and the mean frequency of CA/aberrant cell in each different group of ARBs in controls/medium respect controls/T-1 were highly increased, finding that the differences were also statistically significant for all the

ARBs studied (Candesartan 11.00±2.00 and 0.11±0.02, respectively; Telmisartan 10.00±4.00 and 0.11±0.05, respectively; Valsartan 11.00±2.00 and 0.13±0.04, respectively; Eprosartan 10.00±2.00 and 0.11±0.03, respectively and Olmesartan (10.00±2.00 and 0.11±0.03, respectively) ($p<0.05$ in all cases).

Table IV. Total number of chromosomal structural aberrations (sCA), percentage of aberrant cells, the mean frequency of CA/aberrant cell and mitotic index (MI). Mean ± SD

Group	sCA			Aberrant cells (%)	CA/aberrant cell	MI
	chtb	chsb	Others			
Patients	374	196	1			
Candesartan	67	27	0	8.80±5.37	0.10±0.07	2.75±0.70
Eprosartan	112	59	0	11.85±4.70	0.14±0.07	3.11±0.83
Olmesartan	74	41	0	10.50±3.78	0.12±0.05	3.09±0.31
Telmisartan	66	24	1	9.22±4.29	0.11±0.06	3.25±0.63
Valsartan	55	45	0	8.62±4.40	0.10±0.06	2.64±0.67
Mean in patients				9.85±4.56[a]	0.11±0.06[a]	2.95±0.68[b]
Controls	34	19	1			
Mean in controls/T-1				5.40±5.00	0.06±0.03	3.61±1.04
Controls/medium	315	235	1			
C/Candesartan	60	47	0	11.00±2.00	0.11±0.02	2.64±0.80
C/Eprosartan	56	50	0	10.00±2.00	0.11±0.03	3.05±1.12
C/Olmesartan	67	39	1	10.00±2.00	0.11±0.03	2.64±0.87
C/Telmisartan	61	46	0	10.00±4.00	0.11±0.05	2.44±1.29
C/Valsartan	71	53	0	11.00±2.00	0.13±0.04	2.98±0.86
Mean in controls/medium				10.30±2.56[c]	0.11±0.03[c]	2.77±0.96[c]

[a] Patients vs. controls/T-1 ($p<0.01$, Student´s *t-test*).

[b] Patients vs. controls/T-1 ($p<0.05$, Student´s *t-test*).

[c] Controls/T-1 vs. controls/medium ($p<0.001$, Student´s *t-test*).

In relation to cytotoxicity of ARBs drugs measured by the mitotic index, the MI values showed significant differences when patients (2.95±0.68) were compared to controls/T-1 (3.61±1.04) ($p<0.05$). In the same way, statistical differences were also found when the mean values of MI were compared between controls/T-1 and controls/medium (2.77±0.96) ($p<0.001$).The mean frequency of MI showed an important variability among the different types of ARBs studied. In patients, when the drugs were analyzed separately and compared to controls/T-1, the MI parameter despite of being decreasing in all the groups, the differences were statistically significant just for Valsartan (2.64±0.67) ($p<0.05$). Contrary, in controls/medium, the mean frequency of MI parameter was statistically decreased for three out of the five ARBs studied: Candesartan (2.64±0.80), Olmesartan (2.64±0.87) and Valsartan (2.98±0.86) ($p<0.05$ in the first two cases and $p<0.01$ in the last case) whereas no statistical differences were found for Eprosartan (3.05±1.12) and Telmisartan (2.44±1.29) ($p>0.05$).

Chromosomal Locations of sCA among Samples

A total of 5,500, 5,000 and 1,000 metaphases from standard culture were analyzed in patients, controls/T-1 and controls/medium, respectively. A total of 779 CA located on 205 chromosomal bands were found in patients, while 67 CA distributed on 50 chromosomal bands and 634 CA located on 178 chromosomal bands could be observed in controls/T-1 and controls/medium, respectively.

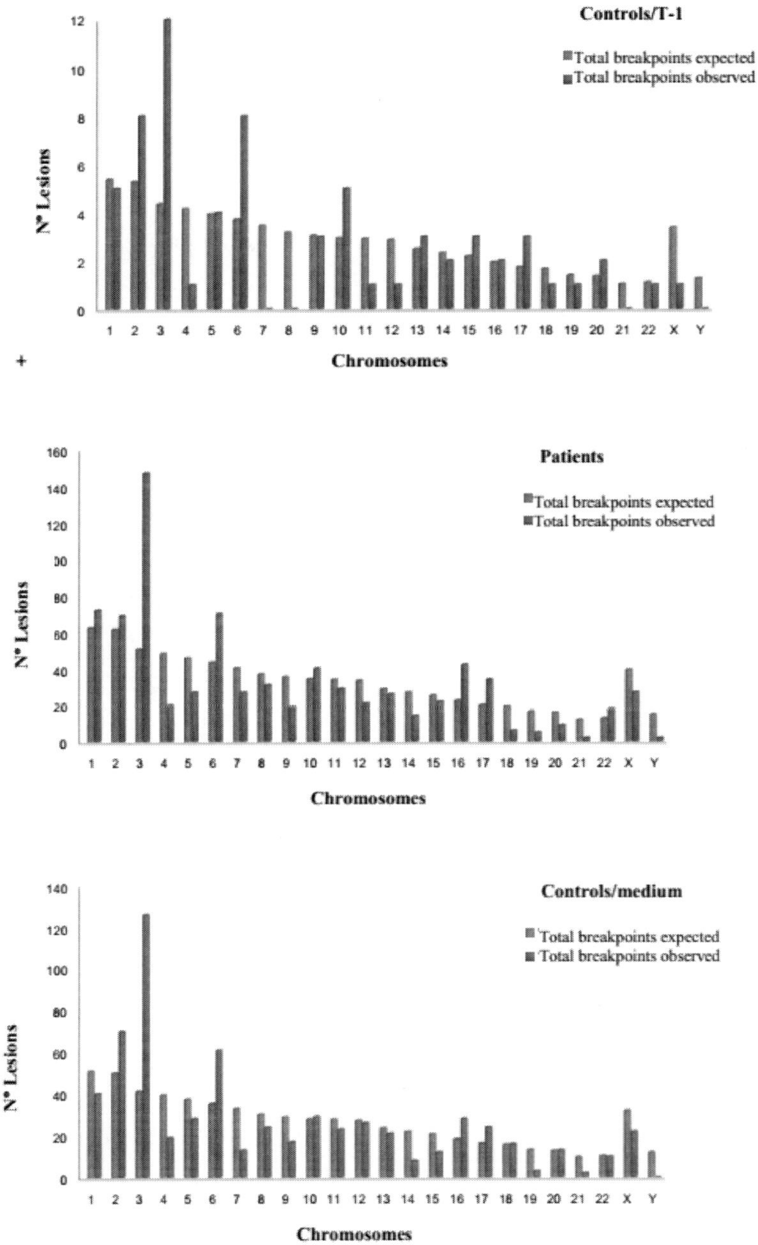

Figure I. Distribution of chromosome breakpoints expected (in grey) and observed (in red) based on their lenght in patients controls/T-1 and controls/medium.

In order to study the possible distribution in the different groups of chromosomes, the frequency of breakpoints in each chromosome were analyzed and compared to the same frequency expected based on their length. Chromosomes involved in a higher level of damage could be observed located mostly on chromosomes 3, 6, 16 and 17 in patients, on chromosomes 2, 3, 6 and 10 in controls/T-1 and on chromosomes 2, 3, 6,16 and 17 in controls/medium as it is shown in Figure I.

Fragile Sites

The FSM method indicated that the minimal number of necessary events at a band to be considered to represent a significantly expressed FS was 4 or more for patients and controls/medium and 3 or more for controls/T-1. The breakpoints distribution in the human ideogram at the 400-band resolution levels is shown in Figure II.

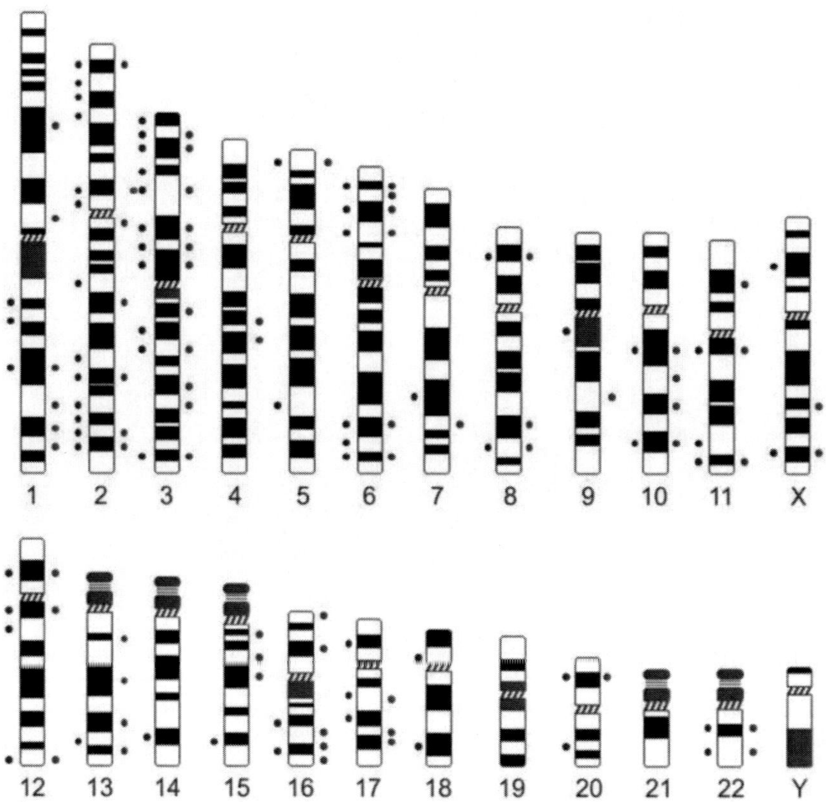

Figure II. Human ideogram showing the distribution of the FS emerged by FSM statistical method in patients (red), controls/T-1 (green) and controls/medium (blue).

In patients, of all the chromosomal bands affected by CA, 67 showed the minimal number to be considered as a FS. The most affected bands were identified as 3p21, 3p14, 6p21, 2q35 and 16q23.

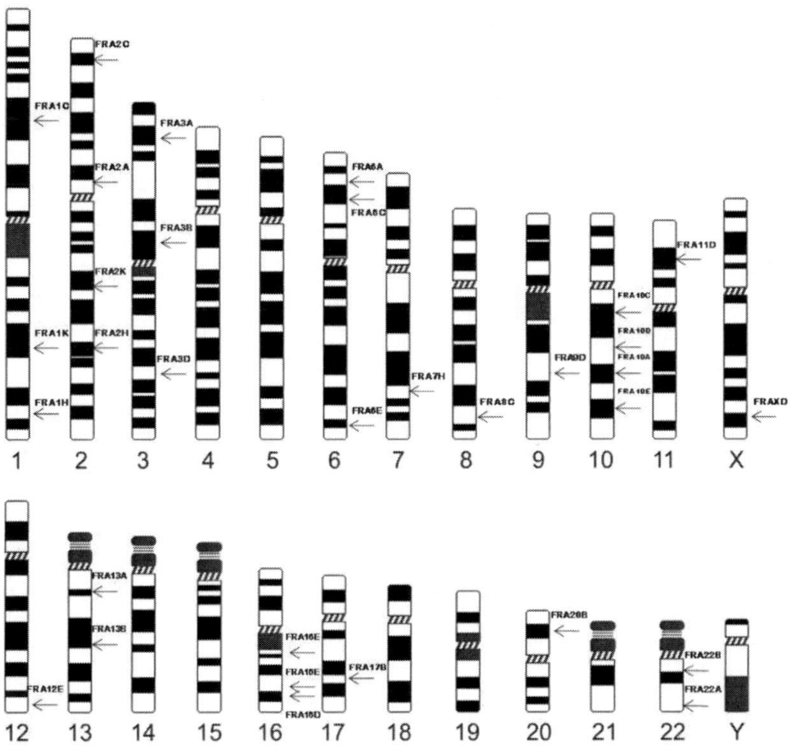

Figure III. Human ideogram showing the distribution of the current recognized FS in patiens.

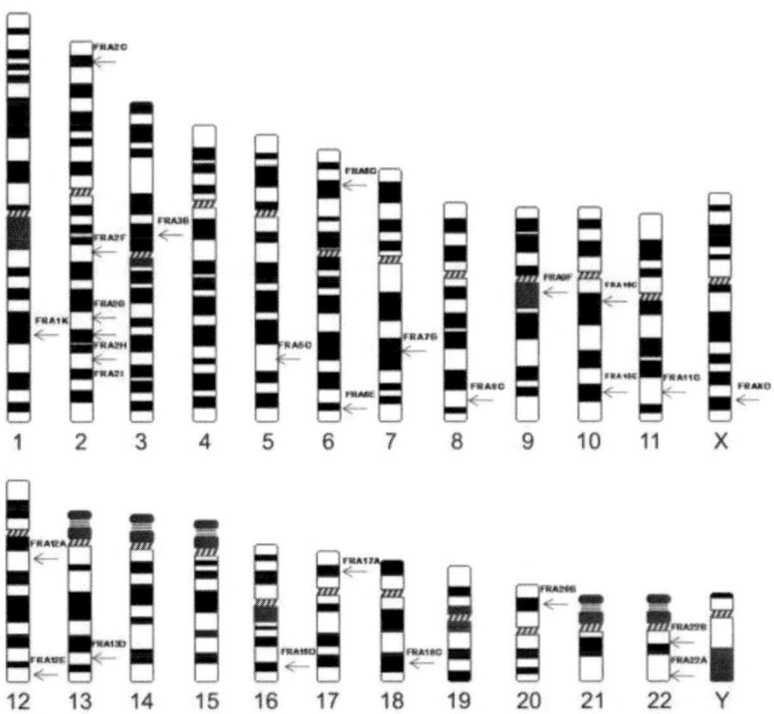

Figure IV. Human ideogram showing the distribution of the current recognized FS in controls/medium.

Of these bands significantly expressed, the 47.76% are currently recognized as FS, corresponding the 81.25% to common fragile sites (cFS) and the 18.75% to rare fragile sites (rFS), as the Figure III shows. In the sample of controls/T-1, just one chromosomal band, concretely 3p21, showed the minimal number of necessary CA need to be consider as FS although nowadays this band is known as a recognized FS.

Finally, in the group of controls/medium, 64 chromosomal bands could be identified as FS of the sample, although only the 40.00% of them are recognized FS which are shown in Figure IV. These well-known FS are classified as cFS, the 66.66%, and rFS, the 33.33%. The chromosomal bands which accumulated the largest number of events in controls/medium are 3p21, 3p14, 16q23, 3p25, 3p24 and 6p22.

4. Discussion

When prescribing an antihypertensive drug, it is fundamental to consider not just its effect in controlling blood pressure but also its potential genotoxicity in humans, so that an antihypertensive drug with negative genotoxicity profile could be prescribed [Snyder and Green, 2001; Bambrilla and Martelli, 2006]. Related to genotoxicity testing applied to ARBs drugs according to regulatory pharmacological agencies worldwide, the majority of the genotoxicity testing has been only tested in bacteria or mammalian cells (rats and hamsters), and besides, several positive results have been emerged [Bambrilla and Martelli, 2006; Bambrilla and Martelli, 2009; Bambrilla and Martelli, 2010]. However, toxicological data from animal experiments can only be used to a limited extend for human risk assessment according to Aaderma [Aaderma et al., 1998]. Regarding this, it is important to underline the importance of our study which contributes to extend the actual information about the genotoxic effects of ARBs drugs providing data on human beings exposed *in vivo* and *in vitro*. Indeed, to our knowledge, this is the first study to thoroughly evaluate the genotoxic potential of ARBs *in vitro* as well as *in vivo*.

To achieve this goal, the following strategies were followed: (1) evaluation of the MN and BNMN frequencies, (2) estimation of the ability of these drugs to induce chromosome loss, (3) determination of the effect of ARBs in the induction of structural chromosomal aberrations, (4) assessment of the nuclear division index and mitotic index as measures of cellular toxicity and (5) identification of most affected chromosomes by CA and possible specific fragile sites on chromosomes of hypertensive patients under treatment with ARBs.

In relation to the first strategy, our results clearly indicated that *in vivo* exposure to the five ARBs led to a statistically significant increase in the frequency of MN and BNMN when patients were compared to controls/T-1. Also after exposure *in vitro* to ARBs drugs, it could be observed a statistically significant enhancement of the two variables studied in the MN assay, even reaching a higher level of significance than in the *in vivo* analysis. These results seem to suggest a genotoxic effect of the ARBs analyzed, mainly *in vitro*.

When the five ARBs chosen were analyzed separately, in the *in vivo* study, a significant increase in the frequencies of MN and BNMN were found in patients treated with Candesartan, Telmisartan and Valsartan compared to controls/T-1. But, on the other hand, *in vitro* in the cultures treated with all the ARBs a genotoxic effect was shown: all the drugs were capable of inducing a significant increase in the frequencies of both variables *in vitro*, although the highest effect could be observed when the Olmesartan drug was tested. Again, this data may indicate an *in vitro* genotoxic effect for the five ARBs studied although it has been corroborated *in vivo* for Candesartan, Telmisartan and Valsartan.

These data are in good agreement with our previous works with antihypertensive agents and previous works on MN assessment in peripheral blood lymphocytes which have shown evidence of genotoxic effect *in vitro* for several other drugs as antineoplastic drugs or clomiphene citrate [Télez et al., 2000; Télez et al., 2001; Cavallo et al., 2005; Yilmaz et al., 2013]. Indeed, non-concordant effects for other antihypertensive drugs have also been described when exposure is *in vivo vs. in vitro*[Morimoto et al., 1993; Télez et al., 2000; Télez et al., 2001; Télez et al., 2010].

Different results *in vivo* and *in vitro* could be explained by the phenomenon of adaptive response to low or chronic doses to the drug *in vivo*. In fact, it may indicate that low and chronic doses of ARBs could induce mechanisms whereby cells became somewhat refractory to the induction of damage by subsequent exposure [Olivieri et al., 1984; Wiencke et al., 1986; Shadley et al., 1994]. This behaviour has been described for patients under other antihypertensive drugs as Atenolol or antileukaemic therapy [Migliore et al., 1991; Télez et al., 2000; Murgia et al., 2007; Krishnaja et al., 2008; Barouki et al., 2010].

With regard to the second strategy, FISH analysis using alpha-satellite probe for all human centromeres showed no statistical differences in the overall frequency of centromere positive MN (CN^+MN) in patients compared to controls/T-1, thus an inability for the ARBs studied to induce chromosome loss *in vivo* could be predicted. Indeed, despite of observing a slight variability among the different antihypertensive drugs analyzed in the frequency of CN^+MN, no statistical significance was found. These result indicate that aneuploidy (chromosome loss) would not be probably the origin of the MN induced *in vivo* by the five ARBs analyzed, although in our previous investigations a more frequent involvement of aneuploidy phenomena in the origin of calcium antagonist and beta blockers antihypertensive drugs-induced MN *in vivo* has been described [Télez et al., 2000; Télez et al., 2001].

In relation to the third strategy, the data indicated that ARBs are capable of inducing sCA (chromosomal and chromatid breaks) in peripheral lymphocytes after the exposure to ARBs because there was a higher expression of sCA *in vivo* and again, mainly *in vitro*. These inductions of sCA may suggest a clastogenic potential for the ARBs analyzed. However, a significantly higher frequency of sCA was shown in the *in vitro* study, fact that leads to indicate a severe cytogenetic damage upon mainly *in vitro* exposure to these antihypertensive drugs.

When the five drugs were compared individually to controls, in the *in vivo* study, significant increases in the percentage of aberrant cells and the mean frequency of CA/aberrant cells were found in patients under treatment with Valsartan, Eprosartan and Olmesartan whereas in the *in vitro* study, the five ARBs analyzed induced a significant increase in the two parameters studied. These results could indicate a remarkable different class effect among ARBs drugs: the five ARBs seem to show a clastogenic activity *in vitro*, although just Valsartan, Eprosartan and Olmesartan maintain this capacity also *in vivo*. However, our results besides of being the first report on monitoring the genotoxic potential of the antihypertensive drugs ARBs following *in vivo* and *in vitro* treatment, they are also the first studies on pointing at a possible inexistence of a class effect among them.

Structural CA are considered to be a highly informative biomarker for detecting adverse health effects, such as the risk of developing cancer [Bonassi et al., 2004; Hagmar et al.,

2004; Bonassi et al., 2008]. Positive results in the CA test were observed for ARBs drugs according to Muller and Kasper and Bambrilla and Martelli, although these positive responses *in vitro* have not been confirmed *in vivo*[Muller and Kasper, 2000; Bambrilla and Martelli, 2006]. To our knowledge there are no published data related to the clastogenic effects of ARBs using CA test in human peripheral lymphocytes. However, our data are in accordance with other several studies which have identified cytogenetic chromosome-damage effects as resulting from the treatment with antihypertensive drugs as Atenolol or Nimodipine, or also treatments with other drugs such as Azathioprine, Amethopterin, Streptonigrine and Phenylbutazone [Cohen et al., 1963; Jensen et al., 1967; Stevenson et al., 1971; Télez et al., 2000; Télez et al., 2001].

The concept of drug class effect is profoundly rooted in medical practice, in which it is usually thought that drugs of the same class have similar clinical effects and therefore are interchangeable. But this premise is based on three important concepts: a similar chemical structure, a similar mechanism of action or similar pharmacological effects [Florez, 2008]. Then, in the case of ARBs, despite of being classified as a same antihypertensive drug class, many authors question the belonging of all of them to the same class according to their chemical differences [Tamargo et al., 2006; Miura et al., 2011]. Based on this, our data suggests that each type of ARB should be analyzed separately thus, our finding require further investigation in order to determinate the inexistence and/or significance of a class effect among ARBs drugs.

To achieve the fourth strategy, nuclear division index (NDI) and mitotic index (MI) are used as indicators of adequate cell proliferation and cytotoxicity in parallel with other biological endpoints. By one hand, the NDI revealed a significant decrease on its values in the *in vivo* study compared to the controls, and this decreasing in cell proliferation was also observed *in vitro* study, although significant differences were just observed in the in *vitro* study. By other hand, the MI showed also a significant decrease on its mean values but this time in the *in vitro* study as well as in the *in vitro* study. Thus, this data indicate that the antihypertensive drugs studied show an effect in decreasing cell proliferation mainly *in vitro*.

In the present study, when the five ARBs were compared individually to controls, the data revealed variation among the five different groups concerning to cytotoxicity. The result suggests that Candesartan, Olmesartan and Valsartan are the ARBs with the highest i*n vitro* cytotoxic potential.

A decrease in MI and/or NDI reflects an inhibition of cell-cycle progression and/or loss of proliferative capacity. Therefore, these results indicate that the analyzed ARB show cellular toxicity *in vitro* [Rojas et al., 1993; Anderson et al., 1988; LópezNigro et al., 2003].Decreases in NDI and MI values were also reported in our previous investigation of the cytotoxic potential of a calcium antagonist antihypertensive drug and no cellular toxicity as observed for a beta-blocker antihypertensive drug. Also Muller and Kasper demonstrated a severe cytotoxicity *in vitro* associated to the intake of ARBs [Muller and Kasper, 2000]. Our study is the first report on human cells and this association between cytotoxicity and ARBs-exposure is also confirmed.

These different results *in vivo* and *in vitro* in genotoxicity and cytotoxicity could be explained by a difference in the metabolism of the compounds *in vivo* [Carr et al., 1996; Ram et al., 2008]. The *in vitro* test is used to quickly test the effects of a presumed genotoxic agent in human cells in short-term cultures. It has the advantage of being able to be used with concentrations that are well-above typical levels but the disadvantages are that the *in* *vitro*assays cannot take fully into account human body absorption, distribution, metabolism and excretion of a pharmaceutical [Aaron et al., 1993; Müller et al., 2000; García-Sagredo et al., 2008]. This may indicate that the cytogenetic effects of the antihypertensive drugs are mainly due to the drugs themselves rather than their metabolites.

Concerning chromosomal breakpoints, distribution was revealed to not be uniform, being chromosomes 3, 6, 16 and 17 affected by a significantly higher number of breakpoints which were expected based on their chromosomal length in patients. Indeed, chromosomes 2, 3, 6 and 16 also showed a higher number of sCA in controls/medium whereas in controls the most affected chromosomes were 3 and 6. Based on these results, it could be deduced that chromosome 16 may be especially sensible to the antihypertensive treatment *in vivo* and *in vitro*. Thus, this increase on genetic damage expressed like a major number of lesions in chromosome 16 seems to be caused by the action of the drug *per se* or even by its metabolites.

Additionally, it is interesting that affected by length in the *in vivo* study with a higher number of lesions chromosome 17 has been identified. Therefore, this chromosome 17 could be associated to the preferential target of ARBs metabolites or even it could be consequence of an increased damage related to the hypertension. In fact, our studies with the alpha beta-blocker Atenolol using the FISH technique with specific chromosome probe also revealed a preferential implication of this chromosome in the MN of hypertensive patients [Télez et al., 2000; Télez et al., 2010].

The FSM method revealed that the 16q23 and 17q21-24 were bands especially related to the antihypertensive drugs or even the hypertension. In patients and controls/medium, the band 16q23 has emerged as FS, so this finding may indicate this band to be particularly sensible to the antihypertensive treatment. It is a know FS called as FRA16D and important genes involved in cellular cycle control as WWOX and FOR are located in this band [Sutherland et al., 2007; Durkin and Glover, 2007].

On other hand, in our patients, the band 17q21-24 has been pointed at a region with a greater propensity to break. This band is a site of the tumour-supression gene BRCA1 (17q21) involved in breast and ovarian cancer, and NF1 (17q21-22.1) [Sutherland et al., 2007; Durkin and Glover, 2007]. Also, the locus 17q21 has been recently proposed as a novel FS designed as FRA17D [Mrasek et al., 2010]. Moreover, reasonable compelling evidence for the existence of a locus in the telomeric q zone of chromosome 17 particularly sensible to hypertension has been recently report [Knight et al., 2003; De Lange et al., 2004; Cheung et al., 2005; Télez et al., 2010]. Our findings support this hypothesis postulated by other studies that suggests the existence of a hypertension susceptibility *locus* on chromosome 17.

Conclusion

In conclusion, our study with patients under antihypertensive treatment with ARBs drugs showed an increased chromosomal damage mainly observed *in vitro*, measured by the CBMN and the CA assays. Thus, our data do not contradict the suggestion previously made that long-term use of ARBs is associated with an increased incidence of cancer occurrence.

However, our results indicated variability among the different ARBs studied in relation to their genotoxicity so a class effect could not be predicted. These results suggested that each type of ARB should be analyzed separately, and subsequently to elucidate this, further investigations are needed, focusing on more epidemiological studies.

Chromosomal location analysis pointed at chromosomes 16 and 17 as preferential targets for the clastogenic effect of ARBs drugs as well as chronic long-term therapy also increased FS expression. Among the several FS emerged as specific, the *locus* 17q21 recently proposed as a new FS, was only expressed in ARBs-treated patients supporting the evidences for a linkage between hypertension and a telomeric *locus* on chromosome 17.

In summary, our study provides evidence for an association among the antihypertensive therapy, arterial hypertension and DNA damage in human lymphocytes, reinforcing the relevance of the biomonitoring of patients chronically exposure to antihypertensive drugs.

Acknowledgments

We thank all patients and controls for their participation in this study. This work was supported by the Vice-Recto rate for research of the University of the Basque Country, Bilbao, Spain (GIU 10/05, UFI 11/32).

References

Aaderma, MJ; Albertini,S; Arni, P; Henderson, LM; Kirsch-Volders, M; Mackay, JM; Sarrif, AM; Stringer, DA; Taalman, RDF. Aneuploidy: a report of an ECETOX task force. *Mutat. Res.* 1998, 410, 3-79.

Aaron, CS; Harbach, PR; Mattano, SS; Mayo, JK; Wang, Y; Yu, RL; Zimer, DM. Risk and benefit evalutation in development of pharmaceutical products. *Environ. Health Perspect.* 1993, 101, 291-295.

Anderson, D; Jenkinson, PC; Dewdeney, RS; Franis, AJ; Godbert, P, Butterworth, KR. Chromosome aberrations, mitogen-inducted blastogenesis and proliferative rate index in peripheral lymphocytes from 106 control individuals of UK population. *Mutat.Res.* 1998, 204, 507-420.

Au, WW. Usefulness of biomarkers in population studies: from exposure to susceptibility and to prediction of cancer. *Int. J. Hyg. Environ. Health.*2007, 210,239-246.

Banegas, JR; Rodriguez-Artalejo, F; de la Cruz Troca, JJ; Guallar-Castillon, P; del Rey Calero, J. Blood pressure in Spain: distribution; awareness; control; and benefits of a reduction in average pressure. *Hypertension.*1998, 32, 998-1002.

Banegas, JR; Rodriguez-Artalejo, F; Ruilope, LM; Graciani, A; Luque, M; de la Cruz-Troca, JJ; Garcia-Robles, R; Tamargo, J; Rey-Calero, J. Hypertension magnitude and management in the elderly population of Spain. *J. Hypertens.* 2002, 20, 2157-2164.

Banegas, JR; Jovell, A; Abarca, B; Aguilar Diosdado, M; Aguilera, L; Aranda, P; Bertomeu, V, Capilla, P; Conthe, P; De Alvaro, F; Fernandez-Pro, A; Formiguera, X; Frias, J; Guerrero, L; Llisterri, JL; Lobos, JM; Macias, JF; Martin De Francisco, AL; Millan, J; Morales, JC; Palomo, V; Roca-Cusachs, A; Roman, J; Sanchis, C; Sarria, A; Segura, J; De La Sierra, A; Verde, L; Zarco, J; Ruilope, LM. Hypertension and health policy in Spain.*Med. Clin.* (Barc). 2009, 132, 222-229.

Barouki, R. Linking long-term toxicity of xeno-chemicals with short-term biological adaptation.*Biochimie.*2010, 92, 1222-1226.

Bender, MA; Preston, RJ; Leonard, RC; Pyatt, BE; Gooch, PC.On the distributions of spontaneous chromosomal aberrations in human peripheral blood lymphocytes in culture.*Mutat. Res.* 1990, 244, 215-220.

Bohm, U; Dahm, PF; McAllister, BF; Greenbaum, IF. Identifying chromosomal fragile sites from individuals: a multinomial statistical model.*Hum. Genet.*1995, 95, 249-256.

Bonassi, S; Znaor, A; Norppa, H; Hagmar, L. Chromosomal aberrations and risk of cancer in humans: an epidemiologic perspective. Cytogenet.*Genome Res.* 2004, 104, 376-382.

Bonassi, S; Norppa, H; Ceppi, M; Stromberg, U; Vermeulen, R; Znaor, A; Cebulska-Wasilewska, A; Fabianova, E; Fucic, A; Gundy, S; Hansteen, IL; Knudsen, LE; Lazutka, J; Rossner, P; Sram, RJ; Boffetta, P. Chromosomal aberration frequency in lymphocytes predicts the risk of cancer: results from a pooled cohort study of 22 358 subjects in 11 countries. *Carcinogenesis.*2008, 29, 1178-1183.

Brambilla, G; Martelli, A. Genotoxicity and carcinogenicity studies of antihypertensive agents.*Mutat. Res.* 2006, 612, 115-149.

Brambilla, G; Martelli, A. Update on genotoxicity and carcinogenicity testing of 472 marketed pharmaceuticals.*Mutat. Res.* 2009, 681, 209-229.

Brambilla, G; Mattioli, F; Martelli, A. Genotoxic and carcinogenic effects of gastrointestinal drugs.*Mutagenesis.*2010, 25, 315-326.

Carr, AA; Prisant, LM. Losartan: first of a new class of angiotensin antagonists for the management of hypertension. *J. Clin. Pharmacol.* 1996, 36, 3-12.

Cavallo, D; Ursini, CL; Perniconi, B; Francesco, AD; Giglio, M; Rubino, FM; Marinaccio, A; Iavicoli, S. Evaluation of genotoxic effects induced by exposure to antineoplastic drugs in lymphocytes and exfoliated buccal cells of oncology nurses and pharmacy employees. *Mutat. Res.* 2005, 587, 45-51.

Cheung, BM; Leung, RY; Man, YB; Wong, LY; Lau, CP. Association of essential hypertension with a microsatellite marker on chromosome 17. J. *Hum. Hypertens.*2005, 19, 407-411.

Chiang, YY; Chen, KB; Tsai, TH; Tsai, WC.Lowered cancer risk with ace inhibitors/ARBs: a population-based cohort study.*J. Clin .Hypertens.* (Greenwich). 2014, 16, 27-33.

Chobanian, AV; Bakris, GL; Black, HR; Cushman, WC; Green, LA; Izzo, JL Jr; Jones, DW; Materson, BJ; Oparil, S; Wright, JT Jr; Roccella, EJ. The National High Blood Pressure Education Program Coordinating Committee: Seventh report of the Joint National Comittee on prevention, detection, evaluation, and treatment of high blood pressure (JNC 7). *Hypertension.*2003, 42, 1206-1252.

Cohen, MM; Shaw, MW; Craig, AP.The effects of streptonigrin on cultured human leukocytes. *Proc. Natl. Acad. Sci. U S A.* 1963, 50, 16-24.

Coogan, PF. Calcium-channel blockers and breast cancer: a hypothesis revived. *JAMA Intern. Med.* 2013, 173, 1637-1638.

De Gasparo, M; Catt, KJ; Inagami, T; Wright, JW; Unger, T. International union of pharmacology. XXIII. The angiotensin II receptors. *Pharmacol. Rev.* 2000, 52, 415-472.

De Lange, M; Spector, TD; Andrew ,T. Genome-wide scan for blood pressure suggests linkage to chromosome 11, and replication of loci on 16, 17, and 22. *Hypertension.*2004, 44, 872-877.

De Miguel, M; Gracía, C; Martín, L; Escribano, M. Guía de desarrollos preclínicos.In CheoMachín. Edited by Gómez, E; Cunchillos, E. GenomaEspaña. 2012.

Decordier, I; Mateuca, R; Kirsch-Volders, M. Micronucleus assay and labeling of centromeres with FISH technique. *Methods Mol. Biol*, 2011, 691, 115-136.

Durkin, SG; Glover, TW.Chromosome fragile sites.*Annu. Rev. Genet.* 2007, 41, 169-192.

Eastmond, DA; Tucker, JD.Identification of aneuploidy-inducing agents using cytokinesis-blocked human lymphocytes and an antikinetochore antibody.*Environ. Mol. Mutagen.* 1989, 13, 34-43.

Fenech, M; Morley, AA.Measurement of micronuclei in lymphocytes.*Mutat. Res.*1985, 147(1-2), 29-36.

Fenech, M. The cytokinesis-block micronucleus technique and its application to genotoxicity studies in human populations.*Environ. Health.Perspect.*1993, 101 Suppl 3, 101-107.

Fenech, M. The advantages and disadvantages of the cytokinesis-block micronucleus method.*Mutat. Res. 1997*, 392, 11-18.

Fenech, M. Cytokinesis-block micronucleus cytome assay.*Nat. Protoc.*2007, 2, 1084-1104.

Florez, J. Farmacología humana.Masson-Salvat. 2008.

Garcia-Sagredo, JM.Fifty years of cytogenetics: a parallel view of the evolution of cytogenetics and genotoxicology. *Biochim.Biophys.Acta.*2008, 1779, 363-375.

Greenbaum, IF; Dahm, PF. A user's guide for FSM: an MS-DOS program for the statistical identification of chromosomal fragile sites. *Technical Report* N. 230; Department 1995.

Greenbaum, IF; Fulton, JK; White, ED; Dahm, PF. Minimum sample sizes for identifying chromosomal fragile sites from individuals: Monte Carlo estimation. *Hum. Genet.*1997, 101, 109-112.

Guler, G; Iliopoulos, D; Han, SY; Druck, T; McCorkell, KA; Huebner, K. Fragile genes at common chromosomal fragile sites: roles in carcinogenesis; In: Arrieta, I; Penagarikano, O,; Télez, T. editors. Fragile Sites: New Discoveries and Changing Perspectives. New York: Nova Science Publishers, Inc. 2007, 223-239.

James, PA; Oparil, S; Carter, BL; Cushman, WC; Dennison-Himmelfarb, C; Handler, J; Lackland, DT; LeFevre, ML; MacKenzie, TD; Ogedegbe, O; Smith, SC Jr; Svetkey, LP; Taler, SJ; Townsend, RR; Wright ,JT Jr; Narva, AS; Ortiz, E. 2014 evidence-based guideline for the management of high blood pressure in adults: report from the panel members appointed to the Eighth Joint National Committee (JNC 8). *JAMA.* 2014, 311(5), 507-520.

Jensen, MK. Chromosome studies in patients treated with azathioprine and amethopterin. Acta Med. Scand. 1967, 182, 445-455.

Kearney, PM; Whelton, M; Reynolds, K; Muntner, P; Whelton, PK; J. He, J. Global burden of hypertension: analysis of worldwide data. *Lancet.* 2005, 365, 217-223.

Kirkland, DJ; Dresp, JH; Marshall, RR; Baumeister, M; Gerloff, C; Gocke, E. Normal chromosomal aberration frequencies in peripheral lymphocytes of healthy human volunteers exposed to a maximum daily dose of paracetamol in a double blind study. *Mutat. Res.* 1992, 279, 181-194.

Kirkland, DJ; Henderson, L; Marzin, D, Muller, L; Parry, JM; Speit, G; Tweats, DJ; Williams, GM. Testing strategies in mutagenicity and genetic toxicology: an appraisal of the guidelines of the European Scientific Committee for Cosmetics and Non-Food Products for the evaluation of hair dyes. *Mutat. Res.*2005, 588(2), 88-105.

Kirsch-Volders, M; Bonassi, S; Knasmueller, S; Holland, N; Bolognesi, C; Fenech, M. Commentary: Critical questions: misconceptions and a road map for improving the use of the lymphocyte cytokinesis-block micronucleus assay for in vivo biomonitoring of human exposure to genotoxic chemicals-A HUMN project perspective. *Mutat. Res*. 2014, 759, 49-58.

Knight, J, Munroe, PB, Pembroke, JC, Caulfield, MJ.Human chromosome 17 in essential hypertension.*Ann. Hum. Genet.*2003, 67, 193-206.

Krishnaja, AP; Sharma, NK.Variability in cytogenetic adaptive response of cultured human lymphocytes to mitomycin C, bleomycin, quinacrinedihydrochloride, Co60 gamma-rays and hyperthermia.*Mutagenesis.*2008, 23, 77-86.

Lindberg, HK; Falck, GC; Jarventaus, H; Norppa, H. Characterization of chromosomes and chromosomal fragments in human lymphocyte micronuclei by telomeric and centromeric FISH.*Mutagenesis.*2008, 23, 371-376.

López-Nigro, MM; Palermo, AM, Mudry, MD, Carballo, MA.Cytogenetic evalutation of two nitroimidazole derivatives.*Toxicol.In vitro*. 2003,17, 35-40.

Mancia, G; De Backer, G; Dominiczak, A; Cifkova, R; Fagard, R; Germano, G; Grassi, G; Heagerty, AM; Kjeldsen, SE; Laurent, S; Narkiewicz, K; Ruilope, L; Rynkiewicz, A; Schmieder, RE; StruijkerBoudier, HA; Zanchetti, A; Vahanian, A; Camm, J; De Caterina, R; Dean, V; Dickstein, K; Filippatos, G; Funck-Brentano, C; Hellemans, I; Kristensen, SD; McGregor, K; Sechtem, U; Silber, S; Tendera, M; Widimsky, P; Zamorano, JL; Kjeldsen, SE; Erdine, S; Narkiewicz, K; Kiowski, W; Agabiti-Rosei, E; Ambrosioni, E; Cifkova, R; Dominiczak, A; Fagard, R; Heagerty, AM; Laurent, S; Lindholm, LH; Mancia, G; Manolis, A; Nilsson, PM; Redon, J; Schmieder, RE; Struijker-Boudier, HA; Viigimaa, M; Filippatos, G; Adamopoulos, S; Agabiti-Rosei, E; Ambrosioni, E; Bertomeu ,V; Clement, D; Erdine, S; Farsang, C; Gaita, D; Kiowski, W; Lip, G; Mallion, JM; Manolis, AJ; Nilsson, PM; O'Brien, E; Ponikowski, P; Redon, J; Ruschitzka, F; Tamargo, J; van Zwieten, P; Viigimaa, M; Waeber, B; Williams, B; Zamorano, JL. Task Force Members: 2007 ESH/ESC Guidelines for the management of arterial hypertension: the Task Force for the management of arterial hypertension of the European Society of Hypertension (ESH) and of the European Society of Cardiology (ESC). *Eur. Heart. J.* 2007, 28, 1462-1536.

Mancia, G; Fagard, R; Narkiewicz, K; Redon, J; Zanchetti, A; Bohm, M; Christiaens, T; Cifkova, R; De Backer, G; Dominiczak, A; Galderisi, M; Grobbee, DE; Jaarsma, T; Kirchhof, P; Kjeldsen, SE; Laurent, S; Manolis, AJ; Nilsson, PM; Ruilope, LM; Schmieder, RE; Sirnes, PA; Sleight, P; Viigimaa, M; Waeber, B; Zannad, F. Task Force Members: 2013 ESH/ESC Guidelines for the management of arterial hypertension: the Task Force for the management of arterial hypertension of the European Society of Hypertension (ESH) and of the European Society of Cardiology (ESC*). J. Hypertens.* 2013, 31, 1281-1357.

Messerli, FH; Williams, B; Ritz ,E. Essential hypertension. *Lancet*. 2007, 370, 591-603.

Migliore, L; Guidotti, P; Favre, C; Nardi ,M; Sessa, MR; Brunori, E. Micronuclei in lymphocytes of young patients under antileukemic therapy. *Mutat. Res*. 1991, 263(4), 243-248.

Migliore, L; Cocchi, L; Scarpato ,R. Detection of the centromere in micronuclei by fluorescence in situ hybridization: its application to the human lymphocyte micronucleus assay after treatment with four suspected aneugens. *Mutagenesis.*1996, 11, 285-290.

Miura, S; Karnik, SS; Saku, K. Review: angiotensin II type 1 receptor blockers: class effects versus molecular effects. *J. Renin. AngiotensinAldosterone Syst.* 2011, 12, 1-7.

Moorhead, PS; Nowell, PC; Mellman, WJ; Battips, DM; Hungerford, DA.Chromosome preparations of leukocytes cultured from human peripheral blood. *Exp. Cell. Res.* 1960, 20, 613-616.

Morimoto, K; Takeshita, T; Take-uchi, T; Maruyama, S; Ezoe, S; Mure, K; Inoue, C. Chromosome alterations in peripheral lymphocytes as indices of lifestyle and genotoxicity. *Int. Arch. Occup. Environ. Health.*1993, 65, S37-41.

Mrasek, K; Schoder, C; Teichmann ,AC; Behr, K; Franze, B, Wilhelm, K, Blaurock, N, Claussen, U, Liehr, T, Weise, A. Global screening and extended nomenclature for 230 aphidicolin-inducible fragile sites, including 61 yet unreported ones. *Int. J. Oncol.* 2010, 36(4), 929-940.

Muller, L; Kasper, P. Human biological relevance and the use of threshold-arguments in regulatory genotoxicity assessment: experience with pharmaceuticals. *Mutat. Res.*2000, 464(1), 19-34.

Murgia, E; Maggini, V; Barale, R; Rossi, AM.Micronuclei; genetic polymorphisms and cardiovascular disease mortality in a nested case-control study in Italy.*Mutat. Res.* 2007, 621(1-2), 113-118.

Norppa, H; Falck, GC.What do human micronuclei contain? *Mutagenesis.*2003, 18, 221-233.

Obe, G; Pfeiffer, P; Savage, JR; Johannes, C; Goedecke, W; Jeppesen, P; Natarajan, AT; Martinez-Lopez, W; Folle, GA; Drets, ME. Chromosomal aberrations: formation; identification and distribution. *Mutat. Res.* 2002, 504, 17-36.

Olin, JL; Veverka, A; Nuzum, DS. Risk of cancer associated with the use of angiotensin II-receptor blockers. *Am. J. Health Syst. Pharm.*2011, 68, 2139-2146.

Olivieri, G; Bodycote, J; Wolff, S. Adaptive response of human lymphocytes to low concentrations of radioactive thymidine.*Science.*1984, 223, 594-597.

Parry, JM; Parry, E. Genetic toxicology. Principles and methods: United Kingdom: Methods in Molecular Biology Springer. 2012.

Pfuhler, S; Albertini, S; Fautz, R; Herbold, B; Madle, S; Utesch, D; Poth ,A; GesellschaftfuerUmwelt-Mutationsforschung: Genetic toxicity assessment: employing the best science for human safety evaluation part IV: Recommendation of a working group of the GesellschaftfuerUmwelt-Mutationsforschung (GUM) for a simple and straightforward approach to genotoxicity testing. *Toxicol. Sci.* 2007, 97, 237-240.

Ram, CV. Angiotensin receptor blockers: current status and future prospects. *Am. J. Med.* 2008, 121, 656-663.

Rojas, E; Herrera, LA; Sordo, M; Gonsebatt, ME; Montero, R; Rodríguez, R; Ostrosky-Wegman, P. Mitotic index and cell proliferation kinetics for the identification of antineoplastic activity. *Anti-Cancer drugs.* 1993, 4, 637-640.

Schaefer, KL; Porter, JA. Angiotensin II receptor antagonists: the prototype Losartan. *Ann. Pharmacother.* 1996, 30, 36-40.

Seabright, M. A rapid banding technique for human chromosomes.*Lancet.*1971, 2(7731), 971-972.

Shadley, JD. Chromosomal adaptive response in human lymphocytes.*Radiat.Res.*1994, 138(1 Suppl), S9-12.

Shadley, JD. Chromosomal adaptive response in human lymphocytes.*Radiat.Res.*1994, 138(1 Suppl), S9-12.

Shaffer, LG; McGowan-Jordan, J; Schimd, M: ISCN 2013: An International System for Human Cytogenetic Nomenclature.Karger, 2013.

Sipahi, I; Debanne, SM; Rowland, DY; Simon, DI; Fang ,JC. Angiotensin-receptor blockade and risk of cancer: meta-analysis of randomised controlled trials. *Lancet Oncol.*2010, 11, 627-636.

Snyder, RD; Green, JW.A review of the genotoxicity of marketed pharmaceuticals.*Mutat. Res.* 2001, 488, 151-169.

Song, JC; White, CM. Pharmacologic; pharmacokinetic; and therapeutic differences among angiotensin II receptor antagonists.*Pharmacotherapy*2000, 20, 130-139.

Stevenson, AC; Bedford, J; Hill, AG; Hill, HF. Chromosomal studies in patients taking phenylbutazone.*Ann. Rheum. Dis.* 1971, 30, 487-500.

Stopper, H; Mulle,r SO. Micronuclei as a biological endpoint for genotoxicity: A minireview. *Toxicol.In Vitro.*1997, 11, 661-667.

Streeten, DH; Anderson, GH Jr; Dalakos, TH. Angiotensin blockade: its clinical significance. *Am. J. Med.* 1976, 60, 817-824.

Sutherland, GR. Fragile sites on human chromosomes. In: Arrieta, I; Penagarikano, O; Télez, M editors. Fragile Sites: New Discoveries and Changing Perspectives. New York: Nova Science Publishers; Inc; 2007, 21-43.

Tamargo, J; Caballero, R; Gómez, R; Núñez, L; Vaquero, M; Delpón, E. Características farmacológicas de los ARA-II. ¿Son todosiguales?*Rev. Esp. Cardiol.*2006, 6, 10-24.

Taylor, AA; Siragy, H; Nesbitt, S. Angiotensin receptor blockers: pharmacology; efficacy and safety. *J. Hum. Hypertens.* 2011, 13, 677-686.

Telez, M; Martinez ,B; Criado, B; Ortega, B; Penagarikano, O; Flores, P; Ortiz-Lastra, E; Arrieta I. Evaluation of the cytogenetic damage induced by the antihypertensive drug nimodipine in human lymphocytes. *Mutagenesis.*2001, 16(4), 345-351.

Telez, M; Martinez, B; Criado, B; Lostao, CM; Penagarikano, O; Ortega, B; Flores, P; Ortiz-Lastra, E; Alonso, RM; Jimenez, RM; Arrieta, I. *In vitro* and *in vivo* evaluation of the antihypertensive drug atenolol in cultured human lymphocytes: effects of long-term therapy. *Mutagenesis.*2000, 15, 195-202.

Telez, M; Ortiz-Lastra, E; Gonzalez, AJ; Flores, P; Huerta, I; Ramirez, JM; Barasoain, M; Criado, B; Arrieta, I. Assessment of the genotoxicity of atenolol in human peripheral blood lymphocytes: correlation between chromosomal fragility and content of micronuclei. *Mutat. Res.* 2010, 695, 46-54.

Tucker, JD; Eastmond, DA; Littlefield, LG. Cytogenetic end-points as biological dosimeters and predictors of risk in epidemiological studies.*IARC Sci. Publ.*1997, 142, 185-200.

Tusell, L; Álvarez, R; Genesca, A; Caballín, MR; Miró, R; Egozcue, J. Analysis of radiation-induced micronuclei in two-cell human-hamster embryos using telomeric and centromeric FISH probes. *Cytogenetic.Cell.Genet.*1996, 74,102-106.

Wang, KL; Liu, CJ; Chao, TF; Huang, CM; Wu, CH; Chen, TJ; Chiang, CE. Long-term use of angiotensin II receptor blockers and risk of cancer: A population-based cohort analysis. *Int. J. Cardiol.* 2013, 165, 2162-2166.

Weinmann, S; Glass, AG; Weiss, NS; Psaty, BM; Siscovick, DS; White, E. Use of diuretics and other antihypertensive medications in relation to the risk of renal cell cancer. *Am. J. Epidemiol.* 1994, 140(9), 792-804.

Wiencke, JK; Afzal, V; Olivieri, G; Wolff, S. Evidence that the [3H]thymidine-induced adaptive response of human lymphocytes to subsequent doses of X-rays involves the induction of a chromosomal repair mechanism. *Mutagenesis.*1986, 1, 375-380.

Wuerzner, G; Burnier, M; Waeber, B. Critical review of cancer risk associated with angiotensin receptor blocker therapy. *Vasc.Health Risk.Manag.*2011, 7, 741-747.

Yilmaz, S; Unal, F; Yilmaz, E; Yuzbasioglu, D; ErkalIlhan, S. Evaluation of the genotoxicity of clomiphene citrate. *Mutat. Res.* 2013, 759, 21-27.

In: Antihypertensive Drugs
Editor: Scott Caldwell

ISBN: 978-1-63463-829-6

Chapter III

Effects of the Polymorphism in Antihypertensive Drugs

Márcia C. de Souza[1*], Weberton R. do Carmo[1], Chris H. J. Franco[1], Luan F. Diniz[1] and Renata Diniz[1]

[1] Grupo de Cristalografia de Pequenas Moléculas (GCPMOL), Departamento de Química, Universidade Federal de Juiz de Fora, Juiz de Fora, Minas Gerais, Brazil

Abstract

Polymorphism, which can be described as the ability of the compound to crystallize in different phases with different crystalline arrangement and / or conformation of the molecules in the crystal lattice, has become a very interesting focus of investigation in the last years. The main purpose of this kind of study is the strategic construction of distinct crystalline arrangements, and the complete comprehension of the connection between structure and physicochemical properties. In recent years, it is a topic of great interest to the scientific community and presents a great challenge for the pharmaceutical industry, since changes in the crystalline arrangement can alter the physicochemical properties of drugs. This chapter will first include a general description about polymorphism and some techniques used in polymorphism characterization. Then, the specific description of some antihypertensive drugs that present polymorphism phenomena will be introduced.

1. Polymorphism

1.1. Definition

The most of drugs used in the hypertension treatment are administered orally in solid form and therefore they can crystallize in different crystalline forms [1]. This phenomenon is

* Corresponding author. Tel: +55 32-2102-3310. E-mail address: marciaphn@gmail.com

known as polymorphism. The term polymorphism comes from the Greek which means "many forms" [2, 3]. Polymorphism in crystalline solids is defined as the ability of the compound to crystallize in different phases with different crystalline arrangement and / or conformation of the molecules in the crystal lattice [2]. The Figure 1 shows two polymorphic forms called hypothetically of polymorphs 1 and 2.

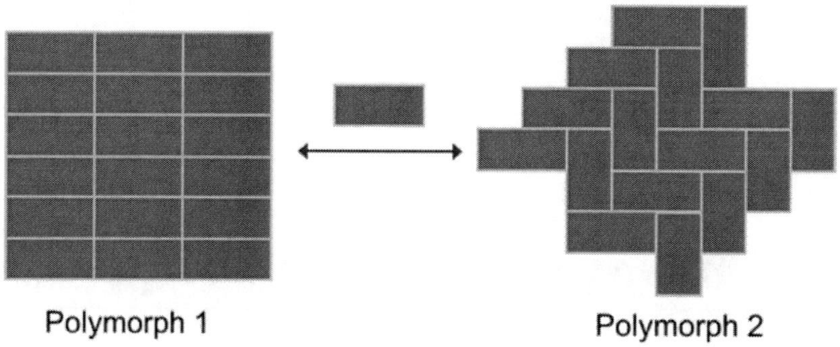

Figure 1. Schematic representation of the structures of two polymorphs.

In pharmaceutical science, polymorphism also is used to designate several solid state forms of active pharmaceutical ingredient (API), including amorphous forms, solvates, hydrates, salts and co-crystals (Figure 2) [4, 5]. For a long time, the term pseudopolymorphism was used to denote the formation of various crystals as the result of solvent molecules being incorporated in the crystal structure [6, 7]. However, more recently this term has become replaced by the term solvatomorphism. When water is the solvent in the crystal lattice, such crystals are known as hydrates [8, 9]. Due to the frequent presence of water in the environment and its use in solvents misture during the crystallization process, the formation of hydrates drugs is very common. Because the water molecule is small and able to form hydrogen bonds, it is easily incorporated into the crystalline lattice of drugs both occupying spaces and stabilizing the structure [4]. Solvates can contain either a stoichiometric or a nonstoichiometric quantity of solvent in the crystal lattice. Normally, desolvation of a stoichiometric solvate results in either a disordered noncrystalline state or a dissimilar crystalline form. Nonstoichiometric solvates comprise solvent molecules that are accommodated in the structure to fill intermolecular voids [10]. A salt refers to a multi-component system where protons are transferred from acid to base in the ionic state. In situation of the API is ionizable, preparation of its salts using pharmaceutically acceptable acids or bases is a common strategy to modulate its solubility, to increase chemical stability or to improve bioavailability [5, 11]. A co-crystal is a stoichiometric multiple component crystal containing an API and one or more unique co-crystal formers in which all components are solids under ambient conditions when in their pure form [10, 12, 13]. Co-crystals can be constructed through several types of interaction, including hydrogen bonding, π-stacking, and van der Waals forces. Co-crystals may include one or more solvent / water molecules in the crystal lattice [14]. When this occurs, it is entitled as co-crystal solvates [15]. The main difference between co-crystals and solvates is the physical state of the isolated pure components and the most important difference between co-crystals and salts is that in salts a proton is transferred from the acidic to the basic functionality of the crystallization partner, while in co-crystals no such transfer occurs [5]. Amorphous solids consist of disordered arrangements of molecules and do not possess a distinguishable crystal lattice. Amorphous solids lack the three-dimensional long-range order of molecular packing or well-defined molecular conformation, but they may have short-range order [5]. As amorphous solid states of an API are far from equilibrium than its crystalline counterparts, they normally have desirable pharmaceutical properties such as higher solubility, faster dissolution rate and improved bioavailability compared to their crystalline counterparts. The higher solubility of amorphous solids is due to their higher energy and molecular mobility compared to their corresponding crystalline counterpart. However, the high energy and molecular mobility also make amorphous solids physically instable and their use for enhancing oral bioavailability has been limited due to the difficulty in preventing recrystallization from the amorphous state during dissolution [5, 8]. In addition, the FDA (Food and Drug Administration) has recently published a Regulatory Classification of Pharmaceutical Co-Crystals in which polymorphs are defined as "Different crystalline forms of the same drug substance (this may include solvation or hydration products and amorphous forms)"; salts as "Any of numerous compounds that result from replacement of part or all of the acid hydrogen of an acid by a metal or a radical acting like a metal: an ionic or electrovalent crystalline compound" and co-crystals as "Crystalline materials composed of two or more molecules in the same crystal lattice" [16]. Though, the definitions for these solid forms are matters of debate among the scientific community, regulatory agencies and industrial groups, without a clear consensus [4].

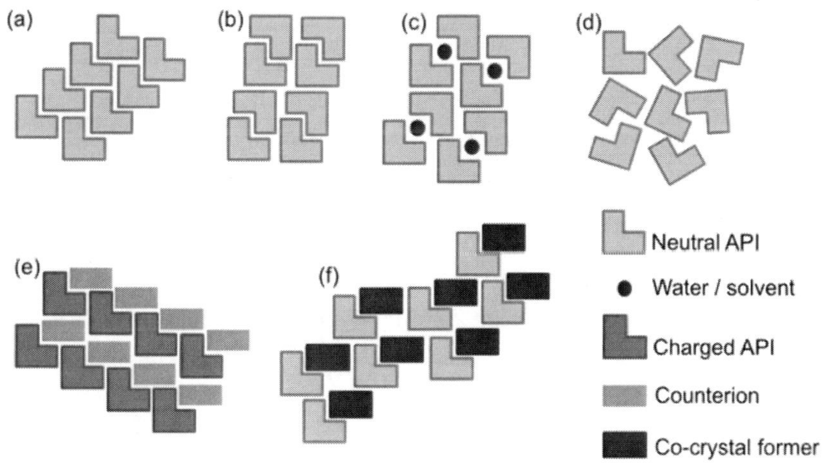

Figure 2. Schematic depiction of various types of solid forms: (a) and (b) polymorphs; (c) solvates; (d) amorphous; (e) salts and (f) co-crystals.

The polymorphic forms of the same compound may differ in properties such as solubility, melting point, crystal shape, refractive index, density, hardness, and others [5]. The change in solubility between different polymorphic forms is particularly important for the pharmaceutical industry, because this factor may affect the bioavailability and consequently the bioequivalence of the drug [8, 17]. Changes in the absorption process caused by factors that alter the solubility can result in therapeutic failure or toxicity representing a risk to the user. It is not uncommon to observe solid-state changes due to extreme conditions used in manufacturing operations, such as extensive mechanical and thermal stress and exposure to solvents [8]. As a result, drug product performance may be significantly altered and / or fail to meet the quality specifications. Thus, polymorphism in drugs is a topic of great interest to the scientific community and presents a great challenge for the pharmaceutical industry, since changes in the crystalline arrangement can alter the physicochemical properties of drugs.

1.2. Classification

1.2.1. Conformational Polymorphism

Conformational polymorphism occurs due to the possible rotation about single bonds in a molecule leading to several possible conformations [2]. Similarly, a nonconformationally rigid molecule can be folded into different arrangements, which subsequently can be packed into alternative crystal structures [18]. In general, flexible molecules with several degrees of torsional freedom and low-energy conformers are more susceptible to exhibit conformational polymorphism [12].

1.2.2. Packing Polymorphism

Packing polymorphism happens when the molecules have similar conformation, but possess different intermolecular interactions, leading to different arrangements between the molecules [2]. It represents instances where conformational relatively rigid molecules can be assembled into different three-dimensional structures through the invocation of different intermolecular mechanisms [18].

1.2.3. Concomitant Polymorphism

Concomitant polymorphism relates to polymorphic crystals that crystallize simultaneously from the same solution and under the same conditions, the latter of which is important and can be interpreted widely [2, 19].

1.2.4. Tautomeric Polymorphism

When different tautomers of a compound crystallize in different crystal forms, they are named as tautomeric polymorphs. Tautomerism occurs when the constitutional isomers of different hydrogen-atom connectivities are in dynamic equilibrium with one another. Tautomers that interconvert in solution or in melt are considered to be the same chemical compound and hence the crystal forms that contain these tautomers can be classified as polymorphs [12].

1.3. Nomenclature

A nomenclature for polymorphs has not been established. Generally, different polymorphic forms of identical molecules are denoted by numerical or alphabetical sequences; the labelling does not follow a terminology rule, and on case uses A, B, C or I, II, III or α, β, γ or 1, 2, 3 to denominate the different polymorphic forms [2, 3]. They can also be differentiated by means of hydration or solvation levels. In general, polymorphs are designated by the chronological order in which they have been reported [4].

2. Polymorphism Characterization

As described above, several pharmaceutical solids can exhibit more than one solid form, crystalline or amorphous, which could modify theirs physical-chemical properties. Due to this fact, is very important the knowledge of the solid form of the API in order to understand the chemical and physical properties of the material [20]. In this sense, there are several techniques that can be used in the physical characterization of the API. Numerous considerations need to be made when the technique is chosen for solid-state characterization of a pharmaceutical entity [20]. The most important used in solid-state investigations are: the spectroscopic techniques as Raman, infrared (IR) and nuclear magnetic resonance (NMR), structural as crystal and powder X-ray diffraction, and thermotechniques as differential scanning calorimetry (DSC) and thermogravimetric analysis (TGA). A general view of these techniques is present below.

2.1. Spectroscopic Techniques

2.1.1. Vibrational Spectroscopy

IR and Raman spectroscopy are used in the identification of molecular vibrations of the molecules and they are methods non-destructive in relation to the samples. The difference between these techniques is the different form of sample and radiation interactions. In IR spectroscopy the radiation modify the electric dipole moment of the molecules and the frequency of absorbed radiation is identical to the dipole variation. On the other hand, in the Raman spectroscopy occurs the inelastic scattering of the radiation, and the frequency of scattering radiation is related to induced dipole moment in the molecule.

Both vibrational spectroscopies can be used in the polymorphism identification. They provide important and useful information in the distinction of polymorphs. In special, the investigation about the lattice vibrations is very important, due to the fact that these vibrations are related to differences in the crystal packing. The bands assigned as lattice modes appears in low frequency in vibrational spectra (100 to 800 cm^{-1}) and are more easy identified in Raman spectra. In the drug characterization is also important the knowledge of the distribution of excipients and API. In this sense, the chemical imaging systems complement the chemical identification by acquiring spatially located spectra that enable visualization of chemical compound distributions [21]. This process has an advantage over classical spectroscopy which is the remaining pixel-to-pixel spectral variation scan that gives more information about the sample or about the ability of the preprocessing method to clean the spectra [21].

2.1.2. Nuclear Magnetic Resonance

The NMR is one of the most important techniques in the polymorphism identification, in particular for API that can not be crystallized to be investigated by single-crystal X-ray diffraction. In general the ^{13}C solid-state NMR are used in the identification of polymorphic forms, but some heteroatoms, like ^{31}P are also investigated in some cases [20]. This technique is normally used in association with other analytical analysis, in special the X-ray diffraction (XRD). The advantages of this technique is that heterogeneous and amorphous samples can be investigated, including qualitative analysis which present less than 1% in the composition [22]. The description of the structure in solid state by NMR is known as NMR crystallography which is the some of the characteristics of high-resolution NMR of solids [22]. However, the great disadvantage is the use of relative quantity of mount required for the analysis (around 200 mg for ^{13}C and 20 mg for ^{1}H) [22].

NMR spectroscopy occurs due to the interaction of magnetic moment of the nuclei with an external magnetic field. The solid-state NMR (ssNMR) is an extremely useful method for characterization of amorphous and insoluble materials. However, due to the low mobility of the particles, the spectra often have low resolution. To minimize this problem in ^{13}C ssNMR, the combination of magic angle spinning, the average of chemical shift anisotropy equal to zero and high power proton decoupling is used to obtain high resolution ^{13}C spectra [23].

For example, in the literature is describing the ssNMR for the molecular complex formed by norfloxacin and β-ciclodextrin with diferents polymorphs of norfloxacin [24]. This API exists in several crystalline forms which include anhydrous, solvates, cocrystals, amorphous and salts [25-27]. In the ^{13}C NMR for two polymorphs of norfloxacin is possible to note the differences in the spectra, mainly among 60-40 ppm in chemical shift [24]. This technique is a powerful tool in characterization of different solid form of API as well as in multicomponent samples of pharmaceutical samples.

2.2. Thermometric Analysis

The analytical techniques that promote a control temperature variation for determine some physico-chemistry properties. The most used thermometric analyses are differential scanning calorimetry (DSC) and thermal gravimetric analysis (TG), which are utilized in the identification of polymorphs, solvates, and in the quality control of API and excipient.

In the TG a thermic profile is obtained and is useful in the determination of the quantity of solvent present in the API and helps in the solvates identification. The DSC measures the heat flow difference between a substance and a reference material as a function of a temperature program. As a result it is possible to determine the temperature change of the endothermic and exothermic phenomena. The use of DSC in polymorphism identification becomes relevant as it is possible to distinguish different crystalline forms through the enthalpy of fusion characteristics.

2.3. X-Ray Diffraction

The X-ray diffraction is the most important technique in polymorphism identification. It is possible to be used in powder and crystal samples and provide detailed information about the solid state, including the molecular description (bond distances and angles) as well the intermolecular interactions and the crystal packing. The interaction occurs between the X-ray radiation and the electron density of the crystalline material given rise to reflection radiation that can be analyzed by the Bragg´s equation [28].

Due to the precise information given by X-ray diffraction (XRD), in special by single-crystal, this technique is able to distinguish one polymorph for another in an efficient way. However, the great difficult is to obtain a single-crystal adequate to XRD. Therefore, the

XRD by powder (XRPD) samples has been used extensively in API characterization, in special in quantitative analyses of drugs as well as in the polymorphism identification. The XRPD can also be used in the determination of cell parameters, space group, crystallinity degree, crystallite size, quali and quantitative analysis in mixtures [28].

The diffraction radiation gives rise to a diffraction pattern, formed by peaks, that is related to crystalline solid organization. This pattern is named diffractogram, and the angular positions of the diffracted peaks as well as their intensities are used in the crystalline phase identification. There are two main methods that can be used in quantitative analysis [23]. The simplest is the use of individual peaks to establish the relationship between phase composition and the individual intensity of the peaks. The second one is the use of all diffraction pattern, as in the Rietveld method [29], to establish the mathematic equation that relate the crystalline phase and its quantity present in the mixtures.

The great disadvantage of XRD is the necessity of the samples present at least one crystalline phase. In quantitative analyses by XRPD the ability to minimize the effects of preferred orientation of the crystallites in the sample is very important to obtain accurate results [23].

The choice of the technique in solid state characterization of API is defined by the objectives of this, the nature of the sample and mainly the where detailed should be the identification of the compound. In Table 1 is displayed the advantages and disadvantages of some techniques used in polymorphism characterization.

In this sense, the following sections presents some antihypertensive drugs that present polymorphism phenomena to illustrate the subjects described above.

Table 1. Main analytical techniques used in the polymorphism investigation [30, 31]

Technique	Application	Advantage	Disadvantage
IR spectroscopy	Polymorph and solvates characterization and identification.	Capable of differentiating polymorphs of solvates/hydrates. Helps in phase identification.	It is possible occurs the loss of information during the sample preparation. The excipients can interfere in the analysis.
Raman spectroscopy	Qualitative and quantitative analysis of polymorphs.	Allows the detection of small quantity of analyte. Great specificity in polymorphism identification.	Interference of excipients.
TGA	Weather thermal behavior of the sample.	Small quantity of sample. Allows the thermal profile of the sample.	Interference of excipients. More useful in investigation of solvates and hydrates.
DSC	Quali and quantitative investigation. Identification of phase transition and purity of the samples.	Phase transition information and API interactions with excipients.	Interference among amorphous and crystalline excipients. Quantification is limited.

Table 1. (Continued)

Technique	Application	Advantage	Disadvantage
ssNMR	Characterization of polimorphs and compounds in general.	Characterization and quantification of crystalline phase. Complements information from X-ray diffraction.	Mistakes in quantitative analysis in solid state.
Single-crystal XRD	Crystal structure determination.	Improved accuracy of information through the elucidation of the crystal structure.	The difficult in the obtainment of the samples.
XRPD	Investigations about polymorphism and crystalline phase.	Crystalline phase identification. Analysis of solid mixture.	Occurrence of preferred orientation. Interference of excipients.

3. Polymorphs of Nifedipine (NIF)

Nifedipine (Figure 3) belongs to group of drugs known as calcium channel blockers (CCBs), used as an antihypertensive agent. This class of drug binds in cardiac sites preventing that Ca ions entry into the cells through L-type Ca channel [32, 33], working as an arterial vasodilator [34, 35], decreasing the risk of heart problems and received the trade name Adalat® with a preparation having commonly 10-20 mg of nifedipine [32, 36]. It is usually recommended for hypertensive patients, however, it is described that CCBs have produced adverse effects such as edema, tachycardia and skin reactions [32, 33].

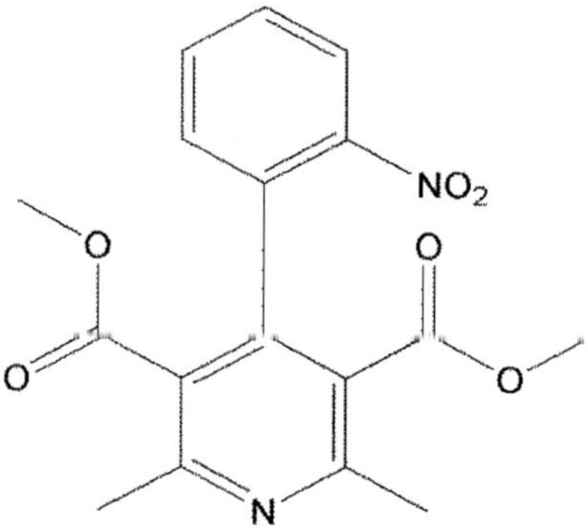

Figure 3. Nifedipine molecular representation.

CCBs can be safely used for the treatment of hypertension, drug effects can be elucidated by many factors such as age, race, sex, food, smoking, drinking habits, disease states and lifestyles that depend on the individual differences in rates of drug metabolism. The response to medicine requires individualization of drug dosage, it defined by doctor responsible [37, 38].

Three polymorphic forms have been reported for nifedipine (NIF) into literature [39], and it were firstly, known as polymorphs forms I, II and III. The deficient of single-crystal X-ray structural data for polymorphs forms of NIF produce a great problem to describe which phase is present in the samples. Thus, early works used different symbols for study of NIF polymorphs forms such as form A, B and C in its place of form I, II and III, respectively [40-42]. It is possible found, other nomenclature system that employed the symbols α, β to refer to forms I and III [43], agreeing with earlier crystallographic data [44]. In this work, we will use A, B and C symbols to report the three polymorphs forms of NIF. Only the structures of form A and form C were solved by single-crystal X-ray diffraction and crystallized in centrosymmetric space groups $P2_1/c$ and $P\text{-}1$, respectively [41, 44, 45]. The polymorph form A is thermodynamically stable at room temperature, and used in pharmaceutical preparations such as capsules, tablets, and solutions [46]. It was crystallized in monoclinic system and space group $P2_1/c$ with crystal data: a = 10.923(5) Å, b = 10.326(6) Å, c = 14.814(7) Å, $\alpha = \gamma$ = 90°, β = 92.70(6)°, Z = 4, V = 1669.03 Å^3. While the polymorphic form C crystallized in the triclinic system and space group $P\text{-}1$ with crystal data: a = 9.666(6) Å, b = 13.701(8) Å, c = 14.118(9) Å, α = 61.028 (3)°, β = 79.631(4)°, γ = 81.904(4)°, Z = 4, V = 1605.89(17) Å^3. The polymorphic forms B and C are metastable and usually may appear during production process and in the presence of molecules like cyclodextrins and polyvinylpyrrolidone [40, 47].

The Figures 4 and 5 show the crystal structures of forms A and C. Both polymorphic forms have the same number of NIF molecules inside the unit cell; however, displaying a molecular packing considerably different. The bond distances and angles are similar and it is possible to see, that acetate group is rotated by 180° in relation to phenyl ring.

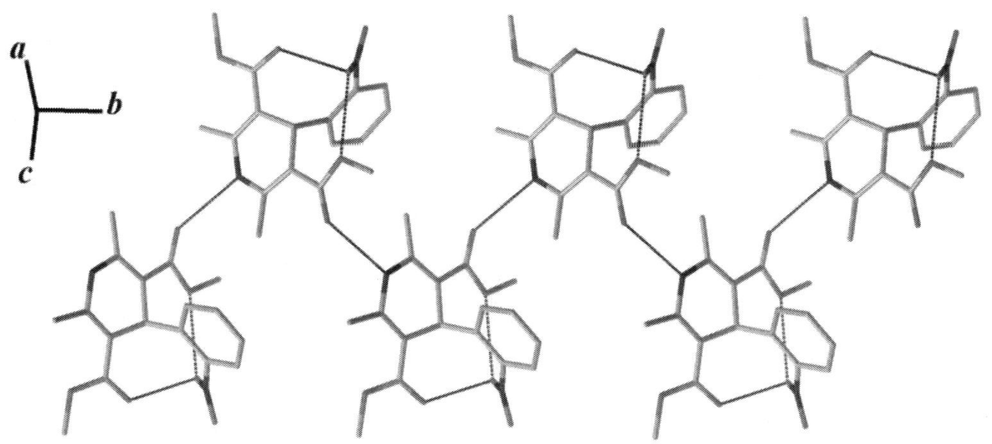

Figure 4. Cristal structure form A of NIF shown along the *b*-axis. Hydrogen bonds between the nifedipine molecules are presented as black dotted lines. Some atoms were omitted for more clarity.

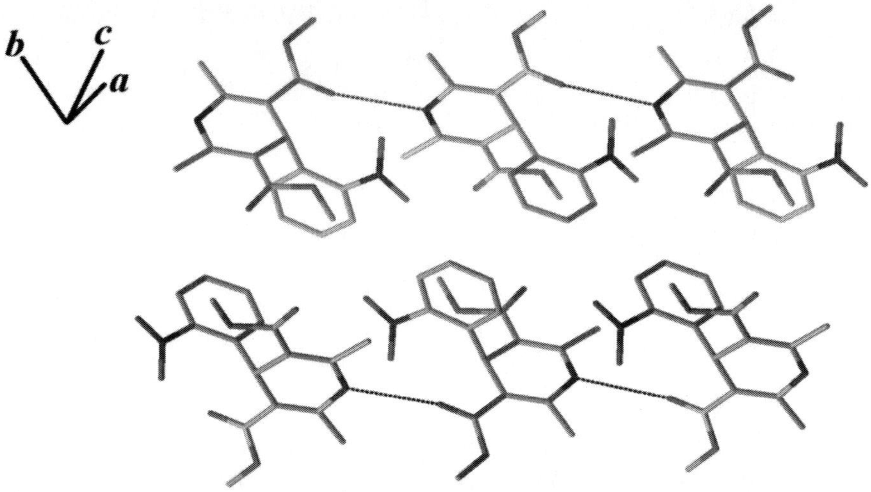

Figure 5. Cristal structure form C of NIF. Hydrogen bonds are show as black dotted lines. Some atoms were omitted for more clarity.

This system shows conformational polymorphism, being the main modification between the polymorphs are the inclinations of phenyl and dihydropyridine rings present in the structures formed. The overlay structures is given in Figure 6 for elucidate differences between the conformational polymorphs forms A and C. The simulated diffraction patterns for forms A and C are shown in Figure 7.

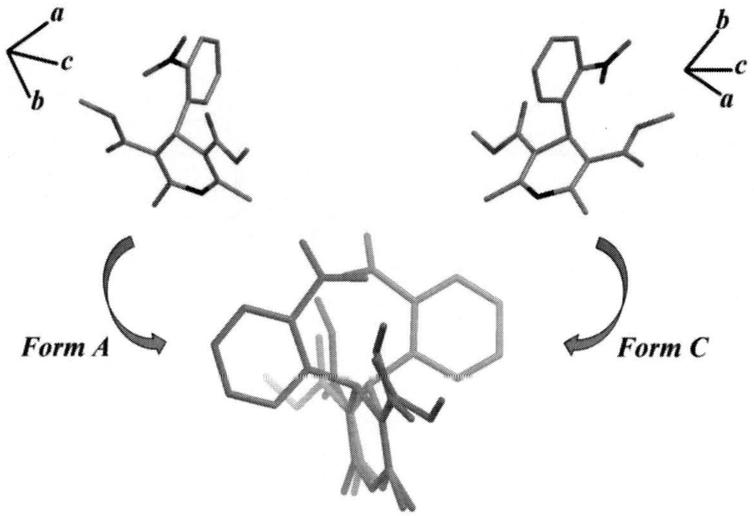

Figure 6. Structural overlay of the NIF in the crystal structures of the form A (left) and form C (right).

The polymorphic forms of NIF can be identified by analysis by powder X-ray diffraction combined with a variety of solid-state analytical techniques [48] such as differential scanning calorimetry (DSC) [42], Fourier transform Raman (FT-Raman), Fourier transform infrared (FT-IR) spectroscopy [43], and by solid-state nuclear magnetic resonance (ssNMR) [49]. The form A has characteristic peaks at 2θ (Cu Kα) in 8.08, 10.45, 16.23 and 24.05 ° while the form C shows peaks at 2θ (Cu Kα) in 7.50, 9.33, 11.54 and 24.54 ° [40, 41, 50]. These peaks are emphasized in the X-ray diffraction patterns in Figure 7. On the other hand, it is observed in the diffraction pattern of metastable form B, four peaks at 2θ (Cu Kα) in 7.32, 9.15, 10.69 and 23.93°, indicating that form B is a polymorph of NIF [40].

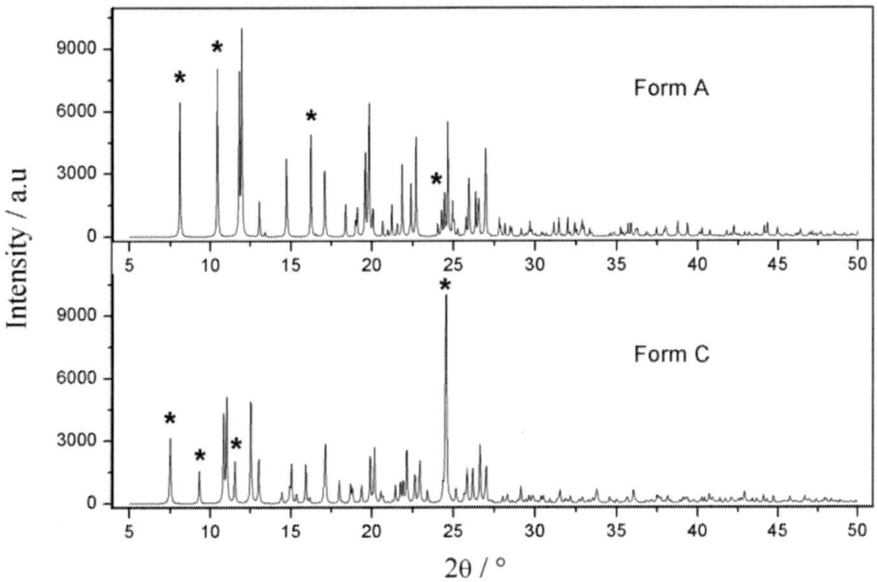

Figure 7. Simulated diffraction patterns for forms A and C of NIF crystals.

The polymorphic forms A, B and C can be distinguished usually by DSC scans of glassy NIF, at a heating rate of 5-10° C.min^{-1} [40, 42, 50]. The DSC measures exhibit endo- and exothermic peaks. The endothermic event at 48°C refers to glassy transition, followed by an exothermic peak at 105°C due to the crystallization process of form B. The exothermic peak at 125 °C is related to polymorphic transition of form B into form A, which melted an endothermic peak at 171°C [42]. When form B is exposed to a cooling and heating cycle by isothermal crystallization method, an endothermic event at 30 °C during cooling and an endothermic event at 60 °C are found. This event displays the polymorphic transformation of form B into form C [51]. The FT-Raman measurements show the structural differences between the three NIF polymorphs forms which can be notable in the region between 1660-1710 cm^{-1}, by associating ester C=O bond stretching modes [43]. The Form A (α-NIF) shows a stretching mode of C=O doublet at 1680 cm^{-1}, this doublet is centred at 1705 cm^{-1} for Form B (γ-NIF) and Form C (β-NIF) exhibits C=O stretching in combination at 1680 and at 1705 cm^{-1} [43].

The form A has a low aqueous solubility (5.42 ± 0.33 μg mL^{-1}, at 30 °C and pH = 1) [46] and irregular bioavailability after oral administration [36]. This may produce a significant alteration of the toxicity characteristic of drug and intensification the adverse effects. Thus, the presence of polymorphism is very important since it affects their physicochemical properties such as solubility, bioavailability and toxicity [34].

Advances in chemistry allow the development of solid-state forms for oral distribution which has objective to improve bioavailability and increase dissolution rate, in many cases, at the cost of the greater physical and chemical stability [52]. The methods to enhance solubility of solids implicate different alterations, such as solid dispersions, solvates and amorphous forms [53, 54]. Natalija Zajc et al. report the use of nifedipine/mannitol solid dispersions to improve a dissolution rate [55]. The mannitol particles are attached on the surface of tinny NIF crystals improving dissolution rate, approximately, in 2.5 times, due wetting of NIF samples, in comparison to pure form A. Other paper in the literature [36], reports the preparation of nifedipine solid dispersions in polymeric matrix system containing Pluronic F68 and Gelucire 50/13. The solubility of these systems is greater than that of the pure NIF sample by a factor of 2.0, simulated gastric fluid at 37 °C. To study of the solid state behaviour of NIF, Maria Klimakow et al. recrystallized glassy NIF samples in various solvent systems [56]. The NIF forms prepared by crystallization process show a strong dependence in relation to the solvent used. For acetonitrile and dichloromethane, it is observed a polymorphic transition of glassy NIF form to form A, and for acetone and ethanol solvents, to form C. When dimethyl sulfoxide (DMSO) and 1,4-dioxane are used as solvent, two novel NIF solvates have been found [46, 57]. The DMSO solvate form of NIF crystallized in the triclinic space group *P-1*, with crystal data: a = 8.0260(6) Å, b = 11.9102(9) Å, c = 12.2806(9) Å, α = 68.282(4)°, β = 76.974(4)°, γ = 81.013(4)°, Z = 2, V = 1059.08(14) $Å^3$. The 1,4-dioxane solvate form crystallizes in the triclinic space group *P-1* and has crystal data: a = 7.6238(2) Å, b = 11.1758(3) Å, c = 11.8898(3) Å, α = 73.524(2)°, β = 73.417(2)°, γ = 75.603(2)°, Z = 2, V = 915.40(4) $Å^3$. The solubility of 1,4-dioxane solvate form was verified at 30 °C and pH = 1 and it was not observed an increase expressively of solubility of the solvate (5.99 ± 0.33 μg mL^{-1}) when compared of Form A [46].

As already cited previously, the use of amorphous forms is another important strategy to improve significantly the oral bioavailability of poorly water soluble drugs. Amorphous solids lack the three-dimensional molecular order and displaying a definite volume with the molecules having an irregular arrangement. Particularly, when using the amorphous phases the aqueous solubility of NIF is increased by factor of 6.0 (35.04 ± 2.51 μg mL^{-1}). These amorphous forms are moderately stable at room temperature; however, it is observed that parts of samples are converted to form A after submitted in different pH conditions [46]. These results may be positive to metabolic properties reducing adverse effects of NIF drug. On the other hand, the amorphous phases show a greater rate and level of photodegradation when exposure to UV–visible radiation (1.8 times larger than Form A), factor is important for drug preparations that utilise the amorphous form [58]. Moreover, the polymorphic modifications of amorphous NIF considering distinct conditions of humidity, temperature and the effect of excipients in the crystallization process have been investigated [43, 59].

A number of explanations may be considered for describing the observed differences in aqueous solubility values from forms of NIF. Crystalline form A and solvates forms of NIF drug are the most stable and shows the lower solubility than that amorphous form due to their low free energy. Thus, crystalline forms have a predisposition to be stable in light, humidity and temperature environments and consequently, they are stable during pharmaceutical development and process of compaction and storage. It is described in the literature, that solvated forms of NIF are generally less soluble than anhydrate forms [46]. The amorphous phases of NIF have high free energy and dissolve faster than their crystalline forms. However, their tending in polymorphic transition to the crystalline form A is a great problem that prevents the utilization as a by-product of industrial fabrication processes.

4. Polymorphs of Valsartan (VAL)

It is known that modifications in the crystalline state of the drugs, especially antihypertensive drugs, lead to changes in their physical and chemical properties [18, 60]. One of antihypertensive drugs that goes through significant changes in solubility and dissolution rate due to the degree of crystallinity in the solid state is the antihypertensive drug Valsartan (Figure 8) [60, 61].

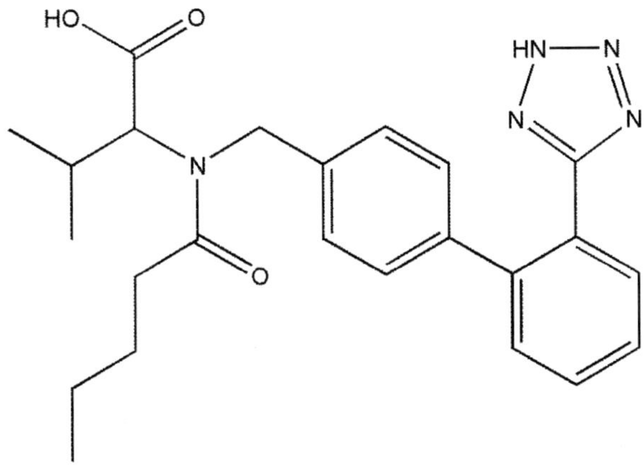

Figure 8. Valsartan molecular representation.

Valsartan (VAL) is selective antagonist of the angiotensin II at the AT_1-receptor that has been widely used in the treatment of mild to moderate hypertension [62, 63]. VAL is formulated as the free acid in capsule and tablet dosage forms, and it was approved by the United States Food and Drug Administration (FDA) in 1996. This drug is normally used in amorphous or low crystallinity form which decreases the chemical and physical stability [64]. VAL presents low stability due to this fact, it needs to be stored under controlled room temperature and protected from humidity and light. However, amorphous forms are generally more soluble and have better dissolution profile than crystalline forms and they have been commercially preferred [62]. Several techniques to obtain solvates of VAL have been used to improve its solubility [60-62, 65].

The recrystallization of the amorphous form of VAL using different organic solvents increases some important pharmacological properties of drug, such as aqueous solubility and *in vitro* dissolution characteristics. The recrystallized products from methanol and acetonitrile had the highest solubility in distilled water, about two times more soluble than VAL whose solubility in water was 0.249 ± 0.020 mg mL^{-1}. All recrystallized products also had *in vitro* dissolution rates higher than antihypertensive VAL [62].

Some patents of polymorphs of antihypertensive drug VAL were deposited in the last decade, WO2004083192, WO2007017897 and WO2012016969 are among the most important, but the amorphous form is most commonly found in pharmaceutical products [61, 62]. The X-ray diffraction pattern of these polymorphs (forms I, II, III, IV, VI, VII, VIII, IX, A, B and C) consists essentially of a crystalline phase contaminated with an amorphous phase. The form D presents degree of crystallinity about 95-98%, and to form E, X-ray diffraction shows that it is anhydrous, althought form F was characterized as a ethanol solvate

[60]. The F and amorphous forms show similar intrinsic dissolution rates, which are 57 and 53 μg cm^{-2} min^{-1}, respectively. However, the pure crystalline form E possesses a lower intrinsic dissolution rate (14 μg cm^{-2} min^{-1}). On the other hand, when formulated into capsules, the dissolution profiles were significant influenced by the solid-state forms used. According to Wang and coworkers, the form E has a dissolution rate 5.5 times greater than that observed for amorphous form [60].

Due to crystal packing, the pure crystalline form E has a surprising chemical and physical stability. It was demonstrated that the form E suffered no degradation when kept under stressful conditions (80 °C / 75% of humidity and 80° C for 6 weeks). Ethanol solvate form F and the amorphous form have suffered thermodecomposition under stressful conditions before 6 weeks [60]. The single crystal structure of form E as well as some interactions (H-bonding) that justify its high chemical and physical stability can be seen in Figure 9. The simulated diffractograms of forms E and F can be seen in Figure 10. The main peaks observed at 2θ (Cu Kα) to form E are: 9.40, 10.84, 11.80, 14.02, 17.82, 18.76, 26.58, and 31.36 °. On the other hand, the main peaks at 2θ (Cu Kα) to form F are: 8.26, 9.72, 11.94, 12.42, 14.62, 17.42, 22.72, and 24.38 °.

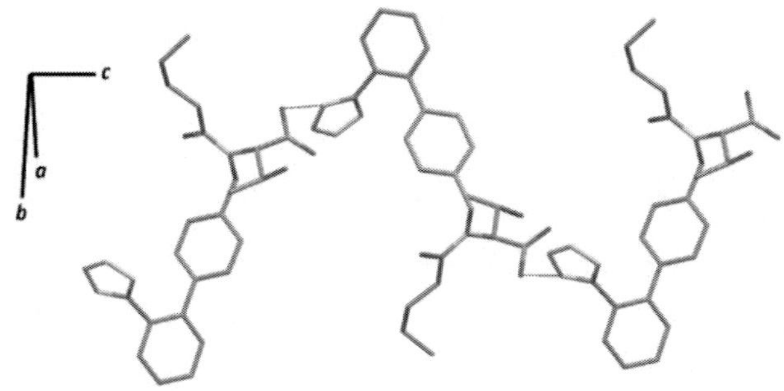

(a)

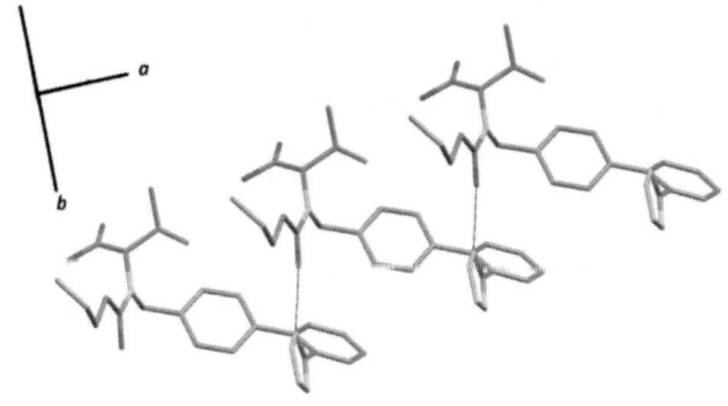

(b)

Figure 9. Crystal structure of form E showing H-bonding between the carboxylic acid and tetrazole ring (a) and the valeryl carbonyl group and the tetrazole ring (b) of VAL.

The crystalline form E of VAL crystallized in orthorhombic system and space group $P2_12_12_1$ with crystal data: a = 7.3516(11) Å, b = 16.346(2) Å, c = 18.801(3) Å, $\alpha = \beta = \gamma = 90$ °, Z = 4, V = 2259.3 (6) Å³. According to crystal structure of form E, the molecules of VAL are connected via two distinctive hydrogen bonds, both associated with the tetrazole moiety. One hydrogen bond is between the carboxylic acid group and the tetrazole ring (Figure 9a) and another one is between the valeryl carbonyl group and the tetrazole ring (Figure 9b). All intermolecular hydrogen bonding interactions provide a high chemical stability in the crystalline structure of VAL [60].

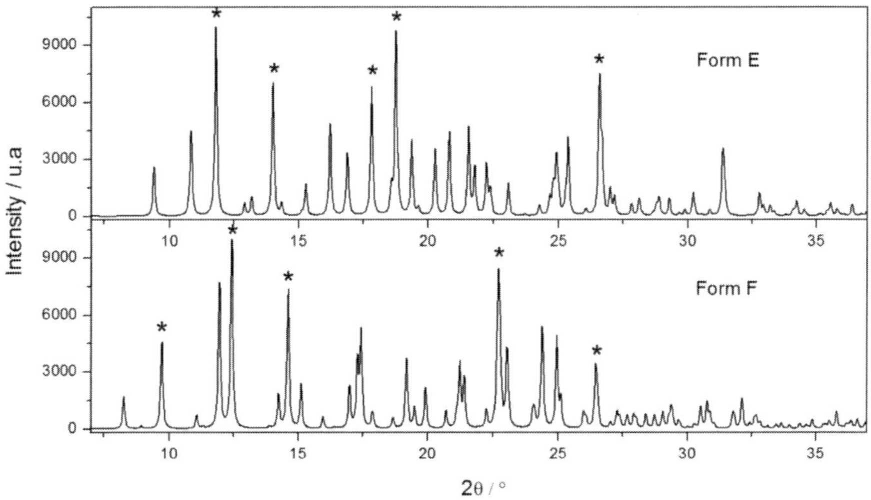

Figure 10. Simulated diffraction patterns for forms E and F of VAL crystals.

5. Polymorphs of Atenolol and Propranolol Hydrochloride

Atenolol also known as 4-[2-hydroxy-3-[(1-methylethyl)amino]propoxy]-benzeneacetamide, Figure 11a, belongs a β-blockers class used as antihypertensive drug [66-68]. There are different subtypes of receptors β (β_1, β_2 and β_3), specifically atenolol is a hydrophilic β_1- adrenergic receptors antagonist, orally administered and excreted in the urine [67]. Atenolol is widely used in the monoterapy and association with others classes of antihypertensive drugs such as diuretic and calcium channel blockers [69].

Atenolol solubility was ascribed by Brazilian pharmacopeia [70] and listed as slightly soluble in water, readily soluble in methanol, soluble in glacial acetic acid and ethanol, slightly soluble in methylene chloride, slightly soluble in acetone, practically insoluble in acetronile. It has oral bioavailability around 50% and half live 6 to 9 hours [71, 72]. Atenolol (2nd generation) was introduced to the market in order to replace propranolol hydrochloride (1st generation), 1-[(2-methylethyl)-amino]-3-(1-naphthalenyloxy)-2-propanol-hydrochloride (Figure 11b), which is a lipophilic β- adrenergic antagonist of the β_1 and β_2-receptors also used in the treatment of hypertension. Propranolol hydrochloride is soluble in water and ethanol, slightly soluble in chloroform and insoluble in ethyl ether [70].

According solubility and gastrointestinal permeability parameters, the Biopharmaceutics Classification System (BCS) divided drugs into four groups: I- High solubility and permeability, II- Low solubility and High permeability, III- High solubility and Low permeability and IV- Low solubility and permeability [73], atenolol and propranolol hydrochloride belongs to the groups III and I, respectively [74].

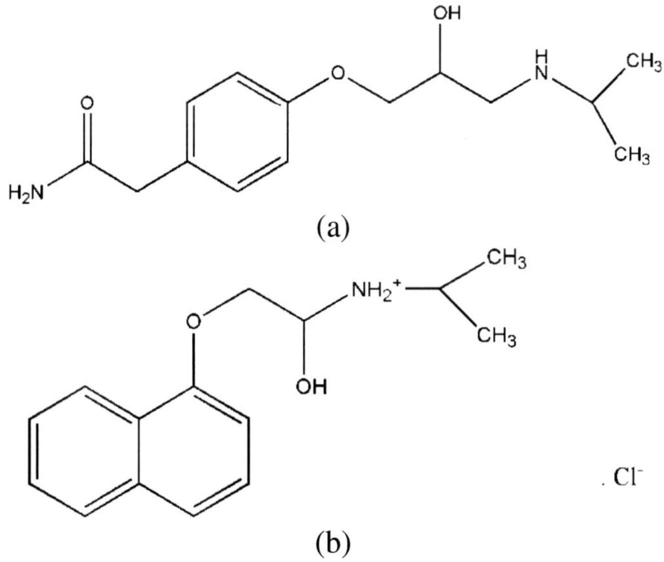

Figure 11. Chemical structure of (a) atenolol and (b) propranolol hydrochloride.

Knowledge of the structure formed in the production of solid drug by pharmaceutical industries is extremely important, since biological activity and physical chemical properties of the drugs depend on the way that the compounds crystallized, as discussed above. So we are doing a brief reviewed about the forms of atenolol and propranolol hydrochloride drugs reported in the literature.

Atenolol synthesis was patented in 1974 [75] but only in 2007 its crystalline structure was first shown to the scientific community [76]. Two crystallographic forms of atenolol were discussed by Esteves de Castro and co-workes [76], specifically (R,S)-atenolol and S-atenolol. Centrosymmetric space group *C2/c* and nonocentrosymmetric space group *C2* were observed for the (R,S) and S forms, respectively. It was observed that asymmetric unit of (R,S)-atenolol have one molecule crystallographically independent and for S-atenolol two molecules crystallographically independent was verified. Despite to positional disorder that appears in two crystalline forms of the drug, the authors suggest two distinct conformation for the (R,S) form called $(R,S)_a$ and $(R,S)_b$ and three conformations to S form (S_a, S_b and S_c), where S_a represents the ordered molecule. It was still observed that the packing of these two forms were very similar and these similarities reflect in unit cell parameters, where cell parameters to the (R,S)-atenolol are a = 55.83(3) Å; b = 5.559(3) Å, c = 9.734(2) Å, $\alpha = \gamma$ = 90° and β = 100.042(6)° and S-atenolol showed the following parameters a = 54.43(3) Å; b = 5.712(3) Å, c = 9.676(2) Å, $\alpha = \gamma$ = 90° and β = 99.510(6)°. The main difference between the forms lies in the molecular tail structure formed by isopropylamino group.

The Figure 12a show the diffractograms of the two samples simulated from the crystalline structure and the main peaks are: (R,S)-atenolol have peaks at 2θ (Cu Kα) 6.43; 9.64; 12.87; 16.11; 17.87; 18.36; 18.49; 18.65; 19.33; 19.50; 20.79; 21.60; 22.37; 22.49; 23.94; 24.43; 24.54; 24.76; 25.63;25.92; 26.47; 26.72; 26.84; 28.42, 29.17; 29.29° and S-atenolol peaks at 2θ (CuKα) 6.59; 9.26; 9.89; 10.34; 13.18; 14.63; 14.83; 15.58; 16.51; 17.57;

18.03; 18.30; 18.68; 19.22; 19.40; 19.55; 20.53; 20.98; 21.54; 22.34; 22.51; 22.78; 23.97; 24.55; 24.92; 25.41; 25.57; 26.65; 26.96; 27.32; 28.27; 28.54; 29.45; 29.62°. Highlight was made in 2θ region 5-17° (Figure 12b) and 17-30° (Figure 12c). Comparing both profile powder patterns, some features can be considered to qualitative analysis, example: the most intense peaks of the S-atenolol form at 2θ 5-17° are displaced by, approximately, 0.16° and 0.25° in comparison to the (R,S) form, Figure 12b. In the 2θ 17-30° region, the displacement for the more intensive peak is 0.24° to the (R,S)-atenolol in comparison to the S form, even in this region, the S-atenolol has a medium intensity peak at 2θ 17.57° which is not observed in the R,S-form, Figure 12c.

Atenolol is a racemic mixture, therefore contains a mixture of two enantiomers. According to pharmacological efficacy, the S(-) form is the more active β-blocker [77].

Propranolol hydrochloride has three polymorphic forms described in the literature, called I, II, III. These polymorphs were exhaustively discussed by Bartolomei and coworkers [78], where differential scanning calorimetry (DSC) data showed endotherms events T_{onset} and fusion enthalpy at: 163.0 ± 0.3 °C and 106.0 ± 0.8 J g^{-1} (form I), 161.8 ± 0.1 °C and 123.8 ± 1.6 J g^{-1} (form II), 144.9 ± 0.4 °C and 77.4 ± 3.4 J g^{-1} (isolated form III from form I in the presence of an alkali halide matrix). The Infrared spectra of forms I and II exhibited significant difference while form I and III showed few subtle difference in fingerprint region [78]. In spectra of form I, a single band at 3337 cm^{-1} was verified while form II showed an intensity band at 3280 cm^{-1} with two shoulders at 3325 cm^{-1} and 3321 cm^{-1} [79].

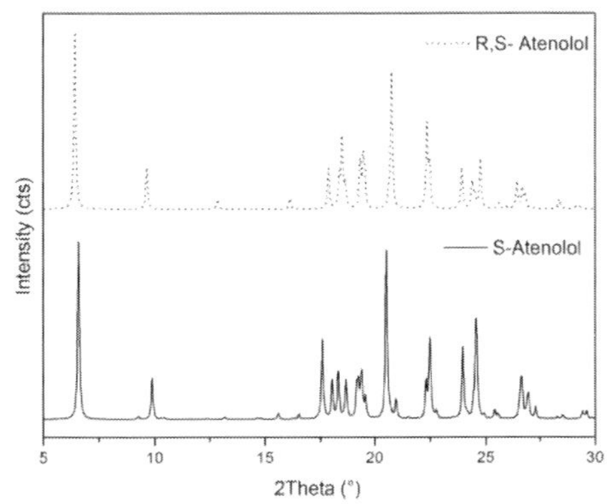

(a)

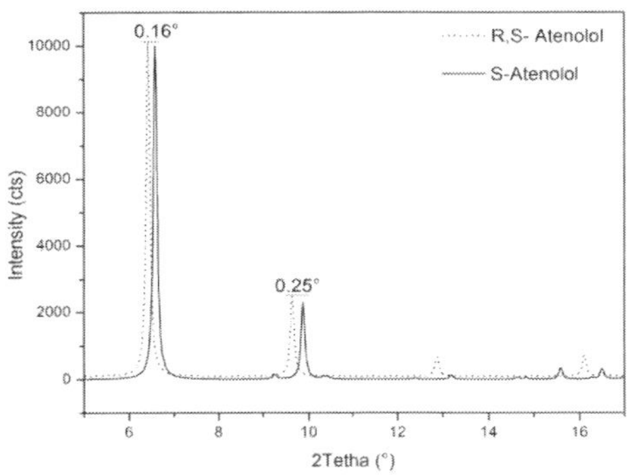

(b)

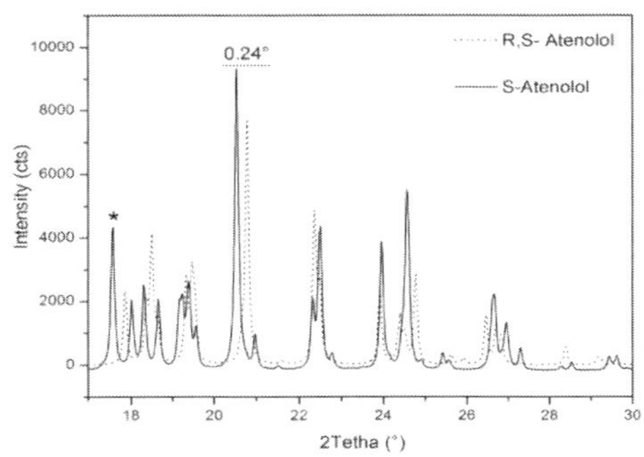

(c)

Figure 12. (a) Diffractograms simulated from crystalline structures of (R,S)-atenolol (Dot line) and S-atenolol (Solid line), (b) Region of 2θ 5-17° and (c) Region of 2θ 17-30°.

Powder pattern diffraction was performed for the forms I and II, where it was observed that profile were different between them, specifically, form I has characteristics peaks at 2θ (CuKα) 23.765, 17.650, 14.255° and form II at 25.085, 17.195, 16.735 and 12.510° [79]. Crystallography structures of propranolol hydrochloride [80-83] are recorded in the literature. From the comparison of powder diffraction data [78, 79], it is possible to conclude that, apparently, the crystalline structure described by Bredikhin and coworkers [83] is associated to the form II. Figure 13 shows the diffractogram simulated from crystalline structures and the main peaks of form II are highlight in asterisk. At room temperature, form II (commercial product) is more stable than form I which is more stable than form III [79]. Solubility and dissolution studies recorded for the polymorphs I and II showed that form I is more soluble and dissolved more faster than form II which is thermodynamically more stable [79].

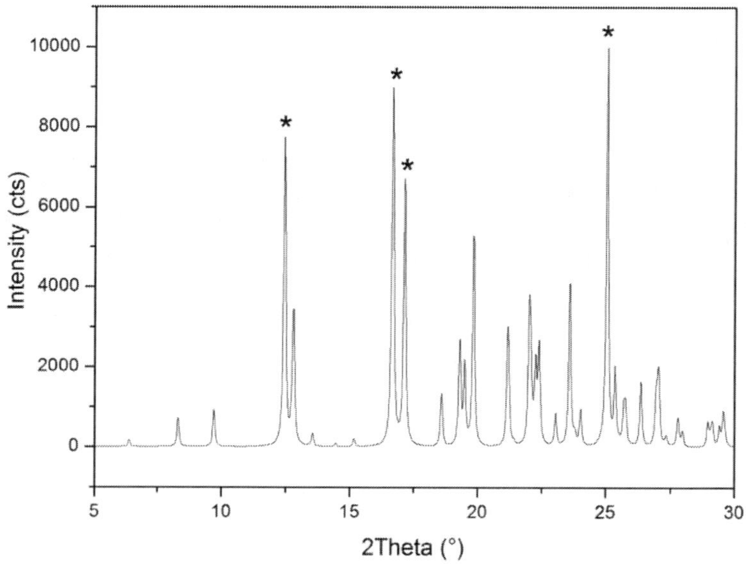

Figure 13. Diffractogram simulated from crystalline structures of propranolol hydrochloride.

Conclusion

The APIs described in this chapter is only a brief demonstration of the importance of polymorphism in the preparation, commercialization and administration of solid pharmaceuticals. The knowledge of each polymorphic form of any API provides relevant information, once some polymorphs should not present similar bioequivalence and / or not be the same therapeutically equivalent.

Acknowledgments

The authors are thankful to the Brazilian Agencies CAPES, FAPEMIG, CNPq for the financial support.

References

[1] Maddileti D., Swapna B., Nangia A. *Crystal Growth & Design.* 2014, 14, 2557-2570.

[2] Brog J.-P., Chanez C.-L., Crochet A., Fromm K. M. *RSC Advances.* 2013, 3, 16905-16931.

[3] Bernstein J. Polymorphism in Molecular Crystals. 2008, New York, USA: *Oxford University Press.*

[4] Santos O. M. M., Reis M. E. D., Jacon J. T., Lino M. E. d.S., Simões J. S., Doriguetto A. C. *Brazilian Journal of Pharmaceutical Sciences.* 2014, 50, 1-24.

[5] Lu J. *African Journal of Pharmacy and Pharmacology.* 2012, 6, 581-591.

[6] Bernstein J. *Crystal Growth & Design.* 2005, 5, 1661-1662.

[7] Seddon K. R. *Crystal Growth & Design.* 2004, 4, 1087.

[8] Chieng N., Rades T., Aaltonen J. *Journal of Pharmaceutical and Biomedical Analysis.* 2011, 55, 618-644.

[9] Bernstein J. *Crystal Growth & Design.* 2011, 11, 632-650.

[10] Brittain H. G. Polymorphism in Pharmaceutical Solids. 2009, New York, USA: Informa Healthcare USA Inc.

[11] Khandavilli U. B. R., Gangavaram S., Goud N. R., Cherukuvada S., Raghavender S., Nangia A., Manjunatha S. G., Nambiar S., Pal S. *Cryst Eng Comm.* 2014, 16, 4842-4852.

[12] Aitipamula S., Chow P. S., Tan R. B. H. *Cryst Eng Comm.* 2014, 16, 3451-3465.

[13] Swapna B., Maddileti D., Nangia A. *Crystal Growth & Design.* 2014, 14, 5991-6005.

[14] Peterson M. L., Hickey M. B., Zaworotko M. J., Almarsson O. *Journal of Pharmaceutical Sciences.* 2006, 9, 317-326.

[15] Srirambhatla V. K., Kraft A., Watt S., Powell A. V. *Cryst Eng Comm.* 2014, 16, 9979-9982.

[16] FDA. U. S. Food and Drug Administration. Guidance for Industry - Regulatory Classification of Pharmaceutical Co-Crystals, 2013. Available at: http://www.fda.gov/downloads/Drugs/Guidances/UCM 281764.pdf. Acessed on: January 2015.

[17] Campeta A. M., Chekal B. P., Abramov Y. A., Meenan P. A., Henson M. J., Shi B., Singer R. A., Horspool K. R. *Journal of Pharmaceutical Sciences.* 2010, 99, 3874-3886.

[18] Vippagunta S. R., Brittain H. G., Grant D. J. W. *Advanced Drug Delivery Reviews.* 2001, 48, 3-26.

[19] Aitipamula S., Chow P. S., Tan R. B. H. *Acta Crystallographica Section B.* 2014, 70, 54-62.

[20] Bugay D. E. *Advanced Drug Delivery Reviews.* 2001, 48, 43-65.

[21] Gendrin C., Roggo Y., Collet C. *Journal of Pharmaceutical and Biomedical Analysis.* 2008, 48, 533-553.

[22] Harris R. K. *Journal of Pharmacy and Pharmacology.* 2007, 59, 225-239.

[23] Stephenson G. A., Forbes R. A., Reutzel-Edens S. M. *Advanced Drug Delivery Reviews.* 2001, 48, 67-90.

[24] Chattah A. K., Mroue K. H., Pfund L. Y., Ramamoorthy A., Longhi M. R., Garnero C. *Journal of Pharmaceutical Sciences.* 2013, 102, 3717-3724.

[25] Barbas R., Marti F., Prohens R., Puigjaner C. *Crystal Growth & Design.* 2006, 6, 1463-1467.

[26] Barbas R., Prohens R., Puigjaner C. *Journal of Thermal Analysis and Calorimetry.* 2007, 89, 687-692.

[27] Puigjaner C., Barbas R., Portell A., Font-Bardia M., Alcobe X., Prohens R. *Crystal Growth & Design. 2010*, 10, 2948-2953.

[28] Newman A. W., Byrn S. R. *Drug Discovery Today.* 2003, 8, 898-905.

[29] Rietveld H. M. *Journal of Applied Crystallography.* 1969, 2, 65-71.

[30] Giron D. *Thermochimica Acta.* 1995, 248, 1-59.

[31] Zhang G. G. Z., Law D., Schmitt E. A., Qiu Y. *Advanced Drug Delivery Reviews.* 2004, 56, 371-390.

[32] Tocci G., Battistoni A., Passerini J., Musumeci M. B., Francia P., Ferrucci A., Volpe M. *Journal of Cardiovascular Pharmacology and Therapeutics.* 2014.

[33] Chung M. W., Bang S., Jin S. K., Woo S. W., Lee Y. J., Kim Y. S., Lee J. K., Lee S. H., Chung H. J. *The Journal of Applied Pharmacology.* 2007, 15, 156-161.

[34] Da Silva Leite R., De Oliveira Macedo R., Torres S., Batista C., De Oliveira Baltazar L., Neto S., De Souza F. *Journal of Thermal Analysis and Calorimetry.* 2013, 111, 2117-2123.

[35] Leonetti G., Cuspidi C., Sampieri L., Terzoli L., Zanchetti A. *Journal of Cardiovascular Pharmacology.* 1982, 4, S325.

[36] Vippagunta S. R., Maul K. A., Tallavajhala S., Grant D. J. W. *International Journal of Pharmaceutics.* 2002, 236, 111-123.

[37] Breimer D. D. *Pharmaceutisch Weekblad Scientific Edition.* 1985, 7, 63-66.

[38] Marsh S., McLeod H. L. *Human Molecular Genetics.* 2006, 15, R89-R93.

[39] Eckert T., Müller J. *Archiv der Pharmazie.* 1977, 310, 116-118.

[40] Hirayama F., Wang Z., Uekama K. *Pharmaceutical Research.* 1994, 11, 1766-1770.

[41] Bortolotti M., Lonardelli I., Pepponi G. *Acta Crystallographica Section* B. 2011, 67, 357-364.

[42] Keymolen B., Ford J. L., Powell M. W., Rajabi-Siahboomi A. R. *Thermochimica Acta.* 2003, 397, 103-117.

[43] Chan K. L. A., Fleming O. S., Kazarian S. G., Vassou D., Chryssikos G. D., Gionis V. *Journal of Raman Spectroscopy.* 2004, 35, 353-359.

[44] Gunn E., Guzei I. A., Cai T., Yu L. *Crystal Growth & Design.* 2012, 12, 2037-2043.

[45] Triggle A. M., Shefter E., Triggle D. J. *Journal of Medicinal Chemistry.* 1980, 23, 1442-1445.

[46] Caira M. R., Robbertse Y., Bergh J. J., Song M., De Villiers M. M. *Journal of Pharmaceutical Sciences.* 2003, 92, 2519-2533.

[47] Raina S. A., Alonzo D. E., Zhang G. G. Z., Gao Y, T.L. S. *Journal Molecular Pharmaceutics.* 2014, 11, 3565−3576.

[48] Chienga N., Radesb T., Aaltonenc J. *Journal of Pharmaceutical and Biomedical Analysis.* 2011, 55, 618-644.

[49] Apperley D. C., Forster A. H., Fournier R., Harris R. K., Hodgkinson P., Lancaster R. W., Rades T. *Magnetic Resonance in Chemistry.* 2005, 43, 881-892.

[50] Grooff D., De Villiers M. M., Liebenberg W. *Thermochimica Acta.* 2007, 454, 33-42.

[51] Zhou D., Schmitt E. A., Zhang G. G., Law D., Vyazovkin S., Wight C. A., Grant D. J. W. *Journal of Pharmaceutical Sciences.* 2003, 92, 1779-1792.

[52] Rodríguez-Spong B., Price C. P., Jayasankar A., Matzger A. J., Rodríguez-Hornedo N.r. *Advanced Drug Delivery Reviews.* 2004, 56, 241-274.
[53] Vasconcelos T., Sarmento B., Costa P. *Drug Discovery Today.* 2007, 12, 1068-1075.
[54] Blagden N., de Matas M., Gavan P. T., York P. *Advanced Drug Delivery Reviews.* 2007, 59, 617-630.
[55] Zajca N., Obrezaa A., Beleb M., Srcica S. *International Journal of Pharmaceutics.* 2005, 291, 51-58.
[56] Klimakow M., Leiterer J., Kneipp J., Rössler E., Panne U., Rademann K., Emmerling F. *Langmuir.* 2010, 26, 11233-11237.
[57] Klimakow M., Rademann K., Emmerling F. *Crystal Growth & Design.* 2010, 10, 2693-2698.
[58] Grooff D., Francis F., De Villiers M. M., Ferg E. *Journal of Pharmaceutical Sciences.* 2013, 102, 1883-1894.
[59] Zhang S.-W., Yu L., Huang J., Hussain M., Derdour L., Qian F., de Villiers M. *AAPS PharmSciTech.* 2014, 15, 1516-1526.
[60] Wang J.-R., Wang X., Lu L., Mei X. *Crystal Growth & Design.* 2013, 13, 3261-3269.
[61] Tran T.-D., Tran P.-L., Park J.-B., Lee B.-J. *Archives of Pharmacal Research.* 2012, 35, 1223-1230.
[62] Nalluri B. N., Krishna M. R., Rao T. P., Crooks P. A. *Journal of Applied Pharmaceutical Science.* 2012, 2, 126-132.
[63] Volpe M. Expert Review of Cardiovascular Therapy. 2012, 10, 1061-1072.
[64] Kshirsagar S. J., Bhalekar M. R., Madgulkar A. R., Sable P. N., Gupta B. K. *Latin American Journal of Pharmacy.* 2010, 29, 393-400.
[65] Chella N., Shastri N., Tadikonda R. R. *Acta Pharmaceutica Sinica B.* 2012, 2, 502-508.
[66] Al-Awadie N. S. T., Khudhair A. F. *Iraqi Journal of Science.* 2014, 55, 12-26.
[67] Larochelle P., Tobe S. W., Lacourcière Y. *Canadian Journal of Cardiology.* 2014, 30, S16-S22.
[68] Tobe S. W. *Canadian Journal of Cardiology.* 2014, 30, S1-S2.
[69] Nobre F., Geleilete T. J. M., Cardoso M. C. M., Coelho E. B. *Revista Brasileira de Hipertensão.* 2003, 10, 270-276.
[70] Farmacopeia Brasileira. Agência Nacional de Vigilância Sanitária, Brasilia: *Anvisa,* 2010, 808.
[71] Kumare M. M., Marathe R. P., Kawade R. M., Ghante M. H., Shendarkar G. R. *Asian Journal of Pharmaceutical and Clinical Research.* 2013, 6, 81-85.
[72] Kuyper L. M., Khan N. A. *Canadian Journal of Cardiology.* 2014, 30, S47-S53.
[73] Amidon G., Lennernäs H., Shah V., Crison J. *Pharmaceutical Research.* 1995, 12, 413-420.
[74] Souza J.d., Freitas Z. M. F., Storpirtis S. *Brazilian Journal of Pharmaceutical Sciences.* 2007, 43, 515-527.
[75] Barrett A., Carter J., Le C. D., Squire C. *Google Patents.* 1974.
[76] Esteves de Castro R. A., Canotilho J., Barbosa R. M., Silva M. R., Beja A. M., Paixão J. A., Redinha J. S. *Crystal Growth & Design.* 2007, 7, 496-500.
[77] Barberich T. J., Bratzler R. L., Young J. W. *Google Patents.* 1992.
[78] Bartolomei M., Bertocchi P., Cotta Ramusino M., Ciranni Signoretti E. *Thermochimica Acta.* 1998, 321, 43-52.

[79] Bartolomei M., Bertocchi P., Cotta Ramusino M., Santucci N., Valvo L. *Journal of Pharmaceutical and Biomedical Analysis*. 1999, 21, 299-309.

[80] Barrans Y., Cotrait M., Dangoumau J. *Acta Crystallographica Section B*. 1973, 29, 1264-1272.

[81] Gadret M., Goursolle M., Leger J. M., Colleter J. C. *Acta Crystallographica Section B*. 1975, 31, 1938-1942.

[82] Ammon H. L., Howe D.-B., Erhardt W. D., Balsamo A., Macchia B., Macchia F., Keefe W. E. *Acta Crystallographica Section B*. 1977, 33, 21-29.

[83] Bredikhin A. A., Bredikhina Z. A., Gubaidullin A. T., Krivolapov D. B., Litvinov I. A. *Mendeleev Communications*. 2004, 14, 268-270.

In: Antihypertensive Drugs
Editor: Scott Caldwell

ISBN: 978-1-63463-829-6

Chapter IV

Management of the Black Hypertensive Patient in a Resource Limited Setting

Ifeoma I. Ulasi,[2,1,3] FWACP, Chinwuba K Ijoma,[1] FMCP, Benedict C. Anisiuba,[1] FMCP, Ngozi A. Ifebunandu,[2,3] FMCP and Uchenna N. Ijoma,[1] FMCP

[1]Department of Medicine, College of Medicine, University of Nigeria Teaching Hospital, Ituku-Ozalla, Enugu State, Nigeria

[2]Department of Internal Medicine, College of Health Sciences, Ebonyi State University, Abkaliki, Ebonyi State, Nigeria

[3]Department of Medicine, Federal Teaching Hospital, Abakaliki, Ebonyi State, Nigeria.

Abstract

Hypertension is by far the most important modifiable risk factor for cardiovascular disease in sub-Saharan Africa. Studies have documented the prevalence of hypertension to be highest in blacks and the incidence and progression of end-organ damage from hypertension are worse in black patients. For example the risk of stroke is double in hypertensive black patients compared with white hypertensive patients. Hypertension in blacks is strongly associated with a lot of other modifiable risk factors for CVD such as obesity, physical inactivity and reduced potassium intake. This observation also applies to black patients in USA and Europe. Consequently, effective treatment of hypertension is particularly important in black patients. Calcium channel blockers and diuretics are effective monotherapy in blacks. Beta blockers, alpha adrenergic blockers, angiotensin converting enzyme inhibitors and angiotensin receptor blockers are less effective as monotherapy. They are however effective as combination therapy which is particularly attractive for black patients. Medical education is important in hypertensive black patients because of the cluster of modifiable risk factors and socioeconomic considerations.

Because of its clinical course, apparent lack of symptoms and association with complications, hypertension has emerged as a major public health concern.

The International Society on Hypertension in Blacks in 2010 recommended antihypertensive therapy for blacks without target organ damage or concomitant cardiovascular diseases at blood pressures greater than 135/85 mmHg, or greater than 130/80 mmHg for those at higher risk.

Current understanding of the underlying pathophysiology of hypertensive disease indicates that the pathophysiology of hypertension in the black is slightly different from those of other races. Black patients with hypertension have enhanced sodium retention, expanded plasma volume, low plasma renin activity and a higher incidence of salt-sensitivity. Consequently, there are differences in the appropriate drugs to use for optimal treatment of hypertension in black patients.

Studies of black hypertensive patients in Africa have documented high prevalence of hypertension and low prevalence of control to target levels. Many factors are responsible including poverty, lack of access to health facilities, poor health seeking behaviours, cultural beliefs including myths and superstition. Attention to all these in addition to education and life style modification and not merely drug therapy will make the necessary change in the current state of hypertension in blacks

In this chapter, the authors will discuss the ethnic/racial peculiarities in the incidence, pathophysiology and management of hypertension in the black hypertensive patient. We shall also review the management of black hypertensive patient in resource limited setting emphasizing the race-related differences in the pathophysiology of hypertension and the need to stream line management taking cognizance of the cost burden of management of hypertension.

Section 1: Introduction and Background

A. Epidemiology, Magnitude and Burden of Hypertension

The prevalence of hypertension is increasing globally. This prevalence is increasing faster in low and middle income economies than in high economy countries [1].

Blacks in diaspora have a higher prevalence of hypertension than whites while the blacks in Africa have a historical progression with the prevalence of hypertension currently approaching that of the whites in Europe. Geographic locations alone may not explain the higher prevalence of hypertension seen in blacks in diaspora.

Blacks in Cuba and other less developed countries do not have a higher prevalence of hypertension than non-blacks [2]. Several factors – lifestyle, environmental and genetic – may be responsible for the disparity in the hypertension prevalence of blacks in various geographic locations. Current data from community studies indicate that two of every five persons have hypertension [3-6].

i. Global Prevalence

Hypertension is the leading cause of cardiovascular disease globally [7, 8]. It is estimated that worldwide, raised blood pressure will cause 7.5 million deaths amounting to about 12.8% of the total number of deaths. Raised blood pressure also accounts for 57 million disability adjusted life years (DALYS), about 3.7% of total DALYS [3]. Blood pressure levels have been shown to be positively and continuously related to the risk for stroke and coronary heart disease.

Hypertension accounts for at least 45% of deaths from heart disease and 51% of deaths from stroke. In 2008, the proportion of adult population aged 25 years and above diagnosed with hypertension was estimated at 40%; documenting an increase in the number of people with hypertension from about 600 million in 1980 to 1 billion in 2008 [4]. Some studies have documented the prevalence of hypertension to be highest in blacks. Similarly, World Health Organization (WHO) noted in its global brief on hypertension in 2013 [4] that the prevalence was highest in Africa (46%) and lowest in the Americas (35%). Worldwide, high income countries have lower prevalence than the middle and lower income countries [3, 6] see Figure 1.

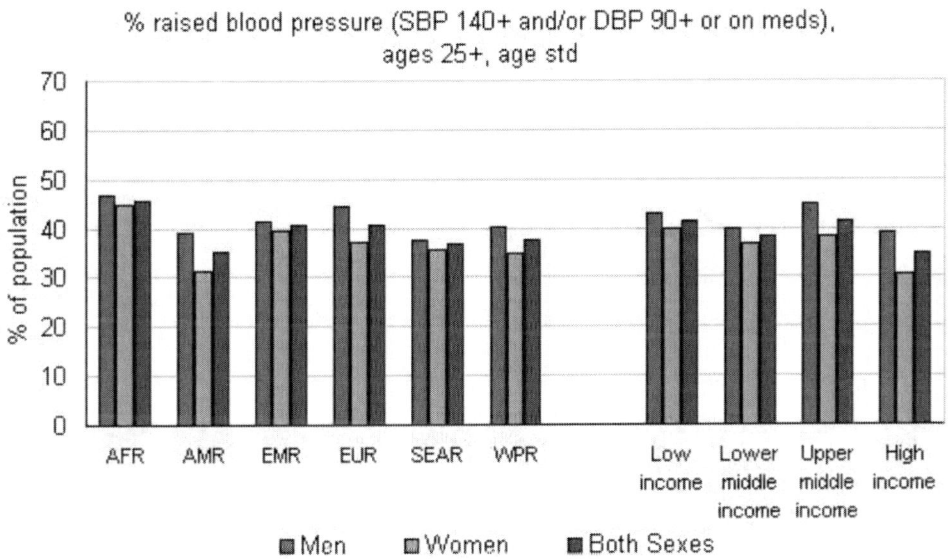

Figure 1. Prevalence of hypertension by world regions and economic status Culled from WHO Global Health Observatory data [3].

ii. Prevalence of Hypertension in Lower and Middle Income Countries (LMICs)

Previously, high blood pressure was associated with more affluent regions of the world [1, 9]. Earlier reports in Africa documented none or very few cases of hypertension [10]. However, the condition is increasing in low and middle-income countries (LMICs) [1] with increasing globalization. For example, the prevalence of hypertension in Nigeria [11] has been increasing steadily from 8.9% (1970 -1979), to 15% (1990 -1999) and 22.5% (2000 – 2009).

The WHO noted that of the 36 million deaths from non-communicable diseases (NCDs) worldwide, 80% i.e. 29 million were in LMICs [6]. Currently, the global burden of hypertension is greatest in LMICs where every 2 in 5 persons in the adult population is affected and this is projected to rise [3, 4, 6]. It is estimated that by 2025, about 3 in 4 persons with hypertension will be living in LMICs [7]. The absolute numbers affected by hypertension in these countries are huge and are likely to increase as the drivers of hypertension (population aging, urbanization with adoption of western lifestyle, reduced physical activity, etc.) burgeon.

iii. Prevalence of Hypertension in Africa

Communicable diseases, maternal, perinatal and nutritional causes of morbidity and mortality accounted for the greatest burden of disease in Africa in the past [12]. Presently and for the foreseeable future, the burden of disease is fast moving towards chronic non-communicable diseases and cardiovascular disease (CVD). This phenomenon was termed the "double burden of disease" by the WHO [13].

In 1929, Donnison described blood pressure patterns in an Africa community where he noted that in 1,800 patients treated in a native hospital over a two-year period, no case of raised blood pressure was seen [10]. Thus, high blood pressure was almost non-existent in African communities in the first half of the twentieth century but current estimates suggest that the highest prevalence of hypertension is in Africa. The increasing prevalence of hypertension in Africa has occurred over a few decades [7, 14]. According to WHO [15] in 2000, there were approximately 80 million adults with hypertension in sub-Saharan Africa (SSA) but their projections from epidemiological data suggest that by 2025 over 150 million of the population will have hypertension. Also, they noted that complications arising from hypertension (stroke and heart failure) were increasingly more common in the continent.

B. Epidemiological Trends

i. Epidemiological Transition

Lifestyle, health and disease patterns change in societies in response to factors such as changes in population structure and economic development resulting in epidemiological transition [16, 17]. Disease patterns transit from infectious and communicable diseases to non-communicable diseases as societies develop, especially in urban and semi-urban populations. This is consequent upon changes in the environmental and behavioral determinants of health and disease. These include growing tobacco use, more fat and calorie consumption, decreasing physical activity and extended exposure to these determinants consequent upon longer life expectancy. The changes in demography, determinants and disease rates in African populations are precipitous, occurring over decades as against those of European and North American populations that occurred over the course of a century or more [18]. As in other parts of the world, the prevalence of hypertension in the sub-Saharan African region has increased as a reflection of the epidemiological transition [19].

Rural to urban migration in most countries in Africa with adoption of western lifestyle accounts for the increasing prevalence of high blood pressure observed in epidemiologic studies [20, 21]. Clustering of risk factors is often associated with clustering of unhealthy lifestyle characteristics and they are more prominent in lower socio-economic groups and in low and middle income (LMI) countries [22]

ii. Urbanization and Westernization

Africa's total population is 1.03 billion and almost 40 percent live in urban areas [7, 23]. The urban population is estimated to rise to 1.23 billion in 2050, by which time 60 percent of all Africans will be living in urban areas [7]. The 2014 revision of the *World Urbanization Prospects* by UN DESA's Population Division [24] noted that Nigeria is one of the three countries projected to have the largest urban growth. The others being India and China. Several cities in Africa such as Lagos, Kinshasa and Luanda are projected to contribute to the urban growth. The increasing urbanization is one of the main reasons for the rising prevalence in hypertension [19]. Largely, levels of hypertension are higher in urban than in rural areas [20, 21] because of socio-behavioral factors associated with urban environments.

iii. Population Aging

People are living longer because of changes in the lifestyle, healthcare and disease management strategies. By the year 2050, the proportion of children is estimated to decline by about a third, so that the population of persons aged 60 years and above will match those of individuals younger than 15 years being about 21 per cent for each group [25]. Though population aging is indeed a global phenomenon, it is important to realize that 73% of this older people will live in LMICs [7].

Despite Africa remaining younger than all other continents, there is currently about 36 million people 65 years and above in Africa (equivalent to 3.6% of the population) but by 2050, the proportion will rise to 10% [26]. This growth will outstrip that of any other world region or any other age group. The enormous shift of demographics will have a strong effect on public health in Africa resulting in growing prevalence of chronic diseases like hypertension and cardiovascular diseases [27].

C. Genetics of and Risk Factors for Hypertension

Essential hypertension is a complex, multifactorial, and polygenic trait. It is thought to result from interactions of multiple genetic and environmental factors. Also, epigenetic inheritance may play a significant role [28]. Familial and twin studies suggest that 30%-50% of the difference in blood pressure readings is due to genetic heritability while about 50% are from environmental factors [29, 30]. Therefore, current knowledge associates hypertension with mainly environmental and lifestyle factors rather than with genetics. Multiple unidentified genetic factors may influence individual susceptibility to diverse aspects of diet and lifestyle. These genetic factors may account for the inter-individual disparities in blood pressure between subjects that display commonalities in behavioral patterns that promote blood pressure rise [31]. Hypertension has a strong relationship and causal link with some social behaviors: use of tobacco, excessive consumption of alcohol, physical inactivity or reduced activity, unhealthy diets (high salt intake, insufficient fruit and vegetable consumption and fatty foods), and obesity. Risk factors leading to hypertension can be modifiable or non- modifiable.

i. Modifiable Risk Factors for Hypertension

Lifestyle factors are very important modifiable risk factors in hypertension, and they are critical determinants of blood pressure levels, operating on the background of genetic susceptibility. For example, excess body fat is a significant cause of hypertension buoyed by additive effects of dietary salt, alcohol, and physical inactivity. Controlled trials in hypertensive patients show blood pressure lowering effects of supplemental potassium, fiber, N-3 fatty acids, diet rich in fruit and vegetables and low in saturated fats [31].

1. Tobacco

Tobacco use is associated with increased risk of developing hypertension and cardiovascular diseases like stroke, thrombosis and heart attack. Smoking causes an immediate increase in blood pressure resulting in higher ambulatory blood pressure levels in smokers than non-smokers. Stopping smoking reduces the overall risk of cardiovascular diseases [32, 33]. Smokeless tobacco has also been associated with hypertension and other diseases like oral cancer, heart disease and other conditions [6]. The prevalence of tobacco use varies widely; in most countries men use tobacco more than women [6]. WHO predictions show that the tobacco companies are moving from high income countries and targeting the LMICs where governmental control may be lax or less rigid [34]. Among men, the highest prevalence of smoking was in LMICs and then declined as country income rises. However, among women higher rates were reported in upper-middle and high-income countries, about five times more than in low- and lower-middle-income countries [6]. There is a controversy about certain aspects of the relationship between hypertension and smoking. Tobacco smoking raises blood pressure acutely and then it decreases in smokers who do not smoke for a week. However, in a study in Israel, men aged 20–39 years and people who smoked >20 cigarettes per day had lowest prevalence of hypertension while never and former smokers had the highest prevalence. This is termed the hypertension-smoking paradox [35]. One reason alluded for this paradox was weight gain after stopping smoking.

2. Alcohol

The association between alcohol and hypertension is well established but the mechanisms involved are yet to be unraveled. Suggested mechanisms include: malfunction of the central nervous system and baroreceptors, rise of sympathetic activity, stimulation of the renin-angiotensin-aldosterone system, and increase in cortisol levels. Others are rise of intracellular calcium levels with associated increase in vascular reactivity, stimulation of the endothelium to release endothelin or inhibition of endothelium-dependent nitric oxide production etc. [36].

The association between alcohol consumption and hypertension was first reported in 1915 by Lian following a study of a group of French servicemen [37]. He found a higher frequency of hypertension in heavy than moderate drinkers. This has since been documented in several other studies [38 - 41]. Studies documenting mean blood pressure levels according to alcohol consumption categories showed blood pressure elevations were 1.6 to 10.9 mmHg higher in the higher consumption groups than in the lower or no alcohol consumption groups. The degree of the increase in blood pressure in heavy drinkers averages about 5 to 10 mmHg, with systolic increases often greater than diastolic increases [42]. However, the Framingham cohort study found no dose-response relationship in alcohol use [42, 43]. But more recently, Panagiotakos et al. (2007) [44] demonstrated that alcohol intake has a semi-parabolic (J-shaped) association with parameters of blood pressure: systolic (P=0.001), diastolic (P=0.02), mean arterial (P=0.001) blood pressures and pulse pressure (P=0.07). They found that intake of 1 to 2 glasses of wine/day lowered likelihood of developing hypertension by 13%. Alcohol intake is relatively common in many countries in Africa and in low resource countries in Europe [45]. There is a direct effect between high levels and specific patterns of alcohol consumption like binge drinking with the risk of hypertension. The influence of heavy drinking on increasing blood pressure levels has been described in Nigeria [46].

3. Insufficient or Inadequate Physical Activity

Inadequate physical activity is the fourth leading risk factor for all-cause mortality. Individuals who do not have adequate physical activity have a 20%–30% increased risk of all-cause mortality compared to those who do at least 30 minutes of moderate intensity physical activity on most days of the week [47]. Studies have demonstrated that adequate physical activity has many health promoting effects [48]. Adequate exercise may have a direct and independent role in reducing hypertension [48]. Africa and most other countries in the LMI economies in the past had high level of physical activity because most people engaged in farming. This high activity was thought in part to explain the low levels of chronic diseases found in Africa. However, the level of physical activity has been decreasing as a result of the high rate of urbanization that has occurred in these regions. WHO STEPS survey has defined adequate physical activity as moderate exercise/activity of more than 150 minutes per week. Participation in this level of physical activity is estimated to reduce the risk of ischemic heart disease by approximately 30%, the risk of diabetes by 27%, and the risk of breast and colon cancer by 21%–25% [48, 49]. It is also known to reduce the risk of hypertension, stroke and depression.

4. Unhealthy Diet

Studies indicate that unhealthy diet enhances morbidity and mortality. For example, approximately 16 million (1.0%) DALYs and 1.7 million (2.8%) of deaths globally are attributable to low fruit and vegetable consumption [49, 50]. Ample consumption of fruit and vegetables is known to reduce the risk for cardiovascular diseases and certain cancers [6]. There is now abundant evidence that dietary and lifestyle factors critically determine an individual's blood pressure levels and the prevalence of hypertension in populations [22]. The DASH (Dietary Approaches to Stop Hypertension) Study Group demonstrated that the use of DASH diet, consisting of foods rich in fruits, vegetables, and low-fat dairy foods, significantly lowered blood pressure [51].

5. High Salt Intake

The quantity of salt in food is a major determinant of blood pressure levels and over-all cardiovascular risk [52]. WHO has recommended intake of less than 5 grams of salt per person per day for prevention of cardiovascular disease (52). Unfortunately, available data show that most populations consume much more salt than recommended (53). It is projected that decreasing dietary salt intake from the current levels of 9–12 grams per day to the WHO recommended level would help reduce blood pressure and cardiovascular disease appreciably (54). Reduced salt intake not only lowers blood pressure and associated CVD risk, it also has other beneficial cardiovascular effects that are independent of and are additive to its blood pressure effect [55]. Such beneficial effects include a direct reduction of stroke, left ventricular hypertrophy, aortic stiffness, chronic kidney disease and proteinuria [56). High intake of sodium is common in countries in Africa and other LMICs mostly from salt used to preserve food or to make it tasty [57]. Intervention studies in Africa show that a reduction in salt intake and an increase in potassium could improve blood pressure in African populations.

In Tanzania, investigators demonstrated that a low sodium diet leading to a low urinary excretion level of 52 mmol per day, lowered blood pressure in normotensive persons appreciably in four to five days [58]. Also, a study in Kenya noted that supplanting sodium with potassium in newly diagnosed patients with hypertension reduced the blood pressure akin to levels achieved with diuretics [59].

6. Insufficient Fruit and Vegetable Consumption

Fruit and vegetable consumption varies among countries and it often reflects the economic, cultural and agricultural production environments [60]. Benefits of fruits and vegetable consumption come from reduction in CVD and hypertension. Compounding the high salt intake, most individuals in LMICs consume insufficient fruits and vegetables resulting in low potassium intake and raised blood pressure. The WHO STEPS surveys reported sufficient fruits and vegetables intake of five or more servings of fruits or vegetables per typical day as very low across countries in Africa. The WHO recommended potassium intake is 90mmol/day [61].

7. High Intake of Fatty Foods

There is convincing evidence that saturated fat and trans-fat increase the risk of coronary heart disease and this risk is reduced when mono-saturated and polyunsaturated fat is used. The analysis of total fats available for human consumption recorded lowest quantities in the South-East Asia Region while the European Region had the highest. For saturated fatty acids (SFAs), the lowest rates were in the African Region, and the highest was in the European Region and the Region of the Americas. Energy from SFAs accounts for a third of the energy from total fat, with the exception of the South-east Asia Region, where SFAs account for over 40% of total fat intake [62]. Some studies reported benefits from consumption of low-fat dairy products [63, 64]. The Seguimiento Universidad de Navarra (SUN) cohort study demonstrated about 54% reduction in incident hypertension among persons who consume low-fat, but not whole-fat, dairy products [63]. In another study, the risk of hypertension inversely correlated with total dairy and low-fat dairy intake [65].

8. Overweight and Obesity

The World Health Organization defines obesity as a condition in which surplus body fat has amassed in the body to such an extent that health may be adversely affected. One of the indices of body weight is the body mass index (BMI) which is the ratio of weight in kilograms to the square of height in meters. BMI is classified as: underweight- BMI <18.5 Kg/m^2 , Ideal weight -BMI 18.5-24.9 Kg/m^2, Overweight -BMI 25-29.9 Kg/m^2, Obesity -BMI 30-39.9 Kg/m^2, Morbid obesity -BMI $\geq$40 Kg/m^2. Therefore using BMI, obesity is defined as BMI greater than 30 kg/m^2. Obesity increases the risk for hypertension, risk for coronary artery disease and some cancers, and reduces life expectancy [66]. There is a high prevalence of overweight and obesity in many LMICs especially among urban women [7]. The mean BMI is significantly higher for women compared to men; the lower male prevalence may be explained by the heavy manual labor men more commonly engage in than women. Also the physiological changes related to pregnancy and childbirth may contribute, and in most cultures in Africa, full-bodied (over-weight and obese) women are preferred. The relationship between overweight or obesity and hypertension is complex [67]. Raised blood pressure is not an invariable consequence of obesity and some suggest that the probable influence of fat on blood pressure is attenuated in obese, hypertensive individuals [67, 68]. Albeit, widespread evidence suggests there is a relationship between obesity and hypertension [67].

9. Socio-Economic Status and Belief System

Blacks in the lower socio-economic class were almost three times as likely to be hypertensive as blacks in the higher status [69]. Low socio-economy is associated with less education. Poor education predisposes individuals to inability to read and understand prescriptions, leading to poor adherence to therapy, poor BP control and more complications [70]. In a recent study in hypertensive African Americans, Ogedegbe et al., noted that while 38% of their patients believed that hypertension can be cured therefore taking anti-hypertensive drugs for life was unnecessary, more than 20% thought that antihypertensive drugs should be taken only when symptomatic [71]. In another study, socio-economy was more strongly associated with hypertension in blacks than in whites. Some investigators have reported that socio-economic disadvantage, less access to best healthcare, etc. are important in causing and sustaining hypertension [72].

ii. Non-Modifiable Risk Factors

Age, race, ethnicity, and heredity have been identified as non-modifiable risk factors for hypertension. Though these factors are not modifiable, their presence helps identify those at greatest risk, enabling institution of strategies that can forestall those risk factors that can be modified. Results of the Framingham Heart Study showed that people who have normal blood pressure by age 55 years have a 90% lifetime risk for the development of hypertension [73]. Isolated systolic hypertension (ISH) has been shown to account for 60% to 70% of all hypertension in people above 60 years of age [74]. The authors of Joint National Committee 7 (JNC 7) recognized and appreciated these age related changes and therefore used them as basis for some of their recommendations [11].

Section II: Pathogenesis and Pathophysiology of Hypertension: Historical Paradigms and Modern Insights

There is yet incomplete understanding of the pathogenesis of hypertension. It is hoped that better understanding of hypertension will lead to more targeted therapies and to greater reduction in hypertension-related cardiovascular disease. This is very germane in hypertension in the black race. It is known that hypertension and its complications disproportionately affect blacks. The reason for this disproportionate affectation could be multifactorial and it is thought to include admix of genetic and environmental nuances.

Historically, blacks had very low prevalence of hypertension [10, 72]. This low prevalence still exists in black communities that have little or no influence of westernization [75]. However, in blacks who are influenced by western life style as typified by the African Americans, the prevalence of hypertension as compared with every other ethnic group in the

US is higher [76, 77]. Hypertension starts early, is more severe, and causes more target organ impairment in blacks.

This section will briefly discuss the pathogenic mechanisms of hypertension and will expatiate on the peculiar mechanisms related to pathogenesis of hypertension as regards blacks.

A. Pathogenic Mechanisms for Hypertension in the General Population

The factors implicated in the genesis of essential hypertension are varied and many. Hypertension is a complex trait arising from interactions of multiple genetic and environmental factors necessary for the regulation and maintenance of blood pressure [28, 78]. The genetic contribution is thought to range from 30% to 50% [79, 80]. There is also some speculation about epigenetic modifications in relation to insulin-like growth factor 2 (IGF2), genotype and blood pressure changes [28]. Essential hypertension has polygenic inheritance meaning that several genes are involved hence no individual gene can be identified as the causative gene. The genetic analysis of hypertension led to complex, unreliable and non-replicable results which made it problematic to draw inferences about the association between specific genes and hypertension [81]. But monogenic forms of hypertension such as Liddle's syndrome, syndrome of apparent mineralocorticoid excess, mineralocorticoid receptor activating mutation, glucocorticoid-remediable aldosteronism, and pseudohypoaldosteronism type II (caused by mutation in WNK kinase family) have simple Mendelian inheritance [78]. These monogenic forms affect common pathways, for example, salt regulation pathway in the kidney suggesting that the kidney may play a significant role in the pathophysiology of hypertension [78, 82]. The association between genetic variation and monogenic forms of hypertension offers great insight into the pathogenic pathway of essential hypertension [78].

The environmental factors known to play a role in development of hypertension include stress, overweight/obesity, a high sodium and low potassium diet, physically inactive/hypo-active, and exposure to toxins (lead, mercury, etc.), pathogens, radiation, and chemicals [83]. Figure 2 shows the determinants in the development of hypertension. Hypertension develops when the balance between the genetic and environmental factors and the modulating activity of the compensatory mechanisms is disrupted. The compensatory factors are defined as vasoactive elements that regulate blood pressure, the ability of the human physiology to regulate BP, and the processes involved in regulation [83, 84].

Other environmental factors such as related to racism (e.g. socioeconomic handicap, poor access to the best health care) play some large role in causation and sustaining raised blood pressure [72]. Africans living in Africa or the West Indies especially individuals living in rural areas have much less hypertension than African Americans [75]. Hypertension prevalence in the rural African communities is still very low and studies show that their blood pressure did not rise with age [75]. Section I of this chapter has discussed the influence of rapid urbanization and westernization on blood pressure pattern in communities in Africa.

The pathways involved in development of hypertension include: increased sympathetic nervous system activity, thought to be related to exaggerated response to psychosocial stress; prolonged high sodium-salt intake; excessive production of sodium-conserving hormones and vasoconstrictors; and inadequate dietary intake of ions like potassium and calcium [85].

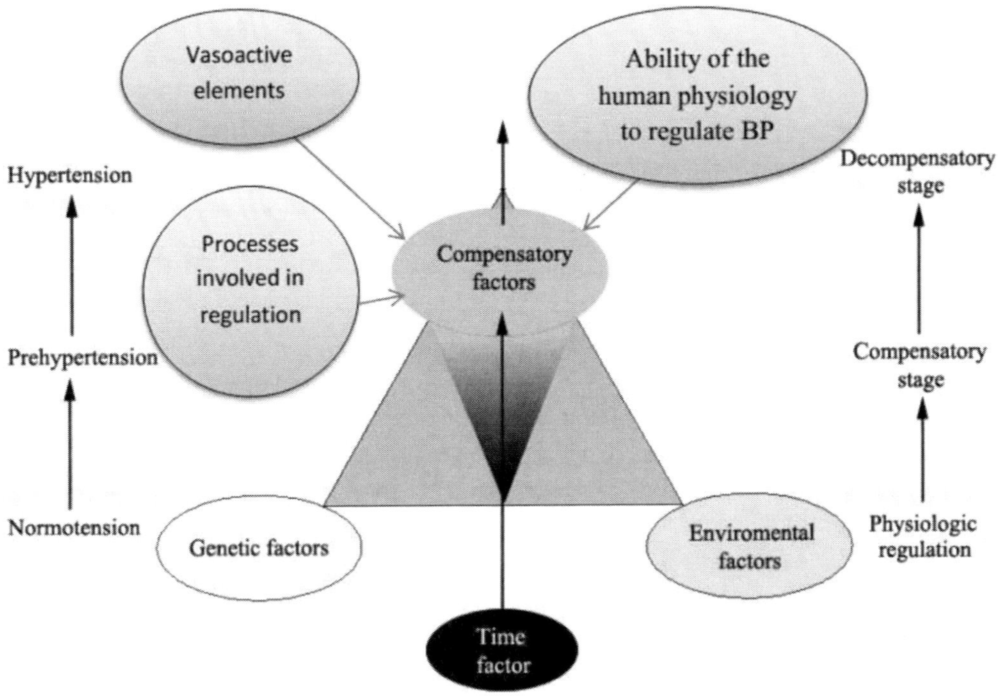

Figure 2. The development and regulation of blood pressure in patients with essential hypertension (modified from Wang and Peng [83]).

The other pathogenic mechanisms are related to imbalance of vasopressor and vasodilator hormones like increased or inappropriate renin secretion with increased release of angiotensin II and aldosterone; reduced vasodilators - such as prostacyclin, nitric oxide, and the natriuretic peptides. There are also changes in the kallikrein–kinin system expression which influences the vascular tone and renal salt handling, abnormalities of resistance vessels, and associated selective changes in the renal microvasculature. Diabetes mellitus, insulin resistance, obesity and elaboration of vascular growth factors have been connected to the pathogenesis of hypertension. Blood pressure is a product of cardiac output and peripheral resistance. Factors that affect the heart like the changes in adrenergic receptors that influence heart rate, inotrope and vascular tone as well as the altered cellular ion transport have been explored to explain hypertension. The more recent concepts are the structural and functional aberrations in the vasculature, including endothelial dysfunction, increased oxidative stress, vascular remodeling, and reduced compliance [85]. As hypothesized by Guyton [82], renal mechanisms may indeed play the primary role in the pathogenesis of hypertension while the other factors augment (sympathetic nervous system activity and vascular remodeling) or buffer (increased natriuretic peptide or kallikrein–kinin expression) the renal mechanisms.

B. Factors Implicated in the Pathogenesis of Hypertension in Blacks

Various mechanisms (genetic and environmental) have been put forward to explain the higher prevalence and severity of hypertension in blacks. Most of the data come from studies in African Americans. Some putative candidate genes such as those encoding constituents of epithelial sodium channels [86], the renin-angiotensin-aldosterone system (RAAS) [87, 88], the kallikrein-kinin system [89], endothelin and endothelin receptors [76], α- and β-adrenergic receptors [90], natriuretic peptides and their receptors [91], and the nitric oxide pathway [92] have been suggested. Although data is sparse, there is some evidence documented for attenuated β-adrenergic vasodilation in African Americans with normal blood pressure [93] and sodium channel sequence variants [86] which are acknowledged hypertension candidate genes. These evidences emanate from small studies.

i. Salt-Dependent Hypertension Hypothesis

It is postulated that Africans living around the Sahara Desert evolved extremely efficient renal re-absorptive mechanisms for sodium [94]. This trait helped them survive the scorch of the desert but exposed them to genetic susceptibility of hypertension when diet high in salt is consumed. More blacks than whites matched for age, gender and blood pressure are salt-sensitive (meaning they have an increase in blood pressure of 5–10 mm Hg over baseline after a brief salt loading) [95]. It is recognized generally that salt sensitivity is more predominant among hypertensive patients than normotensives suggesting that some of the salt sensitivity may well be consequent upon hypertension instead of being the cause [95]. So far, nine forms of hypertension and eight forms of hypotension inherited as Mendelian traits have been identified [76]. They are rare and denote the extremes of human blood pressure variation. Whether variations in sequencing of any of these genes can explain in part or wholly, pathogenesis of primary hypertension is yet to be elucidated.

Mendelian forms of hypertension have revolutionized our knowledge of blood pressure and volume regulation [96, 97]. All the known Mendelian forms of human hypertension are related somewhat to the RAAS [76, 96]. For example, the mutations in the mineralocorticoid receptor genes have opened up the area of mineralocorticoid-induced hypertension [96]. The findings have expounded how mutations may modify the receptors that were once antagonists assuming agonistic action. The epithelial sodium-channel (ENaC) has been explicated; gain-of-function mutations in the β and γ subunits of ENaC lead to Liddle's syndrome and loss-of-function mutations in all three subunits of ENaC on the other hand cause hypotension (pseudohypoaldosteronism type I). Hence, the subunits can mutate to cause hypertension or hypotension.

Usually, the action of aldosterone on the mineralocorticoid receptor stimulates the transcription factors that lead to activation of the ENaC which culminates in the reabsorption of the last 2% of the filtered load of sodium from the distal nephron [76]. Excessive ENaC activity leads to increased sodium reabsorption and expansion of the effective blood volume, resulting in salt-sensitive low-renin hypertension [76]. Such individuals respond to treatment with two classes of potassium sparing diuretics – ENaC antagonist, amiloride and mineralocorticoid receptor antagonist spironolactone. Some reports advocate that some resistant cases of primary hypertension could be obscure mutations of the ENaC i.e. gain-in-function mutations [76]. The ENaCs are construed to be the point to start the search for candidate genes for salt sensitivity as they play a central role in renal sodium handling [98]. While the α-subunit of ENaC is associated with sodium conductance, the β and γ subunits are associated with the structure and regulatory functions of the channel [99]. It is postulated that genes encoding this pathway may be responsible for the heterogeneity in the blood pressure responses to dietary sodium in humans [98].

Furthermore, several single nucleotide polymorphisms have been isolated in the β subunit of ENaC (SCNN1 β gene) - G589S, T594M, R597H, R624C, E632G, G442V, and V434M [76]. But one, T594M, the threonine to methionine mutation at position 594 is linked to hypertension. This variant has been found in 6.1% of African Americans but not in Caucasians (in a study of 231 African American vs 192 Caucasian subjects) [86]. Some controversy still exists about the relationship of this gene variant to hypertension. A study in the US found a frequency of 5%-6% of T594M variant documenting no difference between normotensive and hypertensive individuals [86]. Another study in the UK recorded a four-fold difference in frequency viz: hypertensive patients 8% vs normotensives 2% [100]. Hypertensive individuals with this variant were found to be sensitive to amiloride monotherapy. They were noted to have 17/8mmHg fall of their blood pressures from baseline [101]. These findings indicate that amiloride sensitive channels may account for the rate limiting step in sodium absorption in the distal tubules [86].

ii. Obesity-Related Hypertension

Obesity is well established as one of the key risk factors for incident hypertension in whites in the US [102]. However, obesity has come into focus as another major contributing factor to hypertension in African Americans. According to the Framingham Study, obesity accounts for more than 50% of hypertension [102]. Without a doubt, the interrelationship between obesity, hyperglycemia, insulin resistance, and hypertension is well recognized [103, 104]. Studies document that weight loss decreases blood pressure even without dietary salt restriction. For example, a meta-analysis by Neter et al. in 2003 [105] involving 25 RCTs and about 5,000 patients clearly showed that weight loss of -5.1 kg (95% confidence interval [CI], -6.03 to -4.25) significantly reduced both systolic -4.44 mm Hg (95% CI, -5.93 to -2.95) and diastolic -3.57 mm Hg (95% CI, -4.88 to -2.25) blood pressures. This strategy is important for the prevention and treatment of hypertension. The role of obesity in hypertension as explained by Landsberg (2001) is mediated by several factors including sympathetic nervous system, insulin and leptin [106]. Obesity clusters with insulin resistance, hyperlipidemia/dyslipidemia and hypertension exposing such individuals to high cardiovascular risk [107 108]. Coronary Artery Risk Development in Young Adults (CARDIA) study of young adult African-Americans and white men and women showed that obesity and fasting insulin levels correlated with blood pressure [109]. It is noteworthy that hypertension prevalence has been found to correlate with body mass index in multiple populations throughout the African diaspora [72].

The relationship between obesity and hypertension is interesting and complex. Excessive sympathetic drive seen in overweight persons is thought to be a compensatory mechanism to burn fat and reduce weight gain at the expense of raised sympathetic discharge culminating in hypertension [106, 110]. This hypothesis has been used to explain the mechanism involved in the young non-obese borderline hypertensive individual. The sympathetically-mediated thermogenic drive is strong enough to compensate for the increased caloric intake, hence enabling these young hypertensive persons to avoid obesity [106]. The original Framingham cohort observed that obesity predicted the development of hypertension and on the flip side, hypertension as well, predicted the eventual development of obesity [106]. The realistic interpretation of these data indicates that as subjects age, the efficiency of the thermogenic mechanisms wanes, obesity develops as a consequence, because the increased caloric intake is no longer effectively protected by the raised sympathetic nervous drive [106]. These hypotheses mentioned earlier were deduced from studies involving white cohorts [106 111]. The predominant opinion is that in African Americans neither obesity nor neurogenic factors contribute much to hypertension, which is attributed mainly to salt/volume-related mechanisms [76]. Nesbitt and Victor [76] further explored the relationship between adiposity and sympathetic nervous drive in African Americans and concluded that there was a major gender difference in the relationship between adiposity and sympathetic nerve activity in African Americans. Whilst hypertension and obesity are more prevalent in African-American women than white women, on the other hand, for men, the prevalence of hypertension is way higher in African-American men than white men of comparable levels of obesity [112]. Further studies using intra-neural microelectrodes to document sympathetic nervous activity in normotensive young African-American and white adults of similar age and BMI revealed that in African American women population, obesity caused sympathetic overdrive whereas in African American men, sympathetic activity was disassociated from adiposity. The implication is that sympathetic overdrive in young adults could explain the high incidence of obesity-related hypertension in African-American women and the unduly high incidence of hypertension in lean African-American men [76]. This is similar to the explanation given by Landsberg [106] for why some young adults do not develop obesity.

iii. Renin-Angiotensin-Aldosterone System

Some workers have documented low circulating renin levels in African-Americans [113]. Studies have also reported reduced efficacy of angiotensin-converting enzyme inhibitors and angiotensin receptor blockers as monotherapy in the black hypertensive patients as compared to whites [114, 115]. These findings probably prompted the popular notion that the RAAS is less active in blacks than in whites [114, 116]. However, this assumption is incorrect and cannot explain the black-white differences in hypertension. In the first instance, lower renin levels are expected to correlate with lower blood pressure levels and therefore less target organ damage in blacks. Paradoxically, blacks have higher complications from hypertension than whites. The explanation is that there is dissociation between tissue renin-angiotensin-system activity and circulating renin levels. This was also observed in the Dahl salt-sensitive rats fed on a high-salt diet which also had low plasma renin but elevated renal tissue RAS activity resulting in hypertension and early onset of renal damage [117]. In addition, increased vascular production of angiotensin II has been demonstrated even in association with low renin levels [114, 118]. Healthy normotensive blacks exhibit a greater activation of the RAAS than whites [119]. Studies reporting reduced efficacy of ACE inhibitors as monotherapy in black hypertensive subjects as compared to whites, is another reason for the assumption that the RAAS is less active in blacks than in whites. There is however, a significant overlap in the black-white responses to monotherapy with ACE inhibitors. For example, the reported average black-white difference is 4.6 mmHg but the standard deviation within each group is 12 to 14 mmHg [120]. Variation in response between blacks and whites is therefore much smaller than the variation observed within each group. In effect, the prominence of the RAS-dependent target organ damage such as albuminuria, kidney damage and left ventricular hypertrophy (LVH) in blacks shows that the role of the RAAS in the black hypertensive is most likely under-estimated and incompletely elucidated.

iv. Genetics

Genetic mutations in the non-muscle myosin heavy chain 9 (MYH9) genes on chromosome 22 are associated with kidney diseases such as hypertension-attributed end-stage kidney disease (H-ESKD) as well as other kidney disorders such as HIV-associated nephropathy and focal-segmental-glomerulosclerosis (FSGS) [121]. This genetic mutation is predominant in blacks and may contribute to the black-white differences in hypertension [122, 123]. Apolipoprotein L-1 (APOL1) gene is also found in the same region as MYH9 on chromosome 22. Mutations in APOL1 gene, especially the G1 and G2 variants are highly associated with H-ESKD and FSGS. The presence of this gene may account for the early onset of severity and rapid progression of hypertensive renal disease to end stage kidney disease [124]. These mutations are not found in whites while 10%-15% of blacks are carriers of both alleles and up to 50% carry at least one of the alleles [121]. However, studies in Africa have documented prevalence of 23% to 28% for APOL1 gene double allele [125, 126]. A molecular variant of angiotensinogen (AGT), M235T, found in 90% of blacks is associated with both higher circulating levels of AGT and hypertension [121]. Evidence points to the fact that blacks have more active phenotypes of Na, K, 2Cl co-transporter (NKCC2) resulting in higher sodium reabsorption in the thick ascending loop of Henle, volume expansion and salt-sensitive hypertension [121]. Epigenetics may also explain the black-white differences in hypertension. Rat models have shown that stress in early life can lead to DNA modification such as methylation resulting in phenotypes with higher vascular reactivity without affecting the DNA sequence. Such changes can be transmitted across generations [121].

v. Abnormal BP Diurnal Variation

Non-dipping nocturnal blood pressure pattern is found more in normotensive and hypertensive blacks [127]. This pattern is associated with obesity, salt sensitivity, high dietary salt intake and other factors that drive the high prevalence of hypertension in blacks [114].

vi. Abnormalities in Resistance Vessels

Vascular abnormalities such as higher intima-media thickness, increased stiffness of large central arteries and reduced response of small resistance vessels have been found in black hypertensive patients [114]. Some of these abnormalities occur through endothelin and endothelin-independent pathways [116]. Endothelin-1 (ET-1) levels are much higher in female and male hypertensive blacks than their white counterparts. ET-1 is a potent vasoconstrictor and may contribute to the difference in hypertension among blacks and whites [128]. Vascular stiffness is associated with target organ damage in hypertensive patients [114].

vii. Socioeconomic Considerations

The relationship between socioeconomic conditions and hypertension is complicated [129]. Generally, hypertension is more prevalent in low socioeconomic conditions because of the prevalence of low awareness of hypertension, poor access to health facilities, low birth weight and other factors [130]. An inverse relationship between socioeconomic status and hypertension was also seen in Tanzania [131]. Sometimes, the relationship is contradictory as in rural versus urban dwelling. Most of these socioeconomic conditions are modifiable and could be a focus for hypertension prevention programs. In some studies, despite similar socioeconomic status, blacks still had a greater prevalence of hypertension and lesser degree of blood pressure control than whites [132].

viii. Underweight Phenotype

Low birth weight (LBW) is associated with glucose intolerance and hypertension in later life [133]. A meta-analysis of 78 studies showed that low birth weight (< 2500 g) was associated with a greater risk of systolic hypertension in later life (OR 1.21, 95% CI) [134]. Low birth weight can result from maternal obesity, a risk factor for pre-pregnancy maternal hypertension, and pregnancy-induced hypertension. Hypertension in pregnancy predisposes the patient to preeclampsia and eclampsia and increases the chances of intra-uterine growth retardation as well as premature delivery. The babies from such pregnancies are likely to have low birth weight. Blacks in US have a higher incidence of LBW babies (12.9%) than the whites (8.5%) [135].

ix. Physical Inactivity

Regular physical exercise is important in maintaining optimal BP [48]. Results from the NHANES III survey (1988-1991) showed that physical inactivity was higher in Africa American men (24%) and women (40%) than their white counterparts (males 13% and females 23%) [136]. Physical inactivity is probably responsible for some of the disparities in the prevalence of hypertension between whites and blacks in America [137].

x. Obstructive Sleep Apnea (OSA)

OSA is increasingly being recognized as a risk factor for cardiovascular morbidity and mortality. It is associated with hypertension, cardiac failure, arrhythmias, pulmonary hypertension, coronary heart disease, strokes and traffic accidents [138]. Nocturnal hypoxia from OSA causes increased stimulation of the sympathetic nervous system, vascular inflammation and oxidative stress. Hypertension then results from the increased sympathetic tone. Blacks have a higher prevalence of OSA and greater apnea-hypopnea index (AHI) than whites and this may partly explain the higher prevalence of hypertension in blacks.

Section III: Antihypertensive Drugs and Efficacy in Black Patients

Ethnic variations in the incidence, pathophysiology and treatment of hypertension in the black patient are well documented [139 – 141]. The difference in racial/ethnic response to antihypertensive agents was suggested by the Veterans Affairs (VA) Cooperative Trial [142], which, indicated that whites of European ancestry had a better antihypertensive response to β blockers than blacks of African ancestry while blacks had a better response to diuretics than whites. Following the introduction of the first angiotensin-converting enzyme (ACE) inhibitor into clinical practice in the 1980s, it was noticed that whites responded more favourably to ACE inhibitors than black patients. Beta blockers, ACE inhibitors, and angiotensin receptor blockers (ARBs) are the most recognized agents with respect to racial differences in response.

These observed differences were supported by a meta-analysis, published in 2004 [143], which evaluated 15 clinical trials published between 1984 and 1998. The study documented efficacy of most antihypertensive drugs in black hypertensive patients. Many antihypertensive drugs lowered SBP and DBP, and reached DBP targets better than placebo in black hypertensive patients. There was no significant difference between β blockers and placebo in reducing SBP; similarly there was no significant difference between ACE inhibitors and placebo in reaching DBP targets. Consideration of race/ethnicity in selection of antihypertensive drugs was first recommended by The Fourth Report of the Joint National Committee (JNC-IV) on the Detection, Evaluation, and Treatment of High Blood Pressure [144], published in 1988. With time, ethnicity became a factor in deciding choice of antihypertensive drug treatment [145]. Generally, blacks are thought to respond more favourably to diuretics and calcium channel blockers, while whites tend to respond similarly to all the drug classes.

A. Antihypertensive Drugs and their Efficacy in Black Patients

Various classes of drugs exist to treat hypertension. The major first-line antihypertensive drug classes include thiazides diuretics, β blockers, calcium channel blockers (CCB), ACE inhibitors, α blockers, and ARBs.

i. Thiazide Diuretics

Thiazide diuretics and related drugs have been a major agent for the treatment of primary hypertension due to their efficacy and cost effectiveness. Hydrochlorothiazide, the most popular agent in this class, was used in high doses of 50 to 100 mg per day in the past and was associated with electrolyte and metabolic complications. Later, low-dose therapy came into common use as it is almost equally efficacious and is associated with fewer side effects. A meta-analysis by Psaty et al. [146] established that low-dose (12.5 - 25 mg/d chlorthalidone or hydrochlorothiazide) reduced blood pressure to the same degree as high dose diuretics (≥50 mg/d of same drugs), but more importantly they had similar protection against cardiovascular and total mortality and more beneficial effect on the incidence of coronary heart disease (CHD).

The mechanism of action of thiazides appears to be initial volume loss. The initial hypotensive response is mediated by a modest reduction in plasma volume and cardiac output [147]. Longer-acting diuretics maintain the reduction in intravascular volume more effectively than short-acting loop diuretics in patients. Thiazide diuretics are effective in lowering blood pressure, and reducing the end organ damage of hypertension. They were found to reduce morbidity and mortality from stroke, heart attack, and heart failure more than β blockers [148]. In a systematic review of 19 randomized controlled trials, thiazide diuretics reduced mortality (RR = 0.89; 95% confidence interval [CI], 0.83 to 0.96), stroke (RR = 0.63; 95% CI, 0.57 to 0.71), CHD (RR = 0.84; 95% CI, 0.75 to 0.95), and cardiovascular events (RR = 0.70; 95% CI, 0.66 to 0.76). In that review, low-dose thiazides (eight RCTs) reduced CHD (RR = 0.72; 95% CI, 0.61 to 0.84), but high-dose thiazides (11 RCTs) did not (RR = 1.01; 95% CI, 0.85 to 1.20) [149].

The ALLHAT study [150] established that diuretic based therapy was superior to CCB, ACE inhibitor and α blockers in preventing one or more major forms of CVD, including heart failure and stroke. In this study, chlorthalidone as compared with lisinopril-based treatment showed no inferiority for primary outcomes (CHD mortality and nonfatal myocardial infarction) and superiority for stroke and heart failure (HF) prevention. In contrast, another study, the Second Australian National Blood Pressure trial (ANBP2) [151] indicated a marginal superiority of enalapril versus hydrochlorothiazide-based treatment on primary end points (all CV mortality [first and recurrent] plus all-cause mortality) with no substantial difference for stroke and HF. This conflicting result may be explained on the bases that the ALLHAT study had a greater number of participants and a greater percentage of blacks.

The JNC-VII [11] recommendations derived from the appreciation that thiazide-type diuretics have been the basis of antihypertensive therapy in most outcome trials and that diuretics have been virtually prominent in preventing the CV complications of hypertension. Furthermore, diuretics can be useful in blood pressure control and also in enhancing the antihypertensive efficacy of multidrug regimens, in addition to its affordability over other antihypertensive agents.

ii. Beta Blockers

The antihypertensive action of β blockers is through attenuation of sympathetic effects on the heart with consequent reduction in cardiac output. Other mechanisms include an effect on vascular resistance, inhibition of renin release from the juxta-glomerular apparatus as well as central effect. Beta-blockers have been widely used in the treatment of hypertension for more than 30 years but they are generally less effective in the black hypertensive patient [152]. As a consequence, recent guidelines (National Institute for Health and Clinical Excellence [NICE] guidelines 2011 [153] and JNC 8 2014 [154]) do not recommend beta blockers as first line drugs for treatment of hypertension. Although β blockers reduce blood pressure compared with placebo, their antihypertensive effect is suboptimal compared with other antihypertensive agents [155].

iii. Calcium Channel Blockers

CCBs are highly effective antihypertensive agents in black patients [156, 157]. The CCBs have been shown to lower blood pressure and significantly reduce left ventricular mass in blacks [158].

CCBs were more effective than thiazides in lowering blood pressure as initial treatment in black subjects with hypertension in a South African study [159]. The vasoconstrictor effect of angiotensin-II is antagonised by CCBs [160] with consequent potentially beneficial effects on kidney disease progression [161]. This is especially important in black patients who have increased risk of hypertensive nephrosclerosis [162].

iv. Angiotensin Converting Enzyme Inhibitors

ACE inhibitors are effective in lowering systolic and diastolic pressures in patients with hypertension. Many RCTs including SOLVD (enalapril in heart failure) [163], and EUROPA (perindopril in stable coronary disease) [164] have also demonstrated efficacy of ACE inhibitors in reducing cardiovascular morbidity and mortality in patients with CVD. A recent meta-analysis, involving about 160,000 patients [165] showed that RAAS inhibitors as a class of antihypertensive drugs caused a 5% relative reduction in all-cause mortality in hypertensive patients when compared with other antihypertensive drugs. However, ACE inhibitors are less effective as antihypertensive agents when used alone in black patients [166] but this is overcome by the addition of a diuretic. Many studies have shown the beneficial effects of ACE inhibitors in diabetic nephropathy, especially with proteinuria [167]. The ACE inhibitors have thus become first-line anti-hypertensive agents in diabetic nephropathy, regardless of ethnicity.

v. Angiotensin Receptor Blockers

Angiotensin receptor blockers (ARBs) are now commonly used for treatment of hypertension. The efficacy of this class of drugs is similar to that of ACE inhibitors. One advantage of the ARBs is their favourable side effect profile and are thus indicated when ACE inhibitors are not suitable.

B. Review of Guidelines on Treatment of Hypertension with Reference to Black Patients

i. ISHIB Guidelines

An Update of the International Society on Hypertension in Blacks: Consensus Statement

The first International Society on Hypertension in Blacks (ISHIB) consensus statement on the management of High Blood Pressure in blacks was published in 2003 [168]. Since then additional information on hypertension in black patients have become available and has necessitated review of the consensus statement. The new statement released in 2010 [114] has recommended that in patients with elevated blood pressure without target organ damage, preclinical or overt cardiovascular disease, the target blood pressure should be <135/85 mm Hg. For those with target organ damage, preclinical cardiovascular disease, and/or a history of cardiovascular disease, target blood pressure should be <130/80 mm Hg. The statement further recommends that monotherapy with a diuretic or a CCB is preferred if blood pressure is ≤10 mm Hg above target levels. A two drug therapy is recommended with CCB or diuretic plus a RAAS blocker if blood pressure is >15/10 mm Hg above target.

ii. The Eighth Report of the Joint National Committee (JNC-VIII) on the Detection, Evaluation, and Treatment of High Blood Pressure 2014 [154]

Recommendation 7

In the general black population, including those with diabetes, initial antihypertensive treatment should include a thiazide-type diuretic or CCB. (*For general black population: Moderate Recommendation – Grade B; for black patients with diabetes: Weak Recommendation – Grade C).*

This recommendation was based on a subgroup analysis of data from a single large trial (ALLHAT) that was rated good (ALLHAT 2002) [150]. In that study, a thiazide-type diuretic was shown to be more effective in improving cerebrovascular, heart failure, and combined cardiovascular outcomes compared to an ACE inhibitor in the black patient subgroup. The subgroup included large numbers of diabetic and non-diabetic participants. Thus, the recommendation is to choose thiazide-type diuretics over ACE inhibitors for black patients. Although a CCB was less effective than a diuretic in preventing heart failure in the black subgroup of this trial, there were no differences in other outcomes (cerebrovascular, CHD, combined cardiovascular, and kidney outcomes, or overall mortality) between a CCB and a diuretic. Therefore, both thiazide-type diuretics and CCBs are recommended as first-line therapy for hypertension in black patients.

Recommendation 8

In the population aged 18 years or older with CKD and hypertension, initial (or add-on) antihypertensive treatment should include an ACE inhibitor or ARB to improve kidney outcomes. This applies to all CKD patients with hypertension regardless of race or diabetes status. *(Moderate Recommendation – Grade B).*

This recommendation applies to CKD patients with and without proteinuria, as studies using ACE inhibitors or ARBs showed evidence of improved kidney outcomes in both groups. It is also based on kidney outcomes as there is poor evidence favouring ACE inhibitor or ARB for cardiovascular outcomes in patients with CKD. Neither ACE inhibitors nor ARBs improved cardiovascular outcomes for CKD patients compared with a β blocker or CCB.

Recommendation 8 is specifically directed at those with kidney disease and hypertension and addresses the potential benefit of specific drugs on kidney outcomes. The AASK study showed the benefits of an ACE inhibitor on kidney outcomes in black patients with CKD and provides additional evidence that supports ACE inhibitor use in that population [169].

iii. 2013 European Society of Hypertension/European Society of Cardiology

(ESH/ESC) Guidelines for the Management of Arterial Hypertension

The current (2013) guidelines by ESH/ESC recommends that diuretics (including thiazides, chlorthalidone and indapamide), β blockers, CCBs, ACE inhibitors and ARBs are all suitable for the initiation and maintenance of antihypertensive treatment, either as monotherapy or in some combinations [170]. However, the guideline did not make any specific recommendation for the treatment of the black hypertensive patient.

C. Levels of Awareness, Treatment and Control of Hypertension in Africa

There is still a high prevalence of hypertension in many African countries. In a 2007 systematic review of population based studies on hypertension in sub-Saharan Africa from 1975 to 2006 by Addo et al. [19], the prevalence of hypertension varied between countries but was generally high. Less than 40% of patients were aware of their hypertension status, and less than 30% were on treatment. Of those on treatment, less than 20% achieved control. Table 1 details some of the studies on prevalence, awareness, treatment and control of hypertension in Africa including more recent surveys. This shows that the prevalence of hypertension varies in different parts of the continent, ranging from 9.8% in Burkina Faso [171] to 47.5% in Cameroon [172]. Hypertension is more prevalent in urban areas than in rural communities [75] and is also higher in the elderly and some special groups like market people who by nature of their work are sedentary, overweight/obese and take a lot of salt laden food from food vendors [173]. There are low levels of awareness of hypertension status across board in Africa, ranging from 7.0% in Algeria [174] to 49.5% in Senegal [175]. About half of patients are on treatment and target control is achieved in approximately a third of the patients. There is thus need for more effort at awareness and treatment of hypertension in Africa.

Table 1. Hypertension Awareness, Treatment and Control in Africa

Country	Location	Age range (yrs)	Sample size (%)	Prevalence (%)	Aware	Treated (%)	Control (%)
Burkina Faso Doulougou et al., 2014 [171]	Community based	Adult	1481	9.8	26.8	75.8	60.0
Ethiopia Tesfaye et al., 2009 [176]	Urban Population based	25-64	3713	31.5	35.2	11.0	28.0
Kenya Van de Vijver et al., 2013 [177]	Urban slums	>18	5190	12.3	19.5	47.0	21.0
Mozambique Damasceno et al., 2009 [178]	Rural and urban	25-64	3081	33.1	14.8	48.1	39.9
Uganda Musinguzi et al., 2013 [179]	Urban and Rural	>15	4563	27.2	28.2	51.6	9.3
Cameroon Dzudie et al., 2012 [172]	Community based	>15	2120	47.5	31.7	59.9	24.6
Algeria Temmar et al., 2007 [174]	Population based	>18	1346	44.0			25.0
Egypt Ibrahim MM, 1995 [180]	Nation wide survey	25-95	7951	36.3	37.5	23.9	8.0
South Africa Steyn K, 2008 [181]	Nation-wide survey	>15	13802	23.9	M 41 F 67	M 39 F 26	M 55 F 38
Nigeria Ulasi et al., 2011 [173]	Market community	>18	731	42.2	29.4		
Ekwunife et al., 2010 [182]			756	21.1	30.0	21.0	9.0
Senegal Duboz et al., 2014 [175]	Urban		600	27.5	27.88	16.97	5.45

Section IV: Management and Challenges of Management of Hypertension in Blacks

Management of hypertension including black patients involves non-pharmacologic and pharmacologic therapy.

A. Non-Pharmacologic Treatment of Hypertension in Black Patients

Non pharmacologic strategies are becoming increasingly important in management of hypertension and other CVDs [183]. Therefore, management of hypertension would be incomplete without non pharmacologic interventions like lifestyle modifications. These changes, in addition to controlling blood pressure, also, help lower cardiovascular risk. Regular exercises with optimal body weight, healthy and low-salt diet, and moderate alcohol consumption help control blood pressure. Albeit, life style modification on its own is insufficient to control hypertension in most cases, therefore pharmacological treatment must be instituted. Guidelines on management strategies for hypertension did not emphasize non-pharmacologic treatment until JNC 7 [11] recommended lifestyle modification for all patients with hypertension and also for prehypertension. The new JNC guidelines, JNC 8 [154] did not consider non-pharmacologic strategies in treatment of hypertension. The World Health Organization recognizes the importance of social behaviors on disease patterns. It reported NCDs (hypertension being the most common) as strongly associated and causally linked with four behaviors: tobacco use, physical inactivity, unhealthy diet and excessive use of alcohol [4, 6]. Though some lifestyle modifications seemingly have only minimal blood pressure–reducing effects, they should not be discountenanced. Even reductions in systolic blood pressure in the range of 5 mm Hg is associated with risk reduction in some observational studies. For example, reductions of 14% in mortality caused by stroke, 9% in mortality caused by heart disease, and 7% in all-cause mortality have been documented [184]. Furthermore, a weight reduction of 4.5 kg in overweight persons can reduce or prevent hypertension [185].

Studies in developing countries also show that non-pharmacologic methods are effective in reducing blood pressure in pre-hypertensive and hypertensive individuals [186, 187].

i. Recommended Lifestyle Modifications

1. The JNC 7 [11] states that implementation of healthy lifestyles by all persons is crucial for the prevention of hypertension hence it is indispensable in the management of patients with hypertension. This recommendation is based on evidence from Whelton et al. [188]. Data from Moore et al. [51] also emphasized the need for inclusion of lifestyle modifications as treatment strategies for hypertension. JNC 7 recommended essentially five lifestyle modifications for controlling blood pressure:

(1) reducing sodium intake,
(2) increasing exercise,
(3) moderating alcohol consumption,

(4) following the Dietary Approaches to Stop Hypertension (DASH) eating plan and losing weight.
(5) cessation of tobacco use

2. World Health Organization: stated in its report [49] that dietary and physical activity recommendations for populations and individuals should include strategies to:

- achieve energy balance and a healthy weight
- reduce energy intake from total fats and shift from consumption of saturated fats to unsaturated fats as well as removal of *trans*-fatty acids
- increase consumption of fruits and vegetables, and legumes, whole grains and nuts
- reduce the intake of free sugars
- eliminate harmful use of alcohol
- eliminate tobacco
- reduce salt (sodium) consumption from all sources and ensure that salt is iodized.
- reduce physical inactivity therefore individuals should engage in at least 30 minutes of regular, moderate-intensity physical activity three days per week.

ii. Lifestyle Modifications

Lifestyle modifications will be discussed under the following subheadings: modifications of diet, physical activity and social habits.

1. Dietary Modification

Modification in diets will include – salt/sodium reduction and increased potassium intake, reduction of fatty foods consumed and shift from saturated to unsaturated fats, and increased fruits and vegetable intake.

a. Salt: Sodium Reduction and Increased Potassium Intake

Some studies indicate that high salt intake is associated with an increased risk of high blood pressure (189) while others show that sodium reduction reduces blood pressure [190]. WHO has recommended salt intake of less than 5g/day [6]. The Trial of Non-pharmacologic Interventions in the Elderly (TONE) Study [191] used 80mmol/l per day of sodium and there was a 2.8 mmHg greater reduction in the blood pressure in the intervention group than the control group. In another study [190], patients were enrolled into three different levels of sodium intake viz: 150, 100, and 50 mmol/l/day signifying typical American diet, the upper limit of recommended intake, and a limited intake, respectively. The authors found graded blood pressure reduction which correlated with reduced sodium intake. The JNC 7 [11] and the World Health Organization/ International Society of Hypertension (WHO/ISH) [192] recommend that patients with hypertension should limit their daily sodium intake to approximately 2.4 g or salt of less than 5gm.

b. Modifications of Fat Intake

There is substantial evidence that the consumption of high levels of high-energy foods (processed foods high in fats and sugars) encourages obesity [6]. The Joint Food and Agriculture Organization (FAO)/WHO Expert Consultation (2008) recommended that maximum total fat intake for adults should be 30 – 35 energy percent (%E) [193]. The saturated fatty acids (SFA) should be replaced by polyunsaturated fatty acids and SFA in diet should not exceed 10%E. The recommended dose for poly-unsaturated fatty acid (PUFA) is 6 – 11%E and trans-fatty acid (TFA) of <1%E.

c. Increased Fruits/Vegetable Consumption

Fruit and vegetable consumption is an important component of healthy diet. Consumption of adequate amount of fruits and vegetables leads to lowering of blood pressure. Diets rich in fruits, vegetables, legumes, and whole grains, including fish, nuts, and low-fat dairy products have protective health effect. JNC 7 [11] advocates Dietary Approaches to Stop Hypertension (DASH) diet which is rich in fruits, vegetables, in addition to low fat dairy products with a reduced content of dietary cholesterol, SFA and total fat.

d. DASH Eating Plan

Moore et al. (2001) [51] reported that the use of DASH diet significantly lowered systolic blood pressure compared with the control diet (-11.2 mm Hg; 95% CI, - 6.1 to - 16.2 mm Hg; *P*,0.001) and the fruits/vegetables diet (-8.0 mm Hg; 95% CI, -2.5 to -13.4 mm Hg; *P*,0.01) in patients with stage 1 systolic hypertension. Generally, blood pressure in the DASH group fell from 146/85 to 134/82 mm Hg. Whilst 78% of the DASH diet group (18 of 23 participants) had their systolic blood pressure below 140 mm Hg, in the control and fruit/vegetable groups 24% and 50% respectively had their systolic blood pressure below 140mmHg. The DASH eating plan was associated with mean reductions of 11 mm Hg in systolic blood pressure and 6 mm Hg in diastolic blood pressure. When combined with other life style modification modalities the blood pressure reduction is even more pronounced.

2. Physical Activity

Based on available evidence regarding decrease in blood pressure with aerobic physical exercise, the JNC 7 advocated that for those who are able, exercising regularly (e.g. brisk walking) for at least 30 minutes per day for most days of the week should be encouraged [194, 195]. Kelley and Kelley (2000) [194] demonstrated from cumulative meta-analysis ranked by year, that following exercise, fall in blood pressure ranged from -2 to -4 mm Hg systolic and -3 to -4 mm Hg for diastolic blood pressure. Their results suggest that progressive resistance exercise give small reductions in resting systolic and diastolic blood pressure. Such reductions have been shown to reduce risks for stroke and coronary heart disease [196]. In another meta-analysis, Whelton et al. (2002) [195] found that aerobic exercise was associated with a significant reduction in mean systolic and diastolic blood pressure (-3.84 mm Hg [95% CI, -4.97 to -2.72 mm Hg] and -2.58 mm Hg [CI, -3.35 to -1.81 mm Hg], respectively). The reduction in blood pressure associated with aerobic exercise was seen in hypertensive, normotensive, overweight and normal-weight participants.

3. Social Habits

Social habits like use of tobacco and excessive consumption of alcohol are associated with raised blood pressure.

a. Cessation of Tobacco Use

Minami et al. (1999) [197] investigated the effect of smoking cessation on ambulatory blood pressure, heart rate, and heart rate variability in habitual smokers. The 24-hour ambulatory blood pressure was significantly lower in the nonsmoking period than in the smoking period, by 3.5±1.1 mm Hg systole (P= 0.01) and by 1.9±0.7 mm Hg diastole (P =0.05), though the nighttime blood pressure did not differ between the two periods. The 24-hour heart rate, plasma levels of epinephrine and norepinephrine were significantly lower in the nonsmoking period than in the smoking period.

b. Alcohol Intake in Moderation

Alcohol intake has a semi-parabolic (J-shape) relationship with all blood pressure measurement parameters [44]. The investigators also noted that alcohol consumption of 1–2 wine glasses/day was associated with 13% (95% CI 2–25%) lesser likelihood of having hypertension, irrespective of other characteristics of subjects or type of alcohol taken. Alcohol intake should be restricted to no more than 1 oz (30 mL) of ethanol (equivalent of two drinks) per day in men and no more than 0.5 oz of ethanol (one drink) per day in women.

c. Behavioural Therapies in Treatment of Hypertension

There are different levels of evidence showing that the behavioral therapies may lower blood pressure. Recently, the American Heart Association [198] issued a scientific statement summarizing available data on the blood pressure–lowering efficacy of the various alternative approaches and providing a class of recommendations for their use in clinical practice. The behavioral therapies were: transcendental meditation and other meditation techniques, yoga and other relaxation therapies and biofeedback approaches, device-guided breathing, acupuncture, exercise-based regimens such as aerobics, dynamic resistance and isometric handgrip modalities. Schneider et al. [199], in an RCT in African Americans demonstrated that transcendental meditation reduced SBP by 10.7 mm Hg and DBP by 6.4 mm Hg much more than progressive muscle relaxation which lowered SBP by 4.7 mm Hg and DBP by 3.3 mm Hg. Another study [200], suggested that transcendental meditation may even reduce mortality in patients with hypertension.

iii. What the Guidelines Say about Lifestyle Modifications

Most guidelines: WHO/ISH, National Institute for Health and Clinical Excellence (NICE), British Hypertension Society (BHS), World Health Organization, European Society of Cardiology, American Society of Hypertension (ASH), the American Heart Association (AHA), and the American Medical Association (AMA) recommend the use of non-pharmacologic strategies in addition to pharmacologic interventions in management of hypertension. There are some minor differences between the guidelines but most advocate regular aerobic exercise, reduction of salt and alcohol, low-calorie diets and cessation of smoking. While NICE promotes 'healthy, low-calorie diets' for 'overweight individuals with raised blood pressure, other guidelines BHS, WHO, ESC, ASH, AHA and AMA recognize the wealth of quality clinical trials that clearly show that diet and behavioral interventions have significant beneficial effect on hypertension, which is not limited to overweight persons [201].

B. Pharmacologic Treatment of Hypertension in Black Patients

i. Medications to Treat High Blood Pressure

The following major drug classes are available for treatment of hypertension: thiazide diuretics, β blockers, CCBs, ACE inhibitors, ARBs and renin inhibitors. However, recent guidelines recognize thiazides, CCBs, ACE inhibitors and ARBs as first line antihypertensive drugs. Other drug classes include β blockers, alpha-beta blockers, central-acting agents, vasodilators and aldosterone antagonists.

ii. Choice of Antihypertensive Drugs in Black Patients

The choice of antihypertensive drugs in black patients is influenced by the presence or otherwise of comorbid conditions. Current guideline from ISHIB [114] for the treatment of hypertension in black patients recommends monotherapy with a diuretic or CCB if blood pressure is less than 10 mmHg above target levels. It also recommends combination drug therapy with two drugs; CCB plus an ACE inhibitor or ARB if the blood pressure is greater than 15/10 mmHg above target level. In an oedematous or volume overloaded patient, it recommends a thiazide plus a RAAS blocker.

The JNC 8 [154] makes specific recommendation for the drug treatment of the black hypertensive patient. It recommends that for these patients, initial antihypertensive treatment should include a thiazide-type diuretic or a CCB. However, a recent trial proved the benefit of newer vs older antihypertensive drugs in terms of blood pressure control, reduction of cardiovascular morbidity and mortality, and metabolic side effects. It also indicated that the majority of hypertensive patients require multiple drugs to achieve control. The study [202] involved comparison of newer (amlodipine/valsartan 5/160mg) versus older (bisoprolol/hydrochlorothiazide 5/6.25mg) drug combinations, the newer drug combination lowered systolic blood pressure more (about 5 mmHg) compared with older drugs and therefore controlled hypertension better in native African black patients.

To summarise, the choice of therapy in black hypertensive patients is influenced by the presence or absence of comorbid conditions as well as the efficacy of the drug employed to attain target blood pressure. The optimal treatment of hypertension in black patients continues to evolve, especially with the introduction of new drugs and the need for prognostic data in this ethnic population. Low-dose thiazide diuretics and CCBs are effective and inexpensive first-line drugs in black hypertensive patients. Recent studies have established the efficacy of ACE inhibitors, and ARBs in BP control in black patients as combination therapy and thus are alternative first line drugs in treatment of hypertension in the black patient. The ISHIB in 2010 [114] recommended antihypertensive therapy for blacks without target-organ damage or concomitant cardiovascular diseases at blood pressures greater than 135/85 mmHg, and for those at higher risk, at blood pressures greater than 130/80 mmHg. It also de-emphasized monotherapy in favour of combination therapy. On the other hand, some other authorities, including various expert panels, did not recommend initiating antihypertensive therapy at lower blood pressure goals in black patients than in other patient groups [203].

It is reasonable to recommend that black patients with hypertension should be treated with a thiazide diuretic, a CCB, or ACE inhibitor as first line drug and a combination of these in severe hypertension or when monotherapy is unable to achieve control. Many patients will require more than one agent to achieve target BP.

C. Challenges of Management in the Hypertensive Black Patient

Despite tremendous advances in the management of hypertension, especially the availability of effective drugs, hypertension remains a major public health problem. Prevalence rates are still high while control rates are low in many parts of the world. In the developing countries, prevalence rates are even increasing [19, 204, 205], mainly driven by the effects of urbanization and associated lifestyle changes especially unhealthy diet and reduced physical activity. Challenges in the management of the hypertensive black patients could be patient-related or healthcare facility or provider related. These challenges include:

i. Access to healthcare
ii. Patient adherence
iii. Paucity of health education/ Health literacy
iv. Lifestyle factors
v. Challenges in the interpretation of BP values
vi. Clinical inertia and inadequate BP measurement
vii. Race-Concordant Patient-Doctor Relationship

i. Access to Healthcare

Blacks in Africa and diaspora have less access to quality healthcare than whites [206]. Lack of antihypertensive drugs in health centers and long distance to a health facilities also make it difficult for some people to access health care [173, 207]. Causes of disparity to access to healthcare include:

Cost of care - Management of hypertension is costly in terms of investigation and long-term drug treatment. Individuals in lower socioeconomic status are less likely to achieve good BP control due to cost of care [206, 208].

Lack of financial resources- Lack of financial resource is a barrier to healthcare for many blacks especially those in poor resource setting and where there is no welfare scheme to help the less privileged. In most countries in sub-Saharan Africa and some countries in Asia, patients pay out of pocket [209, 210]. In the US, access to healthcare is reduced among minority populations such as the black population [72].

Lack of health insurance - Many LMICs have fledgling health insurance schemes and even in countries where there is health insurance, many minorities including blacks do not have access to insurance [211]. In the US, racial and ethnic minorities are often given a health insurance plan that restricts the number and amount of services available to them as well as the number of providers they can use.

Other factors include - distance from healthcare facilities, poor transportation system and language barrier.

ii. Patient Adherence

Adherence refers to the extent a patient's behavior coincides with the medical advice in terms of medications, clinic visits and lifestyle modifications [212]. Non-adherence leads to poor BP control and contributes to the high prevalence of hypertension and its complications. Practically, adherence to medications is defined as taking the medications correctly 80% of the time. Measurement of adherence is difficult. Assay of drug levels in body fluids such as blood, saliva or urine is expensive and often impracticable. Self-reporting by patients and counting of drugs during follow-up visits are alternative methods but are subjective. Some patients may not even procure the prescribed medications at all. Patients may forget to take the prescribed medications, or take them at the wrong time, or take lower dosages than recommended. Therefore, non-adherence takes various forms. Adherence is influenced by health literacy [213] and health seeking behavior [214]. Some people in LMICs still believe in and access unorthodox healthcare. They consult traditional healers and spiritual healing homes, often times in consonance with orthodox healthcare services. Additionally, certain belief systems can impede management of hypertension. Such beliefs among blacks reported by Ogedegbe et al. [215] included that anti-hypertensive medication should be taken only when one is symptomatic while others believed that lifelong anti-hypertensive therapy was not necessary and for others, their belief was that hypertension was curable. Health education is needed to overcome such belief systems.

Multidisciplinary approach involving the doctor as well as the patient and the relatives improve adherence. This approach also reduces clinical inertia. Home BP monitoring, cheaper medications, simpler dosage schedules and frequent clinic visit improve patient adherence. Reasons for non-adherence vary from patient to patient and do not necessarily depend on age or availability of health insurance, level of education, information about hypertension, gender or socioeconomic status. The presence of unhealthy habits such as sedentary lifestyle and excessive alcohol and tobacco use predict non-adherence.

iii. Paucity of Health Education/Health Literacy

Studies have demonstrated the benefit of knowledge about hypertension in the adherence to treatment and reduction of complications [216]. The objective is to encourage patients to participate actively in the decisions regarding hypertension management. Two models for health education have been proposed [217]: the Chronic Care Model with the patient as the main collaborator in the decision-making and the Ecological Model in which the patient is at the center but the decision-making process involves the family members and the larger society. Generally, the success of any educational program must take into consideration the patient's cultural background and socioeconomic conditions. In addition, appropriate health policy by the government is indispensable [218].

iv. Lifestyle Factors

Many unhealthy lifestyle factors contribute to the high prevalence of hypertension, especially among African Americans and in the LMICs. Such factors include obesity, high salt intake, excessive alcohol consumption, smoking and sedentary lifestyle [114]. Therapeutic lifestyle changes (TLC) are important in the prevention and long-term management of hypertension [217]._Factors that pose a challenge to the implementation of healthy lifestyle are mainly patient related factors (unfamiliar nutritional requirements and methods of cooking, diet different from that of the rest of the family and cultural values). Challenges related to the health provider include lack of knowledge of current therapeutic guidelines and therapeutic inertia. Some challenges may be from the patient's environment such as transportation problems, lack of safe environment for physical exercise, cost of care and lack of health insurance. Multiple concomitant interventions such as cessation of smoking, complicated diet regimen (for multiple risk factors) as well as physical exercise may be a barrier to effective therapeutic lifestyle changes. Other medical conditions such as arthritis may limit physical exercise [217].

v. Challenges in the Interpretation of Blood Pressure Values

The measured blood pressure is an inherently variable hemodynamic phenomenon. Each heart beat produces a different BP. Additionally, certain factors such as age and hypertension reset the baroreceptors and leads to higher BP variability. As a result, the value of office BP alone in the diagnosis of hypertension has been challenged since the availability of 24-hour BP monitoring [219] which identified certain patterns of BP variability that affect the diagnosis of hypertension. For example, white coat hypertension describes a condition where the office BP is high while the home BP is not elevated. This is not benign and patients with this condition need to be identified and treated. On the other hand, masked hypertension represents a situation where the office BP is normal while the home BP is elevated. This is not a benign condition and patients with this condition need to be identified and treated. The implication is that if one wants to identify the 'real' BP of the patient, 24-hour ambulatory BP monitoring, or at least, home BP monitoring is needed. This poses a challenge in the diagnosis and management of hypertension.

vi. Clinical Inertia and Inadequate Blood Pressure Measurement

Clinical inertia among physicians is an important challenge in achieving target BP goals. It is defined as a condition in which clinicians fail to initiate or intensify treatment when the goals of treatment have not been met [220]. Inadequate knowledge of the therapeutic guidelines may be one of the reasons for clinical inertia. This is one area of intervention that can improve BP control. Some clinicians do not repeat BP measurements especially when the first reading is normal. This practice is inadequate in view of the phenomenon of BP variability. Unduly long follow-up appointments for borderline BP may also delay treatment and constitute a challenge to adequate BP control.

vii. Race-Concordance

Additionally, race-concordance in doctor-patient relationships appears to lead to better patient satisfaction, especially for blacks in diaspora [114]. This may not be applicable to blacks in Africa where black patients prefer white doctors (personal experience).

D. Economics of Hypertension in Blacks

Untreated hypertension imposes enormous burden on the population in terms of the direct and indirect cost of treating the complications such as stroke, heart failure, kidney diseases and ischemic heart disease. Direct cost includes the cost of medications and investigations. Indirect cost includes the cost of hospital visits and the man hours lost during such visits. Anti-hypertensive therapy for the primary and secondary prevention of these conditions is cost-effective [221, 222]. In the US, the cost of primary treatment of hypertension ranges from $10, 000 per quality adjusted life years (QALY) to $100,000.00 per QALY depending on the type of medications used [221]. A study in rural Nigeria showed that the mean monthly cost of antihypertensive medication was \$9.6 ± 3.7. In the study, up to 52.8% of the families studied spent more than 10% of their monthly income on antihypertensive medications [208].

A number of strategies are available to improve the cost-effectiveness of antihypertensive therapy [223]. Lifestyle modification before initiating antihypertensive therapy may identify patients who may not need drug therapy. One should prescribe drugs that are cheaper but effective especially in resource-poor settings. Combination drugs should include those with complementary rather than similar modes of action to improve efficacy. The goal of therapy is to prevent complications of hypertension which are costly to manage. Adherence to therapy should be emphasized to improve outcomes and reduce cost. Cost effectiveness is higher in patients with higher risk. Therefore risk stratification is important in selecting those who will benefit from intensive therapy. Treating patients with white coat hypertension is not cost-effective and home BP monitoring or ambulatory BP monitoring should be used to identify such patients where necessary.

Renin-guided selection of antihypertensive medication has been found to improve cost effectiveness [224]. This is based on the premise that long-term BP elevation involves either volume expansion (associated with low renin levels), or vasoconstriction (with high renin levels). Estimation of plasma renin activity (PRA) level will guide therapy: diuretics are preferred in low renin states and RAAS inhibitors in the high renin states. It is expensive giving antihypertensive medications to all individuals with hypertension. Guidance is needed in selecting the most cost-effective therapy.

Section V: Complications of Hypertension and Drug Therapy in Blacks

Complications of hypertension include those due to the disease per se and those emanating from the drug therapy. Severe or prolonged hypertension causes target organ damage involving primarily the cardiovascular, nervous and genito-urinary systems. Complications of hypertension occur more frequently in the black patient and it is associated with a higher incidence/prevalence of cerebrovascular and renal complications [225]. Stroke from hypertension is commoner in the black hypertensive patient [226]. End-stage kidney disease occurs 20 times more frequently in black patients than non-black [227]. Similarly, black hypertensive patients develop left ventricular hypertrophy more commonly than non-blacks. For example, black patients with mild hypertension where found to have a two-fold higher prevalence of LVH compared to non-black patients with comparable blood pressure levels [228]. However, studies show that on the contrary, the overall risk for CHD in black male population is lower than in white males [229] and Indo-Asians [230]. One of the reasons adduced for the favorable statistics for black male patients in this area, is that black males tend to have higher high-density-lipoprotein (HDL) cholesterol levels and lower plasma triglycerides [229].

Functional and anatomic vascular abnormalities in hypertension are commoner in blacks [231, 232]. This population has more micro and macro-vascular structural and functional abnormalities than whites even when normotensive. Greater intima/media thickening of large resistance vessels such as the carotid artery has been observed. Functional abnormalities seen more in blacks include greater stiffness of large central arteries, impaired endothelium-dependent and endothelium-independent vascular functions such as reduced capacity of resistance vessels to dilate on exposure to vaso-dilatory stimuli [233, 234]. These abnormalities have been associated with greater pressure-related target organ damage [235]. Therefore, even with mild hypertension, blacks have more vascular damage than whites and this may be related to increased micro-particles from tumor necrosis factor α and interleukin-6 [236] Generalized arteriolosclerosis and acceleration of atherogenesis have been observed in hypertensive patients. Arteriolosclerosis is characterized by media hypertrophy, hyperplasia plus hyalinization which are particularly apparent in small arterioles in the eyes and kidneys [237]. These changes result in narrowing of arteriolar lumen causing more hypertension and a vicious cycle sets in, culminating in target organ damage [238].

A. Complications from the Disease

Hypertension affects target organs in some systems of the body and they include: cardiovascular system (heart and vessels), the nervous system (brain and eyes) and genito-urinary system (kidneys).

1. Cardiovascular Complications.

The cardiovascular complications of hypertension include effect on the heart (left ventricular hypertrophy, heart failure, coronary heart disease and arrhythmias) and peripheral vascular diseases (ischemia and gangrene). Currently the leading causes of hospital admissions and in-hospital mortality in sub-Saharan Africa are cardiovascular and infectious diseases [239]. Hypertension-related admissions account for 23.7% - 30.9% of hospital admissions in Nigeria [240, 241]. African American hypertensive patients have a higher risk of cardiovascular complications such as heart disease death (1.5-fold) and heart failure (1.7-fold) than whites [242]. Hypertension is the commonest risk factor for heart failure in Nigeria [204].

i. Cardiac Complications

Coronary heart disease in Africans is more commonly associated with hypertension (53%) followed by diabetes (41%), smoking (39%) and elevated cholesterol (29%) [243]. It is also the most important risk factor for cardiac events in black physicians while in white physicians, smoking, dyslipidemia and a family history of coronary heart disease predominate [244]. Left ventricular hypertrophy (LVH) is more prevalent in African American hypertensive subjects compared to whites [245]. In Nigeria, echocardiographically-determined LVH was found in 30% – 60% of hypertensive subjects [246]. Systolic BP was a stronger correlate of LVH in the CARDIA study than the diastolic BP [247]. A study in Nigeria found that the diastolic BP was an independent predictor of LVH [248]. Atrial and ventricular arrhythmias are under-appreciated as complications of hypertension [204]. Anisiuba et al. studied the ECG of 860 Nigerians seen at the University of Nigeria Teaching Hospital, Ituku/Ozalla and found that 10 out of the 30 of patients (33.3%) who had atrial fibrillation, had hypertension.[249]. Other workers [250] also agree that hypertension is the most important cause of atrial fibrillation. These cardiovascular complications of hypertension contribute in no small measure to the excess mortality from cardiovascular disease seen in blacks. Gillum [251] in a study in 1976 described the death rates from cardiovascular disease in African Americans as probably the highest in the world.

ii. Peripheral Vascular Complications

Hypertension is a common and important risk factor for all vascular disorders, Peripheral vascular disease (PVD) inclusive [252, 253]. At presentation about 2% - 5% of the hypertensive patients have intermittent claudication. On the other hand, 35% – 55% of patients presenting with PVD have hypertension [254, 255]. Hypertension is implicated in the pathogenesis of atherosclerosis which is the pathological basis for PVD.

2. Nervous System – Brain and Eyes

Neurological complications of hypertension may be acute or chronic. Acute complications include hypertensive encephalopathy and subarachnoid hemorrhage. Chronic complications include transient ischemic attack, ischemic stroke, hemorrhagic stroke, cognitive decline and dementia. Hypertension also affects the eyes giving some lesions in the retina, optic nerve and choroid.

i. Effects on the Brain

a. Ischemic Stroke

Hypertension is a major risk factor for ischaemic stroke, accounting for more than half of stroke patients [256]. Although the prevalence of hypertension increases with age, the risk of ischemic stroke from hypertension actually reduces with advancing age [257]. Transient ischaemic attack and ischaemic stroke classically present with acute onset of focal neurological features which differ according to affected brain region. The usual presentation is monoparesis or hemiparesis. Other features include visual impairment, visual field deficits, double vision, aphasia, ataxia, dysarthria, vertigo, seizure, or sudden deterioration in level of consciousness. Stroke is associated with raised blood pressure which frequently normalizes within two weeks of the event. The clinical features also vary depending on the mechanism of stroke.

b. Intracerebral Haemorrhage.

Stroke from intracerebral haemorrhage accounts for 10%-30% of all cases of stroke and is the next most common type of stroke after ischaemic stroke. Hypertension is a major risk factor for haemorrhagic stroke [258] and it is associated with a four-fold increase in risk of haemorrhagic stroke. Relatively young people (<55 years of age), cigarette smokers and patients not adhering to antihypertensive medications are particularly susceptible to haemorrhagic stroke [259, 260]. Intracerebral haemorrhage usually presents with headache, nausea, vomiting, impaired consciousness and sometimes seizures. The blood pressure is often elevated. The site of the haemorrhage determines the specific symptoms and signs.

c. Subarachnoid Haemorrhage (SAH)

Subarachnoid hemorrhage is a fairly common condition with an incidence of about 10 per 100,000 yearly. The condition is associated with high morbidity and mortality. Rupture of intracranial aneurysm accounts for most of the cases. Although some connective tissue disorders, including Ehlers-Danlos syndrome and Marfan syndrome are associated with intracranial aneurysms, some cases are known to occur de novo. Other risk factors for intracranial aneurysms include hypertension and cigarette smoking [261]. A community based study of 27,161 individuals by Isaksen et al. in 2002, showed that cigarette smoking and hypertension are significant independent risk factors for aneurysmal SAH [262]. The usual presentation of subarachnoid hemorrhage is sudden onset of a severe headache which typically peaks within minutes and may last for over one hour [263]. Patients may have impaired consciousness, nausea, vomiting, meningism, and focal neurologic deficits.

d. Hypertensive Encephalopathy

This is a form of posterior reversible encephalopathy syndrome that is due to accelerated hypertension. It is associated with cerebral edema in the subcortical white matter, especially in the occipital and parietal lobes. The condition presents with headache, nausea, vomiting, visual disturbances, anxiety, agitation, impaired consciousness, and seizures. The changes are reversible with treatment but may result in some irreversible damage, such as infarction or haemorrhage.

e. Cognitive Decline and Dementia

The relationship between blood pressure and dementia was noted by Skoog and colleagues [264]. In this study, people aged 70 -85 years were stratified according to age group and followed for 15 years. The investigators found that the risk of dementia was associated with increased blood pressure. Treatment of hypertension was associated with a reduced risk for dementia and cognitive decline in another study [265]. In a study of elderly people in Nigeria followed for 6 years by Ogunniyi et al. in 2011, dementia was more prevalent in the hypertensive patients than non-hypertensive patients [266].

f. Vascular Dementia and Alzheimer Disease

Alzheimer disease is a neurodegenerative dementia with neuritic plaques and neurofibrillary tangles in the brain. It is the most common type of dementia and it is followed by vascular dementia. Vascular dementia on the other hand, is impairment in cognitive function resulting from lesions in the cerebral or cardiac blood vessels. In Europe and North America [267], Alzheimer disease is two times more common than vascular dementia while in Japan and China [268], vascular dementia accounted for about 50 % of all dementias. A study in America by Miles et al. [269] noted that vascular dementia is more prevalent in African America than in Caucasians.

ii. Effects of Hypertension in the Eyes

Hypertension affects the retina, optic nerve head and choroidal circulation causing 3 separate and independent manifestations: hypertensive retinopathy, hypertensive optic neuropathy and hypertensive choroidopathy [270].

a. Hypertensive Retinopathy

Hypertensive retinopathy is classified using the Keith Wagener Barker classification viz.: 0 – no changes, 1 – mild generalized arteriolar narrowing, 2 – focal narrowing and arteriovenous nipping, 3 - features in 1 & 2 plus retinal hemorrhages, exudates and cotton wool spots, 4 – severe grade 3 and papilloedema.

Hypertensive retinopathy includes two disease processes. Autoregulatory mechanisms are responsible for the vasospasms that occur in the retina in response to hypertension [270]. The chronic effects are caused by arteriosclerosis [270] and it predisposes patients to visual loss following vascular occlusions or macroaneurysms which may occur. Usually, arterioles develop vasoconstriction to reduced blood flow because of the elevated luminal pressure. The increased pressure causes endothelial damage. There is degeneration of the arteriolar smooth muscle which causes stretching of the endothelium with affectation of integrity of the wall resulting in leakage of plasma into the vessel wall. Eventually, clotting of plasma within the vessel wall produces mural thickening and luminal narrowing a process termed fibrinoid necrosis [271].

Retinal hemorrhages result when necrotic vessels bleed into the nerve fiber layer (flame shaped hemorrhage) or into the inner retina (dot blot hemorrhage). Cotton wool spots are caused by ischemia to the nerve fiber layer following fibrinoid necrosis and luminal contraction. Persistent ischemia to the nerve fibers eventuates in reduced axoplasmic flow, nerve swelling, and fluffy opacification. Exudates then follow late in the course of disease due to lipid accumulation. Papilledema occurs because of the leakage and ischemia of arterioles supplying the optic disc which have fibrinoid necrosis. Ischemia leads to optic nerve swelling and blurred disc margins and the leakage leads to hemorrhages and disc edema [271].

b. Hypertensive Optic Neuropathy

This is papilloedema or bilateral disc swelling which represents grade IV hypertensive retinopathy in the Keith-Wagener-Barker classification. Papilloedema is thought to be a poor prognostic sign. The pathogenesis of papilloedema from systemic hypertension is controversial and several theories have been postulated. It is thought to be due to ischaemia, raised intracranial pressure, or could occur as part of hypertensive retinopathy or encephalopathy. But certain studies have documented ischaemia to be the possible underlying mechanism [272, 273].

c. Hypertensive Choroidopathy

The choroidal lesions occur as consequence of raised blood pressure and are not as well recognized as those due to retinopathy in current literature. The underlying mechanism is thought to be choroidal ischemia and its subsequent effects on the retina and pigment epithelium [274].

3. Genitourinary System – Kidney

Hypertension ranks in the first three commonest causes of chronic kidney disease in most countries. Both benign and malignant forms of hypertension have adverse effects on the kidney. The risk of renal complication is thought to be more related to systolic than to diastolic blood pressure [275]. Ethnicity and gender are also known to influence the risk of renal complication in hypertension. Black men are at greater risk of developing kidney complications than white men at every level of blood pressure [276].

In benign hypertension, the vascular lesions which result from atherosclerosis and direct effect of blood pressure on the kidney primarily affect the pre-glomerular arterioles [275], thereby causing ischemic changes in the glomeruli and post-glomerular structures. Experimental and clinical data indicate that morphologic changes in the kidney follow functional impairment and vasoconstriction of the afferent arterioles. High pressures are transferred to the arterioles due to alterations in the autoregulation of renal blood flow. Glomerular hyperperfusion following hemodynamic changes due to hypertension also contributes to the glomerular injury and this eventually progresses to glomerulosclerosis [277]. There are changes in the arterioles due to intimal thickening giving arteriolar stiffness, afferent arteriolar hyalinosis and smooth muscle atrophy. Impaired autoregulation in association with hypertrophy and hyperfiltration, and focal segmental glomerulosclerosis give nephrosclerosis. The parenchymal hypoxia from the ischemic glomerulosclerosis leads to tubular atrophy and interstitial fibrosis. There is however a weak correlation between hypertension, and vascular and glomerular lesions [278]. Usually, similar lesions found in nephroslerosis occur in normotensive patients. They may also be found in age-related changes which vary in severity depending on race.

The renal lesion in malignant hypertension consists of fibrinoid necrosis of the afferent arterioles [279], which extends into the glomerulus leading to focal necrosis of the glomerular tuft [280].

Clinically, macroalbuminuria (a random urine albumin/creatinine ratio > 300mg/g) or microalbumiuria (a random urine albumin/creatinine ratio 30–300 mg/g) are early markers of renal injury. These are also risk factors for renal disease progression and for cardiovascular disease [281]

B. Complications of Drug Therapy

Generally, several complications arise from use of antihypertensive drug therapy. The side effects are either a class effect or peculiar to specific drugs. For example, vasodilators as a class cause hypotension, reflex tachycardia and ankle edema while ACE inhibitors cause cough and angioedema.

1. Diuretics

Thiazides came into use in clinical medicine during the 1970s with relatively high doses (150 mg/d of hydrochlorothiazide). This dose was associated with high incidence of side/adverse effects [282]. Lower doses have been found to be as potent as higher doses in blood pressure reduction and are less likely to induce adverse effects [146]. Electrolyte disturbances associated with thiazide diuretic use include hypokalemia, hyponatremia, hypercalcemia, and hypomagnesemia. Other side effects or complications of thiazide diuretics are hyperuricemia, hyperglycemia, hyper/dyslipidemia, etc.

i. Electrolyte Disturbances:

a. Hypokalaemia

In the present era of using low dosages of thiazide diuretics (hydrochlorothiazide and chlorthalidone 12.5 mg and 25 mg) in treatment, the most common side effect of thiazide treatment is hypokalemia. The thiazides do not affect K+ transport directly [283] but rather they do so indirectly though the following mechanisms:

- Increased delivery of sodium to the collecting ducts leads to increased uptake of sodium by the ENaCs and in turn the Na+/K+ exchanger becomes more active resulting in loss of K+.
- Activation of RAAS following the diuretic induced hypovolemia, with the increased aldosterone produced; there is further stimulation of the Na+/K+ exchanger.
- Also the increased nephron flow rate following diuresis reduces K+ concentration in the lumen hence increasing K+ gradient.
- Lastly, thiazides lower the luminal calcium concentration along the distal tubules. This activates the ENaCs inhibited by calcium enhancing K+ secretion [284].

Some observational studies report that diuretic induced hypokalemia may be associated with an increased incidence of arrhythmias [285–287]. In the Multiple Risk Factor Intervention Trial, thiazides were associated with sudden death in hypertensive men who had some electrocardiographic abnormalities. However, later analysis did not prove that thiazides were associated with ventricular ectopy or sudden death [288].

b. Hyponatremia

Hyponatremia may also occur with thiazide therapy. This condition though not very common is potentially fatal and it is often missed [289]. A review showed that of 129 cases reported between 1962 and 1990 with severe treatment-induced hyponatremia, 94% was attributed to thiazide therapy [290]. Risk factors that predispose to hyponatremia were increased water intake, older age and female sex.

ii. Metabolic Side Effects

a. Hyperglycaemia

Thiazide diuretics exhibit some non-renal effects. The non-diuretic thiazide diazoxide, induces hyperglycemia by hyperpolarizing the islet cell membrane in the pancreas leading to inhibition of calcium (Ca2+) influx and Ca2+ dependent release of insulin [291]. The diuretic thiazides (hydrochlorothiazide, hydroflumethiazide, and indapamide) are also thought to exhibit these effects [292]. Another mechanism implicated for the hyperglycemic effect, is that thiazides increase serum glucose through activation of the RAAS. Thiazide diuretics may increase the incidence of new-onset diabetes, especially when combined with β blockers therefore caution is advised in using both in patients who are at high risk of developing diabetes [293].

b. Hyperuricemia

Hyperuricemjia occurs because there is proximal tubular urate reabsorption following increased proximal tubular Na reabsorption consequent upon extracellular fluid volume depletion. There is also thiazide induced reduced uric acid secretion. A retrospective cohort study demonstrated that the use of hydrochlorothiazide at doses of 25 mg daily or more was associated with increased risk of the initiation of anti-gout therapy [294].

c. Hyper/Dyslipidaemia

Changes in lipid profiles have been documented in various studies. These studies show increases in lipid profiles - increased total cholesterol, LDL and triglycerides with thiazide use [295, 296]. The ALLHAT study [295] showed that cholesterol was significantly higher in the chlorthalidone group than in the amlodipine and lisinopril groups at 2 and 4 years. Also, more patients in the chlorthalidone group had total cholesterol higher than 240 mg/dl than was documented in the amlodipine group at 2 years and in the lisinopril group at 2 and 4 years.

iii. Hypotension

Hypotension as a complication of thiazide diuretic therapy is not a major problem in clinical practice. However, when used in excess or in patients prone to volume depletion, such as the elderly or individuals with impaired sympathetic reflex or in combination with sodium restriction, diuretics can cause orthostatic hypotension [297]

2. ACE Inhibitors And Angiotensin Receptor Blockers (ARBs)

The side effects of ACE inhibitors and ARBs may be due to interference with the activity of the RAAS in the maintenance of blood pressure and serum potassium. These side effects can be due to class effect or drug specific. Class related side effects are due to interference with the activity of RAAS. These effects are shared with ARBs since they arise from the reduction in levels of Angiotensin 1I. They include hypotension, early decrease in glomerular filtration rate [GFR] and hyperkalemia [298].

i. Cough

Cough has been reported as a side-effect of at least four ACE inhibitors (299-301], and is likely to be a general class effect of these agents. The size of the problem is not known but it is reported to vary from 0.2% [302] to 33% [303]. The cough is more frequent in women [299] who account for approximately 66% of cases. There is no relationship between the occurrence of cough and age, drug dose or heart failure [299].

The pharmacology of ACE inhibitors can explain the side-effects seen with ACE inhibition. Angiotensin converting enzyme has effects other than the conversion of angiotensin I to angiotensin II. It is the same enzyme as kininase II which is responsible for the breaking down of bradykinin [304] and other tachykinins such as substance P in the lungs [305]. Thus, the action of ACE/Kininase II allows accumulation of these substances. Bradykinin and other tachykinins are relevant to the pathogenesis of cough. Bradykinin stimulates the unmyelinated afferent sensory c-fibres via type J receptors [306], and through a local axon reflex leads to the release of tachykinins [307]. Stimulation of type J receptors by bradykinin [308], or the specific c-fibre stimulant, capsaicin [309], is responsible for the non-productive cough. In addition to cough, bradykinin inhalation causes bronchoconstriction in asthmatic patients [308].

There are suggestions that ACE inhibitor-induced cough may be different from bradykinin-induced cough. While the cough due to ACE-inhibition is counteracted by prostaglandin synthetase inhibitors [310], the cough induced by bradykinin responds to sodium cromoglycate and anticholinergics [308]. Another mechanism to explain the pathogenesis of cough is prostaglandins activity. ACE inhibitors may cause increased prostaglandin production via bradykinin [304]. Prostaglandin E2 (PGE2) can excite the unmyelinated afferent c-fibres causing cough [311]. The neural pathways (the type J receptor) complete the local axon reflex with the unmyelinated c-fibres.

Since only a minority of people develop cough side effect, it is evident that there may be individual susceptibility [312]. Women, individuals with ACE genotype II, and those of black or Asian ethnicity have increased risk of ACE inhibitor-induced cough. ACE inhibitor induced-cough is four times commoner in blacks suggesting a racial/ethnic predisposition [313].

ii. Hypotension

Hypotension results from excessive reduction of blood pressure. It presents with weakness, dizziness or syncope. First dose hypotension (hypotension after initiation of therapy) is more marked in patients with hypovolemia such as those with congestive cardiac failure, hyponatremia and dehydration, and with high baseline renin levels [314, 315]. This side effect is minimized by withholding ACE inhibitor therapy in volume-depleted patients and discontinuing diuretics for 3-5 days, then re-introducing ACE inhibitor at a lower dose.

Glomerular filtration rate is reduced within 3-5 days of initiating ACE inhibitor therapy, but this normalizes later. This is the basis for KDOQI guidance 11 which emphasizes the importance of monitoring eGFR [316]. The reduction in GFR is seen mostly in patients with compromised renal blood flow as occurs in bilateral renal artery stenosis, heart failure and CKD [298, 314].

iii. Hyperkalemia

Angiotensin II and hyperkalemia are major factors that increase aldosterone release. They are also major stimulus for renal potassium excretion. Inhibition of both systemic and local angiotensin II by ACE inhibitors leads to impaired potassium excretion with consequent hyperkalemia [298, 313, 317]. This is more marked in patients with renal insufficiency, diabetic patients, and concomitant use of potassium sparing diuretics, non-steroidal anti-inflammatory drugs (NSAIDs) or in the elderly.

iv. Angioedema

Angioedema is the swelling of deep dermis, subcutaneous, or submucosal tissue due to vascular leakage [318]. In the OCTAVE trial, African-Americans had greater incidence of ACE inhibitor-associated angioedema than Caucasians. Angioedema was three times commoner in blacks compared to whites for those subjects on enalapril [319]. The ALLHAT study [320] also documented higher prevalence of angioedema in blacks than non-blacks. This study observed that 0.7% (23 of 3,210) blacks as opposed to 0.32% (15 of 5,844) non-blacks who were placed on lisinopril had angioedema. These studies also showed that African Americans had more florid angioedema compared to whites. The risk of angioedema was not related to dose, specific ACE inhibitor or concomitant medication [321].

Bradykinin has been implicated in the pathogenesis of angioedema. Usually urinary kallikrein levels are lower in African Americans suggesting low blood levels of kallikren. The sudden increase in bradykinin level from inhibition of kininase II following ACE inhibitor therapy, may be responsible for onset of and severity of angioedema [322]. Genetic polymorphisms of the genes encoding ACE, angiotensinogen and AT1 receptors may be involved in the pathogenesis of cough and angioedema [298].

Another side effect of ACE inhibitors and ARBs is anaphylactoid reaction, and this like cough is due to accumulation of kinins.

3. Calcium Channel Blockers

The CCBs are made up of drugs that are chemically heterogenous but majority of their side effects or adverse reactions are predictable from their pharmacological actions. The side effects [323] fall into the following:

Vasodilatation - headaches, flushing, palpitations, peripheral edema, and hypotension;

Negative inotropy - verapamil has the greatest inotropic effect, followed by diltiazem and the last is nifedipine. These drugs are therefore contra-indicated in patients with severe left ventricular dysfunction or sick sinus syndrome and second or third degree atrioventricular block;

Conduction disturbances such as supraventricular tachyarrhythmia: verapamil and diltiazem have significant effect on cardiac conduction but nifedipine does not when given in therapeutic doses.

Gastrointestinal effects - constipation, diarrhea, nausea, dry mouth, gastroesophageal reflux disease (GERD);

Metabolic effects - not much of metabolic effects is seen in this group but nifedipine, verapamil, and diltiazem in high doses may inhibit release of insulin.

Drug interactions - occur when given in association with cardiac glycosides and β blockers. CCBs may be of benefit in hypertensive patients with normal heart function but should be avoided when there is impairment of cardiac function. These drugs also interact with grapefruits, grapefruit juice and alcohol.

Others side effects are fatigue and skin rash.

4. Beta Blockers

The side effects are widespread because of the sympathetic nervous system involved in the control of physiological and metabolic functions [324]. The side effects of β blockers can be divided into two groups [324]: Those arising from the pharmacological effect of β-adrenergic receptor blockade: they include cold extremities, peripheral edema, bronchospasm, heart failure, prolonged hypoglycemia, bradycardia, heart block, intermittent claudication, and Raynaud's phenomenon. Others are the neurological effects such as hallucinations, insomnia, depression, fatigue, muscle cramps, reduced libido and erectile dysfunction, and nightmares. Other miscellaneous side effects include diarrhea, nausea, constipation, flatulence and gastric pain.

The other reactions that do not seem to result from β-adrenergic receptor blockade: these are rare and include oculomucocutaneous reactions. Beta blockers may interact with other drugs to increase toxicity. There have been suggestions of carcinogenesis with β blockers. Beta blockers interact with a lot of drugs: CCBs, aminophylline, cimetidine, anti-diabetic agents, quinidine, clonidine, cardiac glycosides, epinephrine, ergot alkaloids, glucagon, indomethacin, lidocaine, α methyldopa, monoamine oxidase inhibitors, phenothiazines, phenytoin, phenylpropranolamine, and many more.

5. Other Drug Groups

The side effects of other drugs groups:

Vasodilators [325]: Vasodilating antihypertensive drugs stimulate the peripheral sympathetic nervous system through the carotid sinus baroreceptor reflex mechanism to cause increase in the heart rate, renin release, and sodium and water retention. Vasodilators can cause various side effects and toxicity and they include: headache, facial changes, hair growth, varying degrees of sodium and water retention, allergic reactions and infrequently systemic lupus erythematosus.

Sympatholytic Antihypertensive Agents [326]: These sympatholytic drugs have side effects such as sedation, altered thought process, depression, and orthostatic or exercise hypotension. Sexual problems are particularly important in men. Several of these drugs also have side effects that are specific to each of them. For example, α-methyldopa may cause hemolytic anemia and idiosyncratic allergic reactions. The allergic reaction manifests with fever, malaise, and abnormalities of liver function and in some cases may result in hepatic necrosis and death [327]. Reserpine causes increased appetite, and therefore may result in weight gain. It may also increase gastric acid production and may exacerbate or produce gastritis and ulcer symptoms.

Section VI: Hypertension in Special Populations: Pregnancy, the Elderly and Children

Hypertension remains an important cause of morbidity and mortality in special populations including the elderly, pregnant women as well as children [328-330]. The unique aspects of hypertension in these populations such as its epidemiology, pathophysiologic mechanisms, diagnosis and therapeutic approaches deserve special mention.

A. Blood Pressures Changes in Pregnancy

1. Blood Pressure Changes in Normal Pregnancy

Significant cardiovascular physiologic changes occur during pregnancy. It is important to recognize these differences between the pre pregnancy and pregnancy states when assessing blood pressure during pregnancy. Usually, diastolic blood pressure drops more than the systolic blood pressure. The reduction is typically 8–10 mm Hg or just less than a 10% decline from pre-pregnancy levels. The fall in blood pressure begins during the luteal phase of menstruation and progresses if pregnancy occurs. Peripheral resistance decreases by up to 25%, blood volume increases by up to 50% and cardiac output increases by 35% - 50% above values prior to pregnancy [331, 332]. There is also an increase in renal blood flow and glomerular filtration rate. The cumulative effect is a fall in blood pressure in the first trimester and a slow rise to pre pregnancy levels by the third trimester. It has been demonstrated that the circadian variations in blood pressure are maintained during pregnancy [333].

2. Hypertension in Pregnancy

Hypertension in pregnancy is defined as systolic blood pressure (SBP) of $\geq$ 140mmHg or diastolic blood pressure (DBP) $\geq$ 90mmHg or increase of SBP $\geq$ 30mmHg or DBP $\geq$ 15mmHg over first trimester or pre-pregnancy values [334]. Hypertension occurs in about 6% to 8% of all pregnancies in high income countries as well as in LMICs, and is one of the leading causes of maternal and perinatal mortality [335]. Despite the significant morbidity and mortality associated with hypertension in pregnancy, its pathogenesis remains incompletely elucidated thus limiting the ability to prevent and treat the disorder.

i. Classification of Hypertension in Pregnancy

The US NHBPEP [335] has classified hypertension in pregnancy as follows:

- Preeclampsia- Hypertension developing after 20 weeks gestation with proteinuria and/or oedema
- Gestational hypertension (also called Transient hypertension of pregnancy)- Hypertension developing after 20 weeks gestation without other signs of preeclampsia
- Chronic hypertension- Hypertension before 20 weeks gestation in the absence of trophoblastic disease.
- Preeclampsia superimposed on chronic hypertension - Preeclampsia developing in a woman with pre-existing hypertension

a. Preeclampsia

Preeclampsia is a systemic disease characterized by hypertension, and/or proteinuria. Usually, resolution of the acute symptoms of preeclampsia follows delivery of the placenta suggesting that the placenta plays a central role in its pathogenesis. During normal pregnancy, the placenta undergoes intense vascularization to enable circulation between the fetus and the mother. Vascularization involves maternal spiral artery remodeling which requires a delicate balance between pro-angiogenic and antiangiogenic factors. The imbalance of these factors triggers disease onset [336, 337]. The underlying genetic explanations for the overproduction of anti-angiogenic factors in preeclampsia are still being proposed.

Some risk factors for the development of preeclampsia have been recognized and include the following:

- Prim gravidae
- Age > 40 years or < 18 years
- Preeclampsia in previous pregnancy
- Chronic hypertension
- Chronic kidney disease
- Antiphospholipid antibody syndrome
- Multiple pregnancies
- Vascular or connective tissue disorder
- Family history of pregnancy induced hypertension
- High BMI
- Male partner whose previous partner had preeclampsia

The pathophysiology of preeclampsia has for long centered on abnormal uteroplacental blood flow. A lot of data to support the hypothesis of reduced uterine blood flow in the etiopathogenesis of this condition have recently emerged. Poor trophoblastic invasion of the uterus seems to be the primary pathology [338]. The reduction of the uteroplacental blood flow emanates from the inability of the cytotrophoblasts to penetrate deep into the uterine wall. This condition is also associated with placental infarcts and resultant intrauterine growth retardation [339]. The maternal endothelium is the tissue chiefly affected in preeclampsia. Abnormal endothelial activation and dysfunction lead to extensive vasoconstriction and end organ ischemia. The imbalance in the production and release of endothelial cell compounds (prostacyclin, prostaglandins, thromboxanes, nitric oxide etc) enhance hypercoagulability leading to the formation of intravascular thrombi [340].

Increased expression of soluble fms-like tyrosine kinase (sFlt1), together with decreased placental growth factor (PGF) and vascular endothelial growth factor (VEGF) signaling, were the first abnormalities described [341, 342]. Studies have implicated abnormal levels of several angiogenic factors (sFlt1, PGF and VEGF, etc.) in the pathogenesis of preeclampsia and eclampsia. In normal pregnancy, components of RAAS are elevated but reduced in preeclampsia and eclampsia [343, 344].

ii. Therapeutic Approaches to Hypertension in Pregnancy

Serious complications including acute kidney injury, cerebral hemorrhage, liver failure, abruptio placentae and increased fetal loss are associated with hypertension in pregnancy. This justifies the need for prompt diagnosis and treatment. The dearth of randomized clinical trials in pregnancy and the established risk of teratogenicity with the use of some antihypertensive agents have limited the options for antihypertensive drugs in this condition.

According to the Working Group Report on High Blood Pressure in Pregnancy recommendation [334], diuretics can be used with caution in women whose hypertension predates pregnancy because they potentiate the effect of other antihypertentive agents as well as reducing the tendency to developing edema and preeclampsia. They are however contraindicated where there is a compromise in utero placental blood flow. Alpha methyl dopa remains one of the drugs of choice for initiating treatment in hypertensive women in pregnancy [345] especially in low resource settings. It has been used extensively without any reported fetal abnormalities [346, 347]. It is however able to cross the placental barrier and appear in cord blood. Most beta blockers reduce placental perfusion and thus are linked to intrauterine growth retardation, prematurity and low birth weight [348]. There is lack of evidence for teratogenicity with use of β blockers but they are best avoided in early pregnancy.

Hydralazine, though not advisable for use in early pregnancy because of arrhythmias and maternal hypotension, may be used in the third trimester. It is however being replaced in recent times by other agents with less side effects [349]. Hydralazine is also useful in preeclampsia/ eclampsia [334]. Labetalol has recently become a first line drug for treatment of hypertension in pregnancy because of its safety and efficacy [350, 351]. Nifedipine, a dihydropyridine CCB has been found to be safe in the 2nd or 3rd trimester in humans. Although administration of a CCB in first trimester demonstrated teratogenicity in some animal studies, a randomized multicenter study in humans showed neither benefit nor harm with exposure to a slow release nifedipine in second trimester of pregnancy [352]. ACE inhibitors and ARBs should be avoided during pregnancy. These drugs interfere with neurological and cardiovascular development of the fetus in the first trimester, and later cause irreversible renal impairment, oligohydramnios, pulmonary hypoplasia, limb defects and growth restrictions [353].

B. Hypertension in the Elderly

The prevalence of hypertension increases with age and affects all races. It is common in the elderly in LMICs with a mean prevalence of 52.9%, and ranges from 32.3% in India to 77.9% in South Africa [354]. The prevalence of hypertension in the age group 80 years and above is more than 60% [355]. It has been projected that 75% of medical practice will be directed at the geriatric age group in the future. Data from the Framingham study showed a linear increase of prevalence of hypertension with age: hypertension was present in 27.3% of individuals younger than 60 years and 63% in people in the age group 60-79 years. In those 80 years and older, hypertension was present in 74%. [356].

The elderly have excessive vascular stiffness often causing falsely high blood pressure recording. Care should therefore be taken when measuring blood pressure in elderly subjects. Blood pressure should also be measured in supine, sitting and standing positions because of relatively high prevalence of orthostatic hypotension in this group.

1. Pathophysiology

The most common type of hypertension in older persons is isolated systolic hypertension, defined as a systolic blood pressure of 140 mm Hg or more and a diastolic blood pressure of less than 90 mm Hg. Beyond the age of 55 years, the level of diastolic blood pressure typically decreases while the level of systolic blood pressure increases progressively resulting in a more widened pulse pressure. The underlying abnormality is accumulation of collagen fibers, loss and degeneration of elastic fibers, and deposition of calcium within the vascular wall resulting in increased stiffness of the vascular wall and reduced vascular compliance. Both the combined (i.e., systolic blood pressure 140 mm Hg or more and diastolic blood pressure 90 mm Hg or more) and isolated systolic types of hypertension are characterized by increased total peripheral resistance.

The elderly also have relatively lower levels of renin and aldosterone and lower plasma volume [191]. In the elderly, there is reduced renal excretion of salt and increased salt sensitivity. Low dietary intake of calcium and increased calcinuria also increase peripheral resistance and contribute to the hypertension in the elderly.

2. Therapeutic Approaches

Lifestyle modification is a key ingredient in management of hypertension in the elderly. Weight Loss and salt restriction can obviate the need for antihypertensive drugs in this population [357, 358]. Drug treatment of hypertension in the elderly should be gradual aiming at not more than 25% decrease initially.

The current guidelines for the treatment of hypertension –JNC 8 2014- [154] recommends targets for control of hypertension in patients over 60 years of age at ≤150 mmHg systolic and ≤90 mmHg diastolic. CCBs have been shown to be effective in reducing morbidity and mortality in these patients and are therefore the recommended class of drugs

[154]. In the absence of compelling indication to the use of another class of drug, a long-acting dihydropyridine CCB is recommended.

C. Hypertension in Children

Largely as a result of obesity in children, hypertension has become a major pediatric health problem. A sharp increase in the prevalence of childhood obesity has been recorded in the last two decades. Hypertension is currently present in 5% of adolescents [359]. A high prevalence of hypertension in children has been recorded in studies in Africa [360, 361]. There is a link between hypertension in childhood and in adulthood. Low birth weight and exposure to the environment are risk factors for development of hypertension. Also socioeconomic status, diet, exercise patterns, body size, and exposure to environmental toxins may all contribute to childhood hypertension. The prevalence of secondary hypertension is higher in children than in adults. Secondary hypertension accounts for 85% to 90% of all children with elevated blood pressure. Thus, identification of underlying diseases contributing to the hypertension in children is a priority. Umbilical artery catheterization is responsible for many cases of neonatal hypertension. Renal artery obstruction from thrombosis is another major cause of secondary hypertension. In children aged 13 years and younger, underlying renal disease is the most common cause of secondary hypertension and accounts for as much as 70% to 80% of all cases of secondary hypertension in children [362].

1. Treatment of Hypertension in Children

Non-pharmacologic and pharmacologic treatments are recommended based on the age of the child, the stage of hypertension, and response to treatment.

i. Nonpharmacologic Treatments

Lifestyle changes including weight loss, exercise, a low-fat and low-sodium diet, smoking cessation, and avoidance of alcohol use are recommended for children and adolescents with prehypertension or stage 1 hypertension.

The risk of development of hypertension rises three-fold with obesity and also leads to insulin resistance, hyperlipidemia, and salt sensitivity [363, 364]. The development of LVH is enhanced by the presence of obesity with and without hypertension. [365]. Exercise has been found to be beneficial in control of hypertension in children.

Sodium restriction is a component of the lifestyle modification for control of hypertension. A sodium intake of 1,200 mg per day is recommended by the NHBPEP. A diet similar to the DASH (Dietary Approaches to Stop Hypertension) food plan with no-salt-added diet and with more fresh fruits and vegetables combined with low-fat dairy and protein is said be successful in lowering blood pressure in children [190]. Increased potassium and calcium intake have also been suggested as nutritional strategies to reduce blood pressure. Family support is pivotal to success in implementation of life style changes in the treatment of hypertension in children.

ii. Pharmacotherapy

Presence of symptoms in a hypertensive child and adolescent, end-organ damage, secondary hypertension, stage 1 hypertension that does not respond to lifestyle changes, and stage 2 hypertension are indications for starting antihypertensive medication. Drug therapy is aimed at reducing blood pressure to less than the 95th percentile for sex, age and height in the absence of end-organ damage or comorbid conditions. When there is end-organ damage or comorbid illness, the blood pressure should be lowered to less than the 90th percentile. Usually, drug therapy should be in addition to lifestyle modification.

For children and adolescents, the recommended first line antihypertensive agents will include diuretics, CCBs, ACE inhibitors, and β blockers. Children and adolescents with kidney disease benefit from use of ACE inhibitors and ARBs. However, because of the potential of teratogenicity in the first trimester of pregnancy with use of these drugs, they should be used with caution in older girls who may be sexually active. There is however paucity of long-term outcome studies on the effects of antihypertensive medication in children.

Conclusion

Hypertension is a major health problem worldwide reaching a global prevalence of 40%. In the past, hypertension was rare in rural African communities but in recent times, its prevalence in Africa has outstripped those of other continents. The 2013 WHO brief on hypertension puts the prevalence of hypertension in Africa at 46%, a figure higher than in any other continent. In addition, awareness is low, a significant proportion is untreated and among the treated, many are not controlled to target. The change in prevalence is attributed to rural-urban migration, adoption of western lifestyle, sedentary lifestyle, obesity and an aging population. Hypertension is not only more prevalent in the black patient; it is associated with more target organ damage.

The pathophysiology of essential hypertension is complex, involving interplay between genetic and environmental factors. In spite of this general mechanism, some subtle differences in pathophysiology between black patients and Caucasians are discernible; essential hypertension in the black patient is predominantly low renin and salt sensitive whereas it is high renin in the white patient.

Many antihypertensive drug classes effectively reduce blood pressure in the black hypertensive patient. Thiazide diuretics and related drugs and CCBs are very efficacious in lowering blood pressure in the black hypertensive patient. On the other hand, β blockers, ACE inhibitors and ARBs are less effective as monotherapy in blacks compared to whites. However, recent studies have demonstrated the efficacy of these agents in the control of blood pressure in the black patient especially as combination therapy. There are many challenges to the effective control of blood pressure in LMICs. These include poverty, poor access to healthcare and poor patient adherence to prescribed regimen, paucity of health education/ health literacy, lifestyle factors, challenges in the interpretation of BP values, clinical inertia and inadequate BP measurement.

Hypertension is associated with serious acute and long term complications involving cardiovascular, nervous and urinary systems. The most common of these are LVH, CCF, stroke, CKD and retinopathy. These significantly affect quality of life.

Lifestyle changes including low salt intake, DASH like type of diet, exercise and weight control, and drug therapy are all essential to proper management of hypertension in LMICs. These measures if properly implemented will change the gloomy picture of hypertension in these regions.

References

[1] Ibrahim MM, Damasceno A. Hypertension in developing countries. *Lancet.* 2012 Aug 11; 380 (9841): 611- 619.

[2] Yancy CW. Heart Disease in Varied Populations. In: Braunwald's Heart Disease. 8th ed. Libby P, Bonow RO, Mann DL, Zipes DP (eds). Philadelphia. *Saunders.* Ch.2. pg. 23.

[3] World health Organization: Global Health Observatory (GHO) data. Raised blood pressure: situation and trends. 2015 WHO. [Online] Available from: http://www.who.int/gho/ncd/risk_factors/blood_pressure_prevalence_text/en/ (accessed 30/01/2015).

[4] World Health Organization. A global brief on hypertension: silent killer, global health crisis. World Health Day 2013. [Online] Available from: http://www.who.int /cardiovascular_diseases/publications/global_brief_hypertension/en/ (accessed 20/01/2015).

[5] Lloyd-Jones D, Adams RJ, Brown TM, Carnethon M, Dai S, De Simone G. et al. American Heart Association Statistics Committee and Stroke Statistics Subcommittee. Executive summary: heart disease and stroke statistics–2010 update: a report from the American Heart Association. *Circulation.*2010; 121: 948–954.

[6] World Health Organization. Global status report on non-communicable diseases 2010. Geneva, World Health Organization. 2011. [Online] Available from: http://whqlibdoc.who.int/publications/2011/ 9789240686458_eng.pdf?ua=1 (accessed 19/01/2015).

[7] van de Vijver S, Akinyi H, Oti S, Olajide A, Agyemang C, Aboderin I, Kyobutungi C. Status report on hypertension in Africa – Consultative review for the 6th session of the African Union conference of ministers of health on NCD's. *PanAfrican Medical Journal* 2013; 16:38. doi:10.11604/pamj.2013.16.38.3100

[8] Lozano R, Naghavi M, Foreman K, Lim S, Shibuya K, Aboyans V, et al. Global and regional mortality from 235 causes of death for 20 age groups in 1990 and 2010: a systematic analysis for the Global Burden of Disease Study 2010. *The Lancet.* 2012; 380(9859): 2095-128.

[9] World Health Organization. Global health risks: mortality and burden of disease attributable to selected major risks. *Geneva, World Health Organization.* 2009. http://www.who.int/healthinfo/global_burden_disease/GlobalHealthRisks_report_full.pdf

[10] *Donnison C. Blood pressure in the African natives: its bearing upon aetiology of hyperpiesa and arteriosclerosis. Lancet. 1929; 1:* 6 – 7.

[11] Chobanian AV, Bakris GL, Black HR, Cushman WC, Green LA, Izzo JL, Jr, Jones DW, Jr, Materson BJ, Oparil S, Wright JT, Jr, Roccella EJ, and the National High Blood Pressure Education Program Coordinating Committee . The Seventh Report of the Joint National Committee on prevention, detection, evaluation, and treatment of high blood pressure: the JNC7 report. *JAMA*. 2003; 289: 2560 –2572.

[12] Lopez AD, Mathers CD, Ezzati M, et al., editors. Global Burden of Disease and Risk Factors. Washington (DC): World Bank; 2006. [Online] Available from: http://www.ncbi.nlm.nih.gov/books/ NBK11819/?report=reader (accessed 19/01/2015).

[13] Boutayeb A. The double burden of communicable and non-communicable diseases in developing countries. *Transactions of the Royal society of tropical Medicine and Hygiene 2006 March*; 100 (3): 191 – 199.

[14] Tibazarwa KB, Damasceno AA. Hypertension in Developing countries. *Canadian Journal of Cardiology* 2014; 30 (5): 527 533.

[15] World health Organization. Chapter 4: Disease threats In The health of the people: what works? Bulletin of World Health Organization 2014. [Online] Available from: http://www.who.int/bulletin/africanhealth2014/978-9290232612-C004.pdf?ua=1 (accessed 19/01/2015).

[16] Omran A. The Epidemiologic Transition: A Theory of the Epidemiology of Population Change. *The Milbank Memorial Fund Quarterly*. 1971; 49(4): 509 - 358.

[17] Caldwell JC. Population health in transition. Bulletin of the World Health Organization 2001; 79 (2). [Online] Available from: http://www.ncbi.nlm.nih.gov/pmc/articles /PMC2566347/pdf/11246833.pdf (accessed 18/01/2015).

[18] Kibirige JS. Population growth, poverty and health. *Soc. Sci. Med.*1997 Jul; 45(2): 247 – 259.

[19] Addo J, Smeeth L, Leon DA. Hypertension In Sub-Saharan Africa A Systematic Review. Hypertension 2007; 50: 1012 – 1018. . [Online] Available from: http://hyper.ahajournals.org/content/50/6/1012.full.pdf+html (accessed 10/01/2015).

[20] Ulasi II, Ijoma CK, Onodugo O. A community-based study of hypertension and cardio-metabolic syndrome in semi-urban and rural communities in Nigeria. *BMC Health Services Research*, 10: 71; 2010. Available at http://www.biomedcentral.com/1472-6963/10/71.

[21] Agyemang C. Rural and urban differences in blood pressure and hypertension in Ghana, West Africa. *Public health. 2006*;120(6):525-33.

[22] Bellini LJ. Lifestyle and hypertension – an overview. *Clin. Exp. Hypertens*. 1999; 21 (5-6): 749 – 762.

[23] UN-habitat. The State of African Cities 2010: Governance, Inequalities and Urban Land Markets. Nairobi: UN-Habitat; 2010

[24] United Nations, Department of Economic and Social Affairs. 2014 revision of the World Urbanization Prospects. UN 2014. [Online] Available from: http://www.un.org/en/development/desa/publications/2014-revision-world-urbanization-prospects.html (accessed 10/01/2015).

[25] United Nations, Department of Economic and Social Affairs. World Population Ageing 1950-2050: III. Changing balance between age groups. United Nations n.d. [Online] Available from: http://www.un.org/esa/population/publications/worldageing19502050 /pdf/81chapteriii.pdf (accessed 10/01/2015).

[26] Nabalamba A, Chikoko M. Aging population challenges in Africa. African Development Bank 2011; 1 (1). [Online] Available from: http://www.afdb.org/fileadmin/uploads/afdb/Documents/Publications/Aging%20Population%20Challenges%20in%20Africa-distribution.pdf (accessed 10/01/2015).

[27] CDC. Public health and aging: trends in aging—United States and worldwide. Mortality and Morbidity Weekly Report 2003 February 14; 52 (06): 101 – 106. [Online] Available from: http://www.cdc.gov/mmwr/preview/mmwrhtml/mm5206a2.htm (accessed 01/02/2015).

[28] Kunes J, Zicha J. The interaction of genetic and environmental factors in the etiology of hypertension *Physiol. Res. 2009;* 58 (Suppl. 2): S33 - S41.

[29] Butler MG. Genetics of hypertension. Current status. *J. Med. Liban* 2010; 58: 175 – 178.

[30] Murugan M, Ramalingam K, Nazzuredin M, Rashed HA, Punamalai G. SNP's and its correlation with hypertension: A comprehensive review. Dentistry and Medical Research 2103 Jul-Dec: 1 (1). . [Online] Available from: http://www.dmrjournal.org/temp/DentMedRes113-1396866_035248.pdf (accessed 10/01/2015).

[31] Bellini LJ, Puddey IB, Burke V. Life style and hypertension. *Am. J. Hypertens.* 1999; 12 (9pt1): 934 – 945.

[32] Rodgers A, Ezzati M, Vander Hoorn S, Lopez AD, et al. Distribution of major health risks: findings from the Global Burden of Disease study. *PLoS Medicine*. 2004 Oct; 1 (1): e27.

[33] Bakhru A, Erlinger TP. Smoking Cessation and Cardiovascular Disease Risk Factors: Results from the Third National Health and Nutrition Examination Survey. *PLoS Medicine* 2005 June; 2 (6): e160.

[34] Drope JM editor. Tobacco control in Africa: people, politics, and policies. London: Anthem Press Ltd; 2011. http://www.idrc.ca/ EN/Resources/Publications/openebooks/510-6/index.html (accessed 29/01/2015).

[35] John U, Meyer C, Hanke M, Vo¨ Lzke H, Schumann A (2006). Smoking status, obesity and hypertension in a general population sample: a cross-sectional study. Q J Med 2006; 99:407–415 doi:10.1093/qjmed/hcl047.

[36] Grogan JR, Kochar MS. Alcohol and hypertension. *Arch. Fam. Med.* 1994 February; 3 (2): 150 – 154.

[37] Gillman MW, Cook NR, Evans DA, Rosner B, Hennekens CH. Relationship of Alcohol Intake With Blood Pressure in Young Adults. Hypertension 1995; 25: 1106 – 1110 doi. 10.1161/01.HYP.25.5.1106

[38] Criqui MH, Wallace RB, Mishkel M, Barrett-Conner E, Heiss G. Alcohol consumption and blood pressure: the Lipid Research Clinics Prevalence Study. *Hypertension.* 1981; 3: 557-565.

[39] Bello S, Fatiregun A, Angela Oyo-Ita A, Ikpeme B. Dose-response relationship between alcohol use and blood pressure among drivers of commercial vehicles in Calabar, Southern Nigeria. *Journal of Public Health in Africa* 2010; 1:e5 doi:10.4081/jphia.2010.e5

[40] Marmot MG, Elliott P, Shipley MJ, Dyer AR, Ueshima H, Beevers DG et al. Alcohol and blood pressure: the INTERSALT study. BMJ 1994 May; 308: 1263 – 1267.

[41] *Klatsky AL, Friedman GD, Siegeland AB, Gerard MJ. Alcohol consumption and blood pressure. N. Engl. J. Med.* 1977*;* 296*:* 1194 – *1200.*

[42] Clark LT. Alcohol-induced hypertension: Mechanisms complications, and clinical implications. *JNMA* 1985; 77 (5): 385 – 389.

[43] Wallace RB, Lynch CF, Pomrehn PR, et al. Alcohol and hypertension: Epidemiologic and experimental considerations. The lipid research clinics program. *Circulation* 1981; 64 (suppl 111): 41 - 47.

[44] Panagiotakos DB, Kourlaba G, Zeimbekis A, Toutouzas P, Polychronopoulos E (2007). The J-shape association of alcohol consumption on blood pressure levels, in elderly people from Mediterranean Islands (MEDIS epidemiological study). *Journal of Human Hypertension*; 21, 585–587; doi:10.1038/sj.jhh.1002187

[45] World Health Organization: MSD/MSB. Global status report on alcohol and Health 2014. World Health Organization Geneva. 2014.

[46] Lawoyin TO, Asuzu MC, Kaufman J, Rotimi C, Owoaje E, Johnson L, et al. Prevalence of cardiovascular risk factors in an African, urban inner city community. *West African journal of Medicine*. 2002 Jul-Sep; 21(3): 208 – 211.

[47] World Health Organization. Global recommendations for physical activity for health. Geneva. 2010. [Online] Available from: http://whqlibdoc.who.int/publications /2010/9789241599979_eng.pdf?ua=1 (accessed 10/01/2015).

[48] US Department of Health and Human Services 2002. Physical activity fundamental to preventing disease. [Online] Available from: http://aspe.hhs.gov/health/reports /physicalactivity/ (accessed 10/01/2015).

[49] World Health Organization. Global Strategy on Diet, Physical Activity and Health Promoting fruit and vegetable consumption around the world. Geneva, World Health Organization, 2004. [Online] Available from: http://www.who.int/dietphysicalactivity /fruit/en/ (accessed 03/02/2015).

[50] World Health Organization. *Diet, nutrition and the prevention of chronic diseases: report of a joint WHO/FAO expert consultation*. Geneva, World Health Organization, 2003.

[51] Moore TJ, Conlin PR, Ard J, Svetkey LP, for the DASH Collaborative Research group. DASH (Dietary Approaches to Stop Hypertension) Diet Is Effective Treatment for Stage 1 Isolated Systolic Hypertension *Hypertension*. 2001; 38: 155-158.

[52] World Health Organization. *Creating an enabling environment for population-based salt reduction strategies: report of a joint technical meeting held by WHO and the Food Standards Agency, United Kingdom*. Geneva, World Health Organization; 2010.

[53] Brown IJ et al. Salt intakes around the world: implications for public health. *International Journal of Epidemiology* 2009; 38: 791 – 813.

[54] He FJ, MacGregor GA. A comprehensive review on salt and health and current experience of worldwide salt reduction programmes. *Journal of Human Hypertension* 2009; 23: 363–384.

[55] Law MR, Frost CD, Wald NJ. By how much does dietary salt reduction lower blood pressure? III--Analysis of data from trials of salt reduction. *BMJ*. 1991 Apr 6; 302 (6780): 819-24.

[56] Beaglehole R, Bonita R, Horton R, Adams C, et al. Priority actions for the non-communicable disease crisis. *The Lancet*. 2011; 377 (9775): 1438 – 447.

[57] Cappuccio FP, Sally MK, Frank BM, Jacob P-R, John BE. A community programme to reduce salt intake and blood pressure in Ghana. *BMC Public Health*. 2006 Jan 24; 6: 13.

[58] Mtabaji JP, Nara YM, Mano MM, Yamori Y. Ethnic differences in salt sensitivity: Genetic or environmental factors. *Clin Exp Pharmacol Physiol Suppl.* 1992; 20: 65 – 67.

[59] Obel AO, Koech DK. Potassium supplementation versus bendrofluazide in mildly to moderately hypertensive Kenyans. *J Cardiovasc Pharmacol.* 1991 March; 3 (17): 504 – 507.

[60] Ness AR, Powles JW. Fruit and vegetables, and cardiovascular disease: A review. *Int. J. Epidemiol.* 1997 Feb;26 (1): 1-13.

[61] Popkin BM. Global nutrition dynamics: The world is shifting rapidly toward a diet linked with non-communicable diseases. *Am. J. Clin Nutr.* 2006 Aug; 84 (2): 289 – 298.

[62] World Health Organization: Global Health Observatory. Unhealthy diet. Geneva, World Health Organization; 2015. [Online] Available from: http://www.who.int/gho /ncd/risk_factors/unhealthy_diet_text/en/ (accessed 10/01/2015).

[63] Alonso A, Beunza JJ, Delgado-Rodríguez M, et al. Low-fat dairy consumption and reduced risk of HTN: The Seguimiento Universidad de Navarra (SUN) cohort. *Am. J. Clin Nutr.* 2005 Nov;82(5):972–979.

[64] McGrane MM, Essery E, Obbagy J, Lyon J, MacNeil P, Spahn J, Horn L. Dairy consumption, blood pressure, and risk of hypertension: evidence-based review of recent literature. *Current Cardiovascular Risk Reports;* 5 (4): 287 – 298.

[65] Toledo E, Delgado-Rodríguez M, Estruch R, et al. Low-fat dairy products and blood pressure: Follow-up of 2290 older persons at high cardiovascular risk participating in the PREDIMED study. *Br. J. Nutr.*2009;101(1):59–67.

[66] Obesity: Preventing and managing the global epidemic. WHO Technical report series 894. Geneva: World Health Organization, 2000.

[67] Kotchen TA (2008). Obesity-Related Hypertension? *Weighing the Evidence Hypertension* 52: 801 – 802.

[68] Cutler JA, Sorlie PD, Wolz M, Thom T, Fields LE, Rocella EJ (2008). Trends in hypertension prevalence, awareness, treatment, and control rates in United States adults between 1988 –1994 and 1999 –2004. *Hypertension.* 52: 818 – 827.

[69] James SA, Strogatz DS, Wing SB, Ramsey DL. Socio-economic status, John Henryism and hypertension in blacks and whites. *Am. J. Epidemiol* 1987; 126: 664 – 673.

[70] Odusola A, Hendriks M, Schultsz C, Bolarinwa OA, Akande T, Osibogun A. Perceptions of inhibitors and facilitators for adhering to hypertension treatment among insured patients in rural Nigeria: a quantitative study. *BMC Health Research Services* 2014; 14 (1): 624.

[71] Ogedegbe G, Tobin JN, Fernandez S, Cassells A, Diaz-Gloster, Khalida C, et al. The counseling African Americans to control hypertension: Cluster-randomized clinical trials main effects. *Circulation* 2014; 129: 2044 – 2051.

[72] Cooper RS, Rotimi CN, Ward R. The puzzle of hypertension in African-Americans. *Sci. Am.* 1999;280:56–62.

[73] Vasan RS, Beiser A, Seshadri S, Larson MG, Kannel WB, D'Agostino RB, Levy D. Residual Lifetime Risk for Developing Hypertension in Middle-aged Women and Men. *JAMA.* 2002;287(8):1003-1010. doi:10.1001/jama.287.8.1003.

[74] Franklin S., Jacobs M., Wong N., L'Italien G., Lapuerta P. Predominance of isolated systolic hypertension among middle-aged and elderly US hypertensives: analysis based

on National Health and Nutrition Examination Survey (NHANES) III. *Hypertension* 2001; 37: 869–874.

[75] Cooper R, Rotimi C, Ataman S, McGee D, Osotimehin B, Kadiri S, et al. The prevalence of hypertension in seven populations of West African origin. *Am. J. Public Health*. 1997; 87: 160 – 168.

[76] Nesbitt S, Victor RG. Pathogenesis of Hypertension in African Americans. *CHF 2004*; 10: 24-29.

[77] Kaplan NM. Ethnic aspects of hypertension. *Lancet*. 1994; 344: 450 – 452.

[78] Tanira MOM, Al Balushi KA. Genetic variations related to hypertension: a review. *Journal of Human Hypertension*. 2005; 19: 7 – 19. doi:10.1038/sj.jhh.1001780

[79] Luft FC, Schuster H, Bilginturan N, et al. Treasure your exceptions: what we can learn from autosomal-dominant inherited forms of hypertension. *J. Hypertens*. 1995; 13(12 pt 2):1535 – 1538.

[80] Timberlake DS, O`Connor DT, Parmer RJ: Molecular genetics of essential hypertension: recent results and emerging strategies. *Curr Opin Nephrol Hypertens*. 2001; 10: 71-79.

[81] Williams SM, Addy JH, Phillips JA 3rd, Dal M, Kpodonu J, Afful J et al. Combinations of variations in multiple genes are associated with hypertension. *Hypertension* 2000; 36 (1): 2 – 6.

[82] Guyton AC. Blood pressure control-special role of the kidneys and body fluids. *Science* 1991; 252: 1813 - 1816.

[83] Wang Z, Peng X. Pathogenesis of essential hypertension: development of a 4-dimensional model. Hypothesis 2013, 11 (1): e3, doi:10.5779/hypothesis.v11i1.303

[84] Loutzenhiser R, Griffin K, Williamson G, Bidani A. Renal autoregulation: new perspectives regarding the protective and regulatory roles of the underlying mechanisms. *Am. J. Physiol. Regul. Integr. Comp. Physiol.* 2006;290:R1153-67. http://dx.doi.org/10.1152/ ajpregu.00402.2005.

[85] Oparil S, Zaman A, Calhoun DA. Pathogenesis of Hypertension . *Ann. Intern Med.* 2003; 139:761 – 776.

[86] Su YR, Rutkowski MP, Klanke CA, et al. A novel variant of the beta-subunit of the amiloride-sensitive sodium channel in African Americans. *J. Am. Soc. Nephrol.* 1996; 7: 2543 – 2549.

[87] Jeunemaitre X, Soubrier F, Kotelevtsev YV, et al. Molecular basis of human hypertension: role of angiotensinogen. *Cell.* 1992; 71(1): 169 – 180.

[88] Rotimi C, Morrison L, Cooper R, et al. Angiotensinogen gene in human hypertension. Lack of an association of the 235T allele among African Americans. *Hypertension.* 1994; 24(5): 591 – 594.

[89] Song Q, Chao J, Chao L. DNA polymorphisms in the 5′-flanking region of the human tissue kallikrein gene. *Hum. Genet.* 1997; 99(6): 727 – 734.

[90] Lockette W, Ghosh S, Farrow S, et al. Alpha 2-adrenergic receptor gene polymorphism and hypertension in blacks. *Am. J. Hypertens.* 1995; 8(4 pt 1): 390 – 394.

[91] Barley J, Carter ND, Cruickshank JK, Jeffry S, Smith A, Charlett A, Webb DJ. Renin and atrial natriuretic peptide restriction fragment length polymorphisms: association with ethnicity and blood pressure. *J. Hypertens.* 1991; 9(11): 993 – 996.

[92] Deng AY, Rapp JP. Locus for the inducible, but not a constitutive, nitric oxide synthase cosegregates with BP in the Dahl salt-sensitive rat. *J. Clin. Invest.* 1995; 95(5): 2170 – 2177.

[93] Lang CC, Stein CM, Brown RM, Deegan R, Nelson R, He HB, Wood M, Wood AJJ. Attenuation if isoproterenol mediated vasodilatation in blacks. *N. Engl. J. Med.* 1995; 333: 155 – 160.

[94] Wilson TW, Grim CE. Biohistory of slavery and blood pressure differences in blacks today. A hypothesis. *Hypertension.* 1991; 17 (1 suppl): I122 – I128.

[95] Weinberger MH. Salt sensitivity of blood pressure in humans. *Hypertension.* 1996; 27: 481 – 490.

[96] Luft FC. Mendelian Forms of Human Hypertension and Mechanisms of Disease. *Clinical Medicine & Research* 2003; 1 (4): 291 – 300.

[97] Lifton RP, Gharavi AG, Geller DS. Molecular mechanisms of human hypertension. *Cell* 2001; 104: 545 – 556.

[98] Fuller PJ. Epithelial sodium channels and hypertension. *J. Hypertens.* 1996; 14(12): 1383 – 1386.

[99] Su YR, Menon AG. Epithelial sodium channels and hypertension. *Drug Metab. Dispos.* 2001; 29(4): 553 – 556.

[100] Baker EH, Dong YB, Sagnella GA, et al. Association of hypertension with T594M mutation in beta subunit of epithelial sodium channels in black people resident in London. *Lancet.* 1998; 351: 1388 – 1392.

[101] Baker EH, Duggal A, Dong Y, et al. Amiloride, a specific drug for hypertension in black people with T594M cariant? *Hypertension.* 2002;40:13–17.

[102] Messerli FH, Mittler BS. Framingham at 50. *Lancet.* 1998; 352 (9133): 1006.

[103] Foster DW. Insulin resistance—a secret killer? *N. Engl. J. Med.* 1989; 320: 733 – 734.

[104] Kaplan NM. The deadly quartet: Upper-body adiposity, glucose intolerance, hypertriglyceridemia, and hypertension. *Arch. Intern. Med.* 1989; 149: 1514 – 1520.

[105] Neter JE, Stam BE, Kok FJ, Grobbee DE, Geleijnse JM. Influence of weight reduction on blood pressure: a meta-analysis of randomized controlled trials. *Hypertension. 2003* Nov; 42(5): 878 – 884.

[106] Landsberg L. Insulin-mediated sympathetic stimulation: role in the pathogenesis of obesity-related hypertension (or, how insulin affects blood pressure, and why). *J. Hypertens*. 2001; 19 (3 pt 2): 523 – 528.

[107] Gillum RF, Mussolino ME, Madans JH. Body fat distribution and hypertension incidence in women and men. The NHANES I epidemiologic follow-up study. *Int. J. Obes*. 1998; 22: 127 – 134.

[108] Haffner SM, Ferrannini E, Hazuda HP, et al. Clustering of cardiovascular risk factors in confirmed prehypertensive individuals. *Hypertension.* 1992; 20: 38 – 45.

[109] Maniola TA, Savage PJ, Burke FL, et al. Association of fasting insulin with blood pressure and lipids in young adults: the CARDIA study. *Arteriosclerosis.* 1990; 10: 430 – 436.

[110] Landsberg L. Hyperinsulinemia: possible role in obesity-induced hypertension. *Hypertension.* 1992; 19: I61 – I66.

[111] Levine JA, Eberhardt NL, Jensen MD. Role of nonexercise activity thermogenesis in resistance to fat gain in humans. *Science.* 1999; 283: 212 – 214.

[112] Neser W, Thomas J, Semenya K, et al. Obesity and Hypertension in a longitudinal study of black physicians. *J. Chronic. Dis*. 1986; 39: 105 – 113.
[113] Luft FC, Miller JZ, Grim CE, Fineberg NS, Christian JC, Daugherty SA, Weinberger MH. Salt sensitivity and resistance of blood pressure. Age and race as factors in physiological responses. *Hypertension*. 1991; 17: I102 – I108.
[114] Flack JM, Sica DA, Bakris G, Brown AL, Ferdinand KC, Grimm RH Jr, Hall WD, Jones WE, Kountz DS, Lea JP, Nasser S, Nesbitt SD, Saunders E, Scisney-Matlock M, Jamerson KA, on behalf of the International Society on Hypertension in Blacks. Management of high blood pressure in blacks: an update of the International Society on Hypertension in Blacks Consensus Statement. *Hypertension*. 2010; 56: 780–800.
[115] Wright JT Jr, Dunn JK, Cutler JA, Davis BR, Cushman WC, Ford CE, Haywood LJ, Leenen FHH, Margolis KL, Papademetriou V, Probstfield JL, Whelton PK, Habib GB. Outcomes in hypertensive black and nonblack patients treated with chlorthalidone, amlodipine, and lisinopril. *JAMA*. 2005; 293: 1595 – 1608.
[116] Flack JM, Nasser SA, Levy PD. Therapy of Hypertension in African Americans. *Am. J. Cardiovasc Drugs*. 2011; 11(2): 83-92.
[117] Kobori H, Nishiyama A, Abe Y, Navar LG. Enhancement of intrarenal angiotensinogen in Dahl salt-sensitive rats on high salt diet. *Hypertension*. 2003; 41: 592 – 597.
[118] Boddi M, Poggesi L, Coppo M, Zarone N, Sacchi A, Tania C, Gastone G, Serneri N. Human vascular renin-angiotensin system and its functional changes in relation to different sodium intakes. *Hypertension* 1998; 31 (3): 836 – 842.
[119] Price DA, Fisher ND, Osei SY,Langsang MC, Hollenberg NK. Renal perfusion and function in healthy African Americans. *Kidney Int* 2001; 59 (3): 1037 – 1043.
[120] Sehgal AR. Overlap between whites and blacks in response to antihypertensive drugs. *Hypertension* 2004; 43: 566 – 572.
[121] Tu W, Pratt JH. A consideration of the genetic mechanisms behind the development of hypertension in blacks. *Curr. Hypertens Rep*. 2013 Apr; 15(2): 108 – 113.
[122] Kao WH, Klag MJ, Meoni LA, Reich D, Berthier-Schaad Y, Li M, et al. Myh9 is associated with nondiabetic end-stage renal disease in african americans. *Nat Genet*. 2008; 40: 1185 – 1192.
[123] Kopp JB, Smith MW, Nelson GW, Johnson RC, Freedman BI. Myh9 is a major-effect risk gene for focal segmental glomerulosclerosis. *Nat Genet*. 2008; 40: 1175 – 1184.
[124] Parsa A, Kao WH, Xie D, Astor BC, Li M, Hsu CY, et al. APOL1 risk variants, race, and progression of chronic kidney disease. *N. Engl. J. Med* 2013; 369: 2183 – 2196.
[125] Ulasi, II, Tzur S, Wasser WG, Shemer R, Kruzel E, Feigin E, et al. High population frequencies of APOL1 risk variants are associated with increased prevalence of non-diabetic chronic kidney disease in the Igbo people from south-eastern Nigeria. *Nephron Clin Pract*. 2013; 123 (1-2): 123 - 128.
[126] Tayo BO, Kramer H, Salako BL, Gottesman O, Mckenzie CA, Ogunniyi A, et al. (2013). Genetic variation in APOL1 and MYH9 genes is associated with chronic kidney disease among Nigerians. *Int. Urol Nephrol*. 2013; 45 (2): 485 - 494.
[127] Harshfield GA, Hwang C, Grim CE. Circadian variation of blood pressure in blacks: influence of age, gender and activity. *Journal of Human Hypertension*. 1990; 4 (1): 43 – 47.
[128] Ergul S, Parish DC, Puett D, Ergul A. Racial Differences in Plasma Concentrations in Individuals with Essential Hypertension. *Hypertension* 1996; 28: 652- 655.

[129] Minor D, Wofford M, Wyatt SB. Does socioeconomic status affect blood pressure goal achievement? *Curr. Hypertens Rep*. 2008 Oct; 10(5): 390 – 397.

[130] Grotto I, Huerat M, Sharabi Y. Hypertension and socioeconomic status. *Curr. Opin. Cardiol*. 2008 Jul; 23 (4): 335 – 339. doi: 10.1097/HCO.0b013e3283021c70

[131] Bovet P, Ross AG, Gervasoni JP, Mkamba M, et al. Distribution of Blood Pressure, Body Mass Index and Smoking Habits in the Urban Population of Dar es Salaam, Tanzania, and Associations with Socioeconomic Status. *Int. J. Epidemiol.* 2002; 31: 240-247.

[132] Sampson UKA, Edwards TL, Jahangir E, Munro H, et al. Factors Associated With the Prevalence of Hypertension in the Southeastern United States Insights From 69 211 Blacks and Whites in the Southern Community Cohort Study. *Circ. Cardiovasc Qual Outcomes*. 2014; 7:00-00.)

[133] Opie LH, Seedat YK. Hypertension in Sub-Saharan African Populations. Circulation. 2005;112:3562-3568. Crespo CJ, Smit E, Andersen RE, Carter-Pokras O, Ainsworth BE. Race/ethnicity, social class and their relation to physical inactivity during leisure time: results from the Third National Health and Nutrition Examination Survey, 1988–1994. *Am. J. Prev. Med.* 2000;18:46–53.

[134] Mu M, Wang S, Sheng J, Zhao Y, Archives of Cardiovascular Disease February 2012; 105(2): 99-113)

[135] Flack JM, Nasser SA, O'Connor SM. Ethnicity and Socioeconomic Status in Hypertension. In: Braunwald's Heart Disease. 8th ed. Libby P, Bonow RO, Mann DL, Zipes DP (eds). Philadelphia. Saunders. Ch. B84, pg. 276.

[136] Crespo CJ, Smit E, Andersen RE, Carter-Pokras O, Ainsworth BE. Race/ethnicity, social class and their relation to physical inactivity during leisure time: results from the Third National Health and Nutrition Examination Survey, 1988–1994. *Am. J. Prev. Med.* 2000;18:46–53.

[137] David R. Bassett, Jr.,*,1 Eugene C. Fitzhugh,† Carlos J. Crespo,‡ George A. King,* and James E. McLaughlin*. Physical Activity and Ethnic Differences in Hypertension Prevalence in the United States. *Preventive Medicine* 34, 179–186 (2002

[138] Olafiranye O, Akinboboye O, Mitchell JE, Ogedegbe G, Jean-Louis G. Obstructive Sleep Apnea and Cardiovascular Disease in Blacks. A Call to Action From the Association of Black Cardiologists *Am. Heart J.* 2013; 165(4): 468 – 476.

[139] Harshfield GA, Hwang C, Grim CE. Circadian variation of blood pressure in blacks: influence of age, gender and activity. *J. Hum. Hypertens*. 1990; 4: 43–47.

[140] Profant J, Dimsdale JE. Race and diurnal blood pressure patterns. A review and meta-analysis. *Hypertension*. 1999; 33: 1099 – 1104.

[141] Kikuya M, Ohkubo T, Asayama K, Metoki H, Obara T, Saito S, Hashimoto J, Totsune K, Hoshi H, Satoh H, Imai Y. Ambulatory blood pressure and 10-year risk of cardiovascular and noncardiovascular mortality: the Ohasama study. *Hypertension.* 2005; 45: 240–245.

[142] Veterans Administration Cooperative Study Group on Antihypertensive Agents. Racial differences in response to low-dose captopril are abolished by the addition of hydrochlorthiazide. *Br. J. Clin. Pharmacol.* 1982; 14(suppl 2):97–101.

[143] Brewster LM, van Montfrans GA, Kleijnen J. Systematic review: antihypertensive drug therapy in black patients. *Ann. Intern Med.* 2004; 141: 614–627

[144] The 1988 Report of the Joint National Committee on Detection, Evaluation, and Treatment of High Blood Pressure. *Arch. Intern Med.* 1988; 148:1023–1038.

[145] Zing W, Ferguson RK, Vlasses PH. Calcium antagonists in elderly and black hypertensive patients: therapeutic controversies. *Arch. Intern Med.* 1991;151:2154 – 2162.

[146] Psaty BM, Smith NL, Siscovick DS, Koepsell TD, Weiss NS, Heckbert SR, et al. Health outcomes associated with antihypertensive therapies used as first-line agents. A systematic review and meta-analysis. *JAMA* 2004; 277: 739–745.

[147] van Brummelen P, Man in 't Veld AJ, Schalekamp MA. Hemodynamic changes during long-term thiazide treatment of essential hypertension in responders and nonresponders. *Clin. Pharmacol. Ther* 1980; 27:328.

[148] Wright JM, Musini VM. First-line drugs for hypertension. *Cochrane Database Syst Rev.* 2009; (3):CD001841.

[149] Quynh BUI. First-Line Treatment for Hypertension. *Am. Famhysician.* 2010 Jun 1;81(11):1333-1335.

[150] ALLHAT Officers and Coordinators for the ALLHAT Collaborative Research Group. The Antihypertensive and Lipid-Lowering Treatment to Prevent Heart Attack Trial: major outcomes in high-risk hypertensive patients randomized to angiotensin-converting enzyme inhibitor or calcium channel blocker vs diuretic. *JAMA.* 2002; 288(23): 2981-2997.

[151] Wing LM, Reid CM, Ryan P, Beilin LJ, Brown MA, Jennings GL, et al. A comparison of outcomes with angiotensin-converting-enzyme inhibitors and diuretics for hypertension in the elderly. *N. Engl. J. Med.* 2003; 348: 583 – 592.

[152] Hypertension Detection and Follow-up Program Cooperative Group. Blood pressure studies in 14 communities: a two-stage screen for hypertension. *JAMA* 1977; 237:2385 –2391.

[153] NICE hypertension guideline 2011: evidence based evolution. *BMJ* 2012; 344:e181 doi: http://dx.doi.org/10.1136/bmj.e181.

[154] James PA, Oparil S, Carter BL, Cushman WC, Dennison-Himmelfarb C, Handler J, et al. 2014 Evidence-Based Guideline for the Management of High Blood Pressure in Adults Report From the Panel Members Appointed to the Eighth Joint National Committee (JNC 8) *JAMA.* 2014;311(5):507-520. doi:10.1001/jama.2013.284427.

[155] Sever PS. The Anglo-Scandinavian Cardiac Outcomes Trial: Implications and Further Outcomes. *Hypertension.* 2012; 60: 248 – 259.

[156] Saunders E, Weir MR, Kong BW, Hollifield J, Gray J, Vertes V, et al. A comparison of the efficacy and safety of a beta-blocker, a calcium channel blocker and a converting enzyme inhibitor in hypertensive blacks. *Arch. Intern Med* 1990; 150: 1707 – 1713.

[157] Materson BJ, Reda DJ, Cushman WC, Massie BM, Freis ED, Kochar MS, et al. Single-drug therapy for hypertension in men. A comparison of six antihypertensive agents with placebo. *N. Engl. J. Med* 1993; 328:914–21.

[158] Carr AA, Prisant LM. The new calcium antagonist isradipine. Effect on blood pressure and the left ventricle in black hypertensive patients. *Am. J. Hypertens* 1990; 3:8.

[159] Pinhas Sareli, MD; Ivelin V. Radevski, MD; Zdravka P. Valtchanova, MD; Elena Libhaber, MSc; Geoffrey P. Candy, MSc; Elly Den Hond, DSc; Carlos Libhaber, MD; Daniel Skudicky, MD; Ji G. Wang, MD; Jan A. Staessen, MD. Efficacy of Different Drug Classes Used to Initiate Antihypertensive Treatment in Black Subjects Results of

a Randomized Trial in Johannesburg, South Africa FREE *Arch. Intern Med.* 2001;161(7):965-971. doi:10.1001/archinte.161.7.965.

[160] Epstein M. Calcium antagonists and the kidney: implications for renal protection. *J. Cardiovasc. Pharmacol.* 1991; 18:S64–S70.

[161] Zucchelli P, Zuccala A, Borghi M, et al. Long-term comparison between coptopril and nifedipine in the progression of renal insufficiency. *Kidney Int.* 1992; 42:452–8.

[162] Bakris GL, Mangrum A, Copley JB, Vicknair N, Sadler R. Effect of calcium channel or beta-blockade on the progression of diabetic nephropathy in African Americans. *Hypertension* 1997; 29:744–50.

[163] The SOLVD Investigators. Effect of enalapril on mortality and the development of heart failure in asymptomatic patients with reduced left ventricular ejection fraction. *N. Engl. J. Med.* 1992; 327: 685 – 691.

[164] Fox KM, Henderson JR, Bertrand ME, Ferrari R, Remme WJ, Simoons ML. The European trial on reduction of cardiac events with perindopril in stable coronary artery disease (EUROPA). *Eur. Heart J.* 1998; 19 Suppl J: J52 –J55.

[165] Laura C. van Vark, Michel Bertrand, K. Martijn Akkerhuis, Jasper J. Brugts, Kim Fox, Jean-Jacques Mourad, and Eric Boersma. Angiotensin-converting enzyme inhibitors reduce mortality in hypertension: a meta-analysis of randomized clinical trials of renin–angiotensin–aldosterone system inhibitors involving 158 998 patients *European Heart Journal.* 2012 doi:10.1093/eurheartj/ehs075.

[166] Drayer JIM, Weber MA. Monotherapy of essential hypertension with a converting-enzyme inhibitor.*Hypertension* 1983; 5(suppl 3):108–13.

[167] Taguma Y, et al. Effect of captopril on heavy proteiuria in azotaemic diabetes. *N. Engl. J. Med.* 1985; 313:1617–20.

[168] Douglas JG, Bakris GL, Epstein M, Ferdinand KC, Ferrario C, Flack JM et al. Management of high blood pressure in African Americans: consensus statement of the Hypertension in African Americans Working Group of the International Society on Hypertension in Blacks. *Arch. Intern Med* 2003 10; 163(5): 525 – 541.

[169] Wright JT Jr, Bakris G, Greene T, et al.; African American Study of Kidney Disease and Hypertension Study Group. Effect of blood pressure lowering and antihypertensive drug class on progression of hypertensive kidney disease: results from the AASK trial. *JAMA*. 2002; 288(19): 2421 – 2431.

[170] Mancia G, Fagard R, Narkiewicz K, Redon J, Zanchetti A, Bohm M et al., on behalf of Task Force Members. 2013 ESH/ESC Guidelines for the management of arterial hypertension: the Task Force for the management of arterial hypertension of the European Society of Hypertension (ESH) and of the European Society of Cardiology (ESC). *J. Hypertens.* 2013 Jul;31(7):1281 - 1357. doi: 10.1097/01.hjh.0000 431740.32696.cc.

[171] Doulougou B, Kouanda S, Ouédraogo GH, Meda BI, Bado A, Zunzunegui MV. Awareness, treatment, control of hypertension and utilization of health care services following screening in the North-central region of Burkina Faso Pan *African Medical Journal*. 2014; 19.259. doi:10.11604/pamj.2014.19.259.4707.

[172] Dzudie A, Kengne AP, Muna WFT, et al. Prevalence, awareness, treatment and control of hypertension in a selfselected sub-Saharan African urban population: a crosssectional study. *BMJ Open* 2012;0:e001217. doi:10.1136/bmjopen-2012- 001217

[173] Ulasi II, Ijoma CK, Onwubere BJ, Arodiwe E, Onodugo O, Okafor C High prevalence and low awareness of hypertension in a market population in Enugu, Nigeria. *Int. J.. Hypertens.* 2011 ;2011():869675.
[174] Temmar M, Labat C, Benkhedda S, Charifid M, Thomas F, Bouafia MT, Beane K, Darne B, Safar ME, Benetos A. Prevalence and determinants of hypertension in the Algerian Sahara. *Journal of Hypertension* 2007; 25: 2218 – 2226.
[175] Duboz P, Boëtsch G, Gueye L, Macia E. Hypertension prevalence, awareness, treatment and control in Dakar (Senegal). *Journal of Human Hypertension* 28, 489-493 (August 2014) | doi:10.1038/jhh.2013.142.
[176] Tesfaye F, Byass P, Wall S. Population based prevalence of high blood pressure among adults in Addis Ababa: uncovering a silent epidemic. *BMC Cardiovascular Disorders* 2009, 9:39 doi:10.1186/1471-2261-9-39.
[177] van de Vijver SJ, Oti SO, Agyemang C, Gomez GB, Kyobutungi C. Prevalence, awareness, treatment and control of hypertension among slum dwellers in Nairobi, Kenya. *J. Hypertens.* 2013 May; 31(5): 1018 – 1024.
[178] Damasceno A, Azevedo A, Silva-Matos C, Prista A, Diogo A, Lunet N. Hypertension Prevalence, Awareness, Treatment, and Control in Mozambique: Urban/Rural Gap During Epidemiological Transition. *Hypertension* 2009; 54: 77 – 83.
[179] Musinguzi G, Nuwaha F (2013) Prevalence, Awareness and Control of Hypertension in Uganda. *PLoS ONE* 8(4): e62236. doi:10.1371/journal.pone.0062236
[180] Ibrahim M M. Epidemiology of Hypertension in Egypt. *Saudi J Kidney Dis Transpl* 1999; 10: 352 – 356.
[181] Steyn K, Gaziano TA, Bradshaw D, Laubscher R, Fourie JM. Hypertension in South African adults: results from the Demographic and Health Survey, 1998. *J. Hypertens* 2001; 19: 1717 – 1725.
[182] Ekwunife OI, Udeogaranya PO, Nwatu IL: Prevalence, awareness, treatment and control of hypertension in a Nigerian population. *Health* 2010; 2(7): 731 – 735.
[183] Appel L. Lifestyle Modification as a Means to Prevent and Treat High Blood Pressure. *J. Am. Soc. Nephrol.* 2003; 14: S99–S102.
[184] Whelton PK, He J, Appel LJ, Cutler JA, Havas S, Kotchen TA, et al. Primary prevention of hypertension: clinical and public health advisory from the National High Blood Pressure Education Program. *JAMA* 2002;288:1882-8.
[185] He J, Whelton PK, Appel LJ, Charleston J, Klag MJ. Long-term effects of weight loss and dietary sodium reduction on incidence of hypertension.*Hypertension* 2000;35:544-9.
[186] Subramanian H, Soudarssanane MB, Jayalakshmy R, Thiruselvakumar D, Navasakthi D, Sahai A, Saptharishi LG. Non-pharmacological interventions in hypertension: A Community -based cross-over Randomized Controlled Trial. *Indian J. Community Med.* 2011 Jul-Sep; 36(3): 191–196. doi: 10.4103/0970-0218.86519.
[187] Sarrafzadegan N, Kelishadi R, Esmaillzadeh A, Mohammadifard N, Roohafza H, Azadbakht L, et al. Do lifestyle interventions work in developing countries? Findings from the Isfahan Healthy Heart Program in the Islamic Republic of Iran. *Bull World Health Ogan* 2009; 87: 39–50 | doi:10.2471/BLT.07.049841.
[188] Whelton PK, He J, Appel LJ, Cutler JA, Havas S, Kotchen TA, et al. Primary prevention of hypertension: Clinical and public health advisory from The National High Blood Pressure Education Program. *JAMA*. 2002; 288: 1882 – 1888.

[189] Stamler J, Rose G, Elliott P, Dyer A, Marmot M, Kesteloot, Stamler R. Findings of the International Coopertaive INTERSALT study. *Hypertension.* 1991; 17 (1 Suppl): 15 – 19.

[190] Sacks FM, Svetkey LP, Vollmer WM, Appel LJ, Bray GA, Harsha D, et al. Effects on blood pressure of reduced dietary sodium and the Dietary Approaches to Stop Hypertension (DASH) diet. *N. Engl. J. Med* 2001; 344: 3 - 10.

[191] Whelton PK, Appel LJ, Espeland MA, Applegate WB, Ettinger WH Jr, Kostis JB, et al. Sodium reduction and weight loss in the treatment of hypertension in older persons: a randomized controlled trial of nonpharmacologic interventions in the elderly (TONE) [published correction appears in JAMA 1998;279:1954]. *JAMA* 1998; 279:839 - 846.

[192] WHO/ISH. Prevention of cardiovascular disease: guidelines for assessment and management of total cardiovascular risk. *World Health Organization.* Geneva 2007.

[193] Joint FAO/WHO Expert Consultation. Interim Summary of Conclusions and Dietary Recommendations on Total Fat & Fatty Acids http://www.fao.org/ag/agn/nutrition/docs /Fats%20and%20Fatty%20Acids%20Summary.pdf

[194] Kelley GA, Kelley KS. Progressive resistance exercise and resting blood pressure: a meta-analysis of randomized controlled trials. *Hypertension.* 2000; 35: 838 – 843.

[195] Whelton SP, Chin A, Xin X, He J. Effect of aerobic exercise on blood pressure: a meta-analysis of randomized, controlled trials. *Ann. Intern Med.* 2002; 136: 493 – 503.

[196] Collins R, Peto R, MacMahon S, Hebert P, Fiebach NH, Eberlein KA, Godwin J, Qizilbash N, Taylor JO, Hennekens CH. Blood pressure, stroke, and coronary heart disease, part 2: short-term reductions in blood pressure: overview of randomised drug trials in their epidemiological context. *Lancet.* 1990; 335: 827 – 838.

[197] Minami J, Ishimitsu T, Matsuoka H. Hypertension Effects of Smoking Cessation on Blood Pressure and Heart Rate Variability in Habitual *Smokers.* 1999; 33 [part II]: 586-590.

[198] Brook RD, Appel LJ, Rubenfire M, Ogedegbe G, Bisognano JD, Elliott WJ, et al.; on behalf of the American Heart Association Professional Education Committee of the Council for High Blood Pressure Research, Council on Cardiovascular and Stroke Nursing, Council on Epidemiology and Prevention, and Council on Nutrition, Physical Activity and Metabolism.Beyond Medications and Diet: Alternative Approaches to Lowering Blood Pressure A Scientific Statement From the American Heart Association. *Hypertension.* 2013; 61: 00-00

[199] Schneider RH, Staggers F, Alexander CN, Sheppard W, Rainforth M, Kondwani K, et al. A randomised controlled trial of stress reduction for hypertension in older African Americans. *Hypertension* 1995; 26: 820 - 827.

[200] Schneider RH, Alexander CN, Staggers F, Rainforth M, Salerno JW,Hartz A, et al. Long-term effects of stress reduction on mortality in persons > or = 55 years of age with systemic hypertension. *Am. J. Cardiol.* 2005; 95: 1060 - 1064.

[201] Nicoll R, Henein MY. Hypertension and lifestyle modification: how useful are the guidelines? British Journal of General Practice, *December 2010* DOI: 10.3399/bjgp10X544014.

[202] J R M'Buyamba-Kabangu, B C Anisiuba, M B Ndiaye, D Lemogoum, L Jacobs, C K Ijoma, L Thijs, H J Boombhi, J Kaptue, P M Kolo, J B Mipinda, C E Osakwe, A Odili, B Ezeala-Adikaibe, S Kingue, B A Omotoso, S A Ba, I I Ulasi and J A Staessen on behalf of the Newer versus Older Antihypertensive Agents in African Hypertensive

Patients Trial (NOAAH) Investigators. Efficacy of newer versus older antihypertensive drugs in black patients living in sub-Saharan Africa. *Journal of Human Hypertension advance online publication* 27 June 2013; doi: 10.1038/jhh.2013.56.

[203] Wright JT, Agodoa LY, Appel L, Cushman WC, Taylor AL, Obegdegbe GG, Osei K, Reed J. New Recommendations for Treating Hypertension in Black Patients Evidence and/or Consensus? *Hypertension.* 2010; 56: 801 – 803.

[204] Ogah OS, Okpechi I, Chukwunonye II, Akinyemi JO, et al. Blood Pressure: Prevalence of Hypertension and Hypertension-Related Complications in Nigerian Africans. A Review. *World J. Cardiol.* 2012 Dec 26; 4(12): 327-340

[205] Cheung BMY, Cheung TT. Challenges in the management of hypertension in Asia. *European Heart Journal Supplements* (2012) 14 (Supplement A), A37–A38

[206] Ferdinand KC. Hypertension in Blacks. In: Hypertension Primer, 4th ed. Ch. B85. Izzo JL, Sica DA, Black HR. eds. Lippincot Williams and Wilkins, Philadelphia. 2008, page 280.

[207] Pires JE, Sebastiao YV, Langa AJ, Nery SV: Hypertension in Northern Angola: prevalence, associated factors, awareness, treatment and control. *BMC Publ Health* 2013, 13(1):90.

[208] Ilesanmi OS, Ige OK, Adebiyi AO. The managed hypertensive: the costs of blood pressure control in a Nigerian town. *The Pan African Medical Journal.* 2012; 12: 96

[209] Onwujekwe O, Hanson K, Ichoku H, Uzochukwu B. Financing incidence analysis of house hold out-of-pocket spending for health: getting more health for money in Nigeria? *Int. J. Health Plann Manage* 2014 April-June; 29 (2): e174 –e185

[210] Chen L-C, Lee Y-Y, Lin T-H, Lee C-S, Li C-J, Wu D-C. How Does Out-of-Pocket Payment Affect Choices When Accessing Health Care?—A Qualitative Study on Hypertensive Outpatients in Southern Taiwan. *VALUE IN HEALTH REGIONAL ISSUES 1* (2012): 105–110.

[211] US Department of Human and Health Services. HHS Action Plan to Reduce Racial and Ethnic Health Disparities: A nation free of disparities in health and health care. (Online). Available from: http://minorityhealth.hhs.gov/npa/files/Plans/HHS /HHS_Plan_complete.pdf

[212] Dennison CR, Miller NH. Adherence to Antihypertensive Therapy. In: Hypertension Primer, 4th ed. Ch. C123. Izzo JL, Sica DA, Black HR. eds. Lippincot Williams and Wilkins, Philadelphia. 2008, page 414.

[213] Parker R. Health literacy: a challenge for American patients and their health care providers. *Health Promotion International* 2000. 15, No. 4: 277 - 283.

[214] FN Chukwuneke, CT Ezeonu, BN Onyire, PO Ezeonu, N Ifebunandu, MC Umeora. Health Seeking Behaviour and Access to Health Care Facilities at the Primary level in Nigeria: our experience. *Ebonyi Medical Journal* 2012; 11 (1-2): 51 - 57

[215] Ogedegbe G, Mancuso CA, Allegrante JP. Expectations of blood pressure management in hypertensive African-American patients: a qualitative study. *J. Natl. Med. Assoc.* 2004; 96:442 – 449.

[216] Ghembaza MA, Senoussaoui Y, Tani MK, Meguenni K. Impact of patient knowledge of hypertension complications on adherence to antihypertensive therapy. *Curr. Hypertens Rev.* 2014;10(1):41 - 48.

[217] Scisney-Matlock M, Bosworth HB, Giger JN, Strickland OL, et al. Strategies for Implementing and Sustaining Therapeutic Lifestyle Changes as Part of Hypertension Management in African Americans. *Postgrad Med.* 2009 May; 121(3): 147–159.
[218] Lemogoum D. Challenge for Hypertension Prevention and Control Worldwide: The Time for Action. *The Journal of Clinical Hypertension August* 2014; 16(8): 554-556.
[219] Mancia G, De BG, Dominiczak A, Cifkova R, Fagard R, Germano G, et al. 2007 ESH-ESC practice guidelines for the management of arterial hypertension: ESH-ESC Task Force on the Management of Arterial Hypertension. *J. Hypertens.* 2007;25:1751–1762. doi: 10.1097/HJH.0b013e3282f0580f
[220] Huebschmann AG[1], Mizrahi T, Soenksen A, Beaty BL, Denberg TD. Reducing clinical inertia in hypertension treatment: a pragmatic randomized controlled trial. *J Clin Hypertens* (Greenwich). 2012 May; 14(5): 322 - 329.
[221] Elliot JW. The Economic Impact of Hypertension. *J Clin Hypertens* 2003; 5(3 suppl 2): 3-13.
[222] Gaziano JM, Manson JE, Ridker PM. Primary and Secondary Prevention of Coronary Heart Disease. In: Braunwald's Heart Disease 8th ed. Libby P, Bonow RO, Mann DL, Zipes DP (eds). Philadelphia. Saunders. Ch. 45:Page 1132.
[223] Elliot WJ. Economic Considerations in Hypertension Management. In:Hypertension Primer, 4th ed. Ch. B102. Izzo JL, Sica DA, Black HR. eds. Lippincot Williams and Wilkins, Philadelphia. 2008. Pg. 333.
[224] Smith SM, Campbell JD. Cost-Effectiveness of Renin-Guided Treatment of Hypertension. *Am. J. Hypertens* Nov 2013; 26(11): 1303-1310.
[225] Gibbs CR, Beevers DG.The management of hypertensive disease in Black patients. QJM 1999; 92 (4): 187 – 192. DOI: http://dx.doi.org/10.1093/qjmed/92.4.187 187-192 First published online: 1 April 1999.
[226] Cruickshank JK, Beevers DG, Osbourne VL, Haynes RA, Corlett JC, Selby S. Heart attack, stroke, diabetes and hypertension in West Indians, Asians and whites in Birmingham, England. *Br. Med. J.* 1980; 281:1108.
[227] Shulman NB, Hall WD. Renal vascular disease in African-Americans and other racial minorities. *Circulation* 1991; 83:1477 – 1479.
[228] Hammond IW, Devereux RB, Alderman MH, Lutas EM, Spitzer MC, Crowley JS, et al. The prevalence and correlates of echocardiographic left ventricular hypertrophy among employed patients with uncomplicated hypertension. *J. Am. Coll. Cardiol.* 1986; 7:639–50.
[229] Zarotti R. A review on ethnic differences in plasma triglycerides and high-density-lipoprotein cholesterol: is the lipid pattern the key factor for the low coronary heart disease rate in people of African origin? *Eur. J. Epidemiol.* 1998; 14 (1): 9 – 21.
[230] Enas E A, Senthilkumar A, Vinod C, Puthumana N. Dyslipidaemia among Indo-Asians strategies for identification and management. *Br. J. Diabetes. Vasc. Dis.* 2005; 5: 81 – 90.
[231] Heffernan KS, Jae SY, Wilund KR, Woods JA, Fernhall B. Racial differences in central blood pressure and vascular function in young men. *Am. J. Physiol. Heart Circ. Physiol.* 2008; 295: H2380–H2387.
[232] Din-Dzietham R, Couper D, Evans G, Arnett DK, Jones DW. Arterial stiffness is greater in African Americans than in whites: evidence from the Forsyth County, North Carolina, ARIC cohort. *Am. J. Hypertens.* 2004; 17: 304– 313.

[233] D'Agostino RB Jr, Burke G, O'Leary D, Rewers M, Selby J, Savage PJ, Saad MF, et al. Ethnic differences in carotid wall thickness: the Insulin Resistance Atherosclerosis Study. *Stroke*. 1996; 27: 1744 – 1749.

[234] Ferreira AV, Viana MC, Mill JG, Asmar RG, Cunha RS. Racial differences in aortic stiffness in normotensive and hypertensive adults. *J. Hypertens.* 1999; 17: 631 – 637.

[235] Neal L, Greene EL. Pathophysiology of chronic progressive renal disease in the African American patient with hypertension. *Am. J. Med Sci.* 2002; 323: 72 – 77.

[236] Brown MD, Feairheller DL, Thakkar S, Veerabhadrappa P, Park J. Racial differences in tumor necrosis factor-α-induced endothelial microparticles and interleukin-6 production. *Vascular Health and Risk Management* 2011:7 541–550.

[237] Brenner BM, Garcia DL, Anderson S. Glomeruli and blood pressure. Less of one, more the other? *Am. J. Hypertens* 1988; 1: 335 - 347.

[238] Cheng C, Daskalakis C, Falkner B. Alterations in capillary morphology are found in mild blood pressure elevation *Journal of Hypertension*: November 2010 - Volume 28 - Issue 11 - p 2258–2266.

[239] Etyang AO, and Scott JAG. Medical causes of admissions to hospital among adults in Africa: a systematic review. *Glob Health Action* 2013, 6: 19090 http://dx.doi.org/10.3402/gha.v6i0.19090].

[240] Kolo PM, Jibrin YB, Sanya EO, M. Alkali M, Peter Kio B, Moronkola RK Hypertension-Related Admissions and Outcome in a Tertiary Hospital in Northeast Nigeria. *International Journal of Hypertension*, Volume 2012 (2012), Article ID 960546, 6 pages http://dx.doi.org/10.1155/2012/960546.

[241] Osuji CU, Onwubuya EI, Ahaneku GI, Omejua EG. Pattern of cardiovascular admissions at Nnamdi Azikiwe University Teaching Hospital Nnewi, South East Nigeria. *The Pan African Medical Journal.* 2014;17:116.

[242] American Heart Association. 2003 Heart Disease and Stroke Statistics—Update. Dallas, TX: American Heart Association; 2002.

[243] Anjorin CO, Buba F, Eneh AC. Myocardial infarction at the University of Maiduguri Teaching Hospital, North Eastern Nigeria: A long term review. *J. Med. Sci.* 2005; 5: 358-362

[244] Thomas J, Thomas DJ, Pearson T, et al. Cardiovascular disease in African American and white physicians: the Meharry cohort and Meharry-Hopkins cohort studies. *J. Health Care Poor Underserved.* 1997;8:270–284.

[245] Flack JM, Ferdinand KC, Nasser SA. Epidemiology of hypertension and cardiovascular disease in African Americans. *J. Clin. Hypertens.* 2003;5(1 suppl 1):5–11.

[246] Adebiyi AA, Ogah OS, Aje A, Ojji DB, Adebayo AK, Oladapo OO, Falase AO. Echocardiographic partition values and prevalence of left ventricular hypertrophy in hypertensive Nigerians. *BMC Med. Imaging* 2006; 6: 10.

[247] Flack JM, Gardin JM, Yunis C, et al., for the CARDIA Research Group. Static and pulsatile blood pressure correlates of left ventricular structure and function in black and white young adults: the CARDIA study. *Am. Heart J.* 1999;138:856–864.

[248] Ogah OS, Bamgboye AE. Correlates of left ventricular mass in hypertensive Nigerians: an echocardiographic study. *Cardiovasc J Afr* 2010; 21: 79-85.

[249] Anisiuba BC, Ejim EC, Onwubere BJC, Ikeh VO, et al. Atrial fibrillation cases seen at the University of Nigeria Teaching Hospital, *Enugu. JCM* Dec 2005; 10(2): 102-106.

[250] Vester EG. Arterial hypertension and cardiac arrhythmias. *Dtsch Med. Wochenschr.* 2008 Dec;133 Suppl 8:S261-5. doi: 10.1055/s-0028-1100958. Epub 2008 Dec 15. (Article in German).

[251] Gillum RF. The epidemiology of cardiovascular disease in black Americans (editorial). *N. Engl. J. Med.* 1996; 335:1597-1598.

[252] Makin A, Lip GYH, Silverman S, Beevers DG. Peripheral vascular disease and hypertension: a forgotten association? *Journal of Human Hypertension* (2001) 15, 447 – 454.

[253] Kannel WB. Role of blood pressure in cardiovascular morbidity and mortality. *Prog. Cardiovasc. Dis.* 1974; 17: 5 – 24.

[254] Violi F, Criqui M, Longoni A, Castiglioni C. Relation between risk factors and cardiovascular complications in patients with peripheral vascular disease. Results from the A.D.E.P. study. *Atherosclerosis* 1996; 120: 25 – 35.

[255] Cheng SW, Ting AC, Lau H, Wong J. Epidemiology of atherosclerotic peripheral arterial occlusive disease in Hong Kong. *World J. Surg.* 1999; 23: 202 – 206.

[256] Droste DW, Ritter MA, Dittrich R, Heidenreich S, Wichter T, Freund M, Ringelstein EB. Arterial hypertension and ischaemic stroke. *Acta Neurologica Scandinavica.* 2003; 107 (4): 241–251 DOI: 10.1034/j.1600-0404.2003.00098.x

[257] Goldstein LB, Adams R, Becker K, et al. Primary prevention of ischemic stroke. *Circulation.* 2001; 103 (1): 163 – 181.

[258] Ferro JM. Update on intracerebral haemorrhage. *Journal of Neurology.* 2006; 253 (8): 985 - 999.

[259] Ariesen MJ, Claus SP, Rinkel GJE, Algra A. Risk Factors for Intracerebral Hemorrhage in the General Population. A Systematic Review. *Stroke.* 2003;34:2060 - 2066.

[260] Qureshi AI, Tuhrim S, Broderick JP, Batjer HH, Hondo H, Hanley DF. Spontaneous Intracerebral Hemorrhage. *N. Engl. J. Med.* 2001; 344:1450-1460. DOI: 10.1056/NEJM200105103441907

[261] Weir BRA, M.D., Gail L. Kongable GL , Kassel NF, , Schultz JR, Truskowski LL Sigrest A. Cigarette smoking as a cause of aneurysmal subarachnoid hemorrhage and risk for vasospasm: a report of the Cooperative Aneurysm Study. *Journal of Neurosurgery September* 1998 ; 89(3): 405 – 411.

[262] Isaksen J, Egge A, Waterloo K, Romner B, Ingebrigtsen T. Risk factors for aneurysmal subarachnoid haemorrhage: The Tromsø study J Neurol *Neurosurg Psychiatry* 2002; 73: 185 – 187.

[263] Al-Shahi R. Subarachnoid haemorrhage. *BMJ* 2006; 333:235.

[264] Skoog I, Nilsson L, Persson G, Lernfelt B, Landahl S, Palmertz B, Andreasson LA, Odén A, Svanborg A15-year longitudinal study of blood pressure and dementia. *The Lancet1996*; 347, (9009): 1141 – 1145.

[265] Peila R, White LR, Masaki K, Petrovitch H, Launer LJ. Reducing the Risk of Dementia Efficacy of Long-Term Treatment of Hypertension. *Stroke;* 2006; 37: 1165 – 1170.

[266] Ogunniyi A, Lane KA, Baiyewu O, Gao S, Gureje O, Unverzagt FW et al. Hypertension and incident dementia in community-dwelling elderly Yoruba Nigerians. *Acta Neurologica Scandinavica* 2011; 124 (6): 396 – 402.

[267] Centers for Disease Control and Prevention. Public health and aging: trends in aging-- United States and worldwide. *JAMA.* 2003; 19; 289 (11): 1371 - 1373.

[268] Sachdev P, Vascular cognitive disorder. *Int. J. Geriatr Psychiatry* 1999; 14: 402 – 403.

[269] Miles PE, Froehlich TE, Borgadus Jnr. ST, Inouye SK. Dementia: Are there differences between Africa American and Caucasians. *Journal of the American geriatric Society*. 2001; 49 (4): 477 – 484.
[270] Chatterjee S, Chattopadhya S, Hope-Ross M, et. al. Hypertension and the eye: changing perspectives. *J. Hum. Hypertens* 2002; 16: 667-675. *Journal of Human Hypertension* (2002) 16**,** 667-675. doi: 10.1038/sj.jhh.1001472
[271] Garner, A. Ashton N. Pathogenesis of hypertensive retinopathy: a review. *J. R. Soc. Med.* 1979; 72: 362 - 365.
[272] Talks SJ, Good P, Clough CG, Beevers DG, Dodson SJ. The acute and long-term ocular effects of accelerated hypertension: a clinical and electrophysiological study. *Eye* 1996; 10 (Pt 3): 321 - 327.
[273] Kishi S, Tso MOM, Hayreh SS. Fundus lesions in malignant hypertension. II. A pathologic study of experimental hypertensive optic neuropathy. *Arch. Ophthalmol.* 1985; 103**:** 1198 - 1206.
[274] Hayreh SS, Servais GE, Virdi PS**.** Fundus lesions in malignant hypertension. V. Hypertensive choroidopathy. *Ophthalmology* 1986; 93: 1383 - 1400.
[275] Marín R, Gorostidi M, Fernández-Vega F, Alvarez-Navascués R. Systemic and glomerular hypertension and progression of chronic renal disease: the dilemma of nephrosclerosis. *Kidney Int.* Suppl 2005; 68 (99): S52 – S56.
[276] Lindhorst J, Alexander N, Blignaut J, Rayner B. Difference in hypertension between blacks and whites: an overview. *Cardiovasular Journal of Africa* 2007; 18 (4): 241 – 247.
[277] Kwoh C, Shannon MB, Miner JH, Shaw A. Pathogenesis of non-immune glomerulopathies. *Annual review of Pathology* 2006; 1: 349 – 374.
[278] Bogomir Žižek (2012). Target Organ Damage in Essential Hypertension, Genetics and Pathophysiology of Essential Hypertension, Prof. Madhu Khullar (Ed.), ISBN: 978-953-51-0282-3, InTech, Available from: http://www.intechopen.com/books/genetics-and pathophysiology-of-essential-hypertension/target-organ-damage-in-essential-hypertension
[279] Muirhead EE, Pitcock JA. Histopathology of severe renal vascular damage in blacks. *Clinical Cardiology* 1989; 12 (12 Suppl 4): IV 58 – 65.
[280] Linz W, Becker RH, Schölkens BA, Wiemer G, Keil M, Langer KH. Nephroprotection by long-term ACE inhibition with Ramipril in spontaneously hypertensive stroke prone rats. *Kidney Int.* 1998; 54 (6): 2037 – 2044.
[281] Levey AS, Cattran D, Friedman A. Miller WG, Sedor J, Tuttle K., et al. Proteinuria as a surrogate outcome in CKD: report of a scientific workshop sponsored by national Kidney Foundation and the US Food and Drug Administration. *Am. J. Kidney Dis.* 2009; 54: 205–26.
[282] Ellison DH, Loffing J. Thiazide Effects and Adverse Effects Insights From Molecular Genetics. *Hypertension* 2009; 54: 196 – 202.
[283] Vela´zquez H, Wright FS. Control by drugs of renal potassium handling. *Ann Rev Pharmacol Toxicol* 1986; 26: 293 – 309.
[284] Okusa MD, Velazquez H, Ellison DH, Wright FS. Luminal calcium regulates potassium transport by the renal distal tubule. *Am. J. Physiol* 1990; 258: F423 – F428.
[285] Myers MG. Diuretic therapy and ventricular arrhythmias in persons 65years of age and older. *Am. J. Cardiol* 1990; 65: 599 – 603.

[286] Siegel D, Hulley SB, Black DM, Cheitlin MD, Sebastian A, Seeley DG, Hearst N, Fine R. Diuretics, serum and intracellular electrolyte levels, and ventricular arrhythmias in hypertensive men. *JAMA 1992;267: 1083 – 1089.*

[287] Siscovick DS, Raghunathan TE, Psaty BM, Koepsell TD, Wicklund KG, Lin X, Cobb L, Rautaharju PM, Copass MK, Wagner EH. Diuretic therapy for hypertension and the risk of primary cardiac arrest. *N. Engl. J. Med.* 1994; 330: 1852–1857.

[288] Papademetriou V: Diuretics, hypokalemia, and cardiac arrhythmia: a 20-year controversy. *J. Clin. Hypertens* (Greenwich) 2006; 8: 86.

[289] Gross P and Palm C: Thiazides: do they kill? *Nephrol. Dial Transplant* 2005; 20: 2299.

[290] Sonnenblick M, Friedlander Y and Rosin AJ: Diuretic-induced severe hyponatremia. Review and analysis of 129 reported patients. *Chest* 1993; 103: 601.

[291] Seino S, Iwanaga T, Nagashima K, Miki T. Diverse roles of K(ATP) channels learned from Kir6.2 genetically engineered mice. *Diabetes*. 2000; 49: 311 – 318.

[292] Gillis KD, Gee WM, Hammoud A, McDaniel ML, Falke LC, Misler S. Effects of sulfonamides on a metabolite-regulated ATPi-sensitive K+ channel in rat pancreatic B-cells. *Am. J. Physiol.* 1989; 257: C1119 – C1127.

[293] Salvetti A, Ghiadoni L. Thiazide Diuretics in the Treatment of Hypertension: An Update. JASN April 2006; 17 (4 suppl 2): S25 - S29.

[294] Gurwitz JH, Kalish SC, Bohn RL, Glynn RJ, Monane M, Mogun H et al.: Thiazide diuretics and the initiation of anti-gout therapy. *J. Clin. Epidemiol.* 1997; 50**:** 953.

[295] Goldman AI, Steele BW, Schnaper HW, Fitz AE, Frohlich ED and Perry HM Jr: Serum lipoprotein levels during chlorthalidone therapy. A Veterans Administration-National Heart, Lung,and Blood Institute cooperative study on antihypertensive therapy: mild hypertension. *JAMA* 1980; 244**:** 1691.

[296] Grimm RH Jr, Leon AS, Hunninghake DB, Lenz K, Hannan P and Blackburn H: Effects of thiazide diuretics on plasma lipids and lipoproteins in mildly hypertensive patients: a double-blind controlled trial. *Ann. Intern Med* 1981; 94**:** 7 - 11.

[297] Morgan T. The use of diuretic drugs and aldosterone antagonists in hypertension. In: Doyle AE, ed. Handbook of Hypertension, vol 5. Amsterdam: Elsevier, 1984:67 – 91.

[298] Expert Consensus Document on Angiotensin Converting Enzyme inhbitors in cardiovascular diseases. The task force on AE Inhibitors of the European Society of Cardiology. *European Heart journal.* 2004; 25: 1454 – 1470.

[299] Coulter DM, Edwards IR. Cough associated with captopril and cnalapril. *Br. Med. J.* 1987, 294. 1521 – 1523.

[300] Doering W, Maass L, Irmisch R, Konig E.- Pharmacokinetic interaction *study with ramipril and digoxin in heallhy volunteers. Am. J. Cardiol.* 1987; 59: 600 – 640.

[301] Bolzano K, Arriaga J, Bemal R, et al. -The antihypertensive effect of lisinopril compared to atenolol in patients with mild to moderate essential hypertension. *J. Cardiovasc. Pharmacol.* 1987; 9 (Suppl. 3): 543 - 547.

[302] Chalmers D, Dombey SL. Lawson OH. Post marketing surveillance of captopril (for hypertension): a preliminary report. *Br. J. Clin. Pharmacol.* 1987; 24; 343 - 349.

[303] Town GI, Hallwright GP, Maling TJB, O'Donnell TV. Angiotensin converting enzyme inhibitors and cough. *NZ Med. J.* 1987; 100: 161 - 163.

[304] Regoli D. Barabe J. - Pharmacology of bradykinin and related peptides. *Pharmacal. Rev.* 1980; 32: 1-46.

[305] Casceiri MA, Bull HO, Murnford RA, et al. - Carboxylterminal tripeptidyl hydrolysis of substance P by purified rabbit lung angiotensin converting enzyme and the potentiation of substance P activity in vivo by captopril and MK 422. *Mol. Pharmacol.* 1984; 25: 287 – 293.

[306] Kaufman MP, Coleridge HM, Coleridge JCO, Baker DO. - Bradykinin stimulates afferent vagal C fibres in intrapulmonary airways of dogs. *J. Appl. Physiol.,* 1980; 48: 511 – 517.

[307] Rossoni 0, Omini C, Vigano T, Mandelli V, Folco GC, Berti F. - Bronchoconstriction by histamine and bradykinin in guinea-pigs: relationship to thromboxane A2 generation and the effect of aspirin. *Prostaglandins* 1980; 20: 547-557.

[308] Fuller RW, Dixon CMS. Cuss FMC, Bames PJ. - Bradykinin-induced bronchoconstriction in humans. *Am. Rev. Respir. Dis.* 1987; 135: 176 – 180.

[309] Fuller RW, Choudry NB. -Increased cough reflex associated with angiotensin converting enzyme inhibitor cough. *Br. Med. J.* 1987; 295: 1025 – 1026.

[310] Morice AH, Brown MJ, Lowry R, Higenbottam T. - Angiotensin-converting enzyme and the cough reflex. *Lancet 1*987; 2: 1116 – 1118.

[311] Coleridge HM, Coleridge JCG, Ginzcl KH, et al.- Stimulation of "irritant" receptors and afferent C fibres in the lungs by prostaglandins. *Nature* 1976; 264: 451 – 453.

[312] Berkin KE. Respiratory effects of angiotensin converting enzyme inhibition. *Eur. Respir. J.* 1989, 2, 198 – 201.

[313] Elliot WJ. Higher incidence of discontinuation of angiotensin converting enzyme inhibitor due to cough in black subjects. *Clin. Pharmacol. Ther* 1996; 60: 582 – 588.

[314] Schoolwerth AC, Sica DA, Ballermann BJ, Wilcox CS. Renal consideration in angiotensin converting enzyme inhibitor therapy. *Circulation* 2001; 104: 1985 – 1991.

[315] Bennet WM. Drug interactions and consequences of sodium restriction. *Am. J. Clin. Nutr.* 1977; 65 (2 Suppl): 687S – 681S.

[316] K/DOQI Clinical Practice Guidelines on Hypertension and Antihypertensive agents in chronic kidney disease. Use of ACE inhibitors and ARBs in chronic kidney disease, 2012. www.kidney.org/professionals/kdoqi/guidelines_bp/guide_11.htm (accessed 4 Feb 2015).

[317] Reardon LC, Macpherson DS. Hyperkalemia in outpatient using angiotensin converting enzyme inhibitors. *Arch. Intern Med.* 1998; 158: 26 – 32.

[318] Wakisaka M, Shuto M, Abe H, Tajima M, Shiroshita H, bandoh T, et al. Computed tomography of the gastrointestinal manifestation of hereditary angioedema *Radial Med. Dec* 2008; 26 (10): 618 – 621.

[319] Kostis JB, Kim HJ, Rusnak J, Casale T, Kaplan A, Corren J, Levy E. Incidence and characteristics of angioedema associated with enalapril. *Arch. Intern Med.* 2005 Jul 25;165(14):1637-42.

[320] The ALLHAT Officers and Cordinators for the ALLHAT Collaborative Research Group. Major outcomes in high risk hypertensive patients randomized to angiotensin converting enzyme inhibitor or calcium channel blocker vs diuretic: the anithypetensive and Lipid Lowering Treatment to Prevent Heart Attack Trial (ALLHAT). *JAMA.*2002; 288: 2981 - 2997.

[321] Slater EE, Merrill DD, Guess HA, et al. Clinical profile of angioedema associated with angiotensin converting inhibition. *JAMA* 1988; 260: 967 – 970.

[322] 34 Baram M, Kommuri A, Sellers SA, Cohn JA. ACE inhibitor induced angioedema. *J. Allergy Clin. Immunol. in Practice* 2013; 1: 442 – 445.

[323] Russel RP. Side Effects of Calcium Channel Blockers. *Hypertension* 1988; 11 [Suppl II]: H-42 – 44.

[324] Frishman WH. β3-Adrenergic receptor blockers: Adverse effects and drug interactions. *Hypertension* 1988; 11 [Suppl II]: II-21 - II-29.

[325] Pettinger WA,. Mitchel HC. Side Effects of Vasodilator Therapy *Hypertension* 1988; 11 [Suppl II]: II-34-II-36.

[326] Engelman K.Side Effects of Sympatholytic Antihypertensive Drugs. *Hypertension* 1988; 11 [Suppl II]: II-30-II-33.

[327] Elkington SG, Schreiber WM, Conn HO. Hepatic injury caused by L-alpha-methyldopa. *Circulation* 1969; 40: 589 - 594.

[328] Amrey A, Brixxo P, Clement D, De Schaepdryver A, Fagard R, Forte J, Henry F et al. Mortalilty and morbidity results from the European working party on high blood pressure in the elderly trial. *The Lancet* 1985; 325 (8442); 1349-1359.

[329] Duley L. Maternal mortality associated with disorders of pregnancy in Africa, Asia, Latin America and the Carribean, *BJOG.* 1992; 99: 547 - 553.

[330] Daniels DS, Meyer RA, Loggie JMH. Determinants of cardiac involvement in children and adolescents with essential hypertension. *Circulation* 1990; 82(4): 1243 – 1248.

[331] National Institute of Health. Working Group Report on high blood pressure in pregnancy. Bethesda: National institutes of Health 2000. *NIH Publication* 00-3029

[332] Report of the National High Blood Pressure Education Program Working Group on High Blood Pressure in Pregnancy. *Am. J. Obstet Gynecol.* 2000; 1831: S1 – 22.

[333] Poppas A, Shroff SG, Korcarz CE, Hibbard JU, Berger DS, Lindheimer MD, et al. Serial assess- ment of the cardiovascular system in normal pregnancy. *Circulation* 1997; 95: 2407 – 2415.

[334] van Oppen AC, Stigter RH, Bruinse HW. Cardiac output in normal pregnancy: a critical review. *Obstet Gynecol.* 1996; 87: 310–318.

[335] Diana E. Ayala, Ramón C. Hermida, Artemio Mojón, José R. Fernández, Manuel Iglesias. Circadian Blood Pressure Variability in Healthy and Complicated Pregnancies. *Hypertension.* 1997; 30: 603-610 doi: 10.1161/01.HYP.30.3.603

[336] Zhou Y, Damsky CH, Fisher SJ: Preeclampsia is associated with failure of human cytotrophoblasts to mimic a vascular adhesion phenotype. One cause of defective endovascular invasion in this syndrome? *J. Clin. Invest.* 1997; 99 :2152 – 2164.

[337] Zhou Y, Fisher SJ, Janatpour M, Genbacev O, Dejana E, Wheelock M, Damsky CH: Human cytotrophoblasts adopt a vascular phenotype as they differentiate. A strategy for successful endovascular invasion? *J. Clin. Invest.* 1997; 99: 2139 – 2151.

[338] Lim KH, Zhou Y, Janatpour M, McMaster M, Bass K, Chun SH, Fisher SJ: Human cytotrophoblast differentiation/invasion is abnormal in pre-eclampsia. *Am. J. Pathol* 1997; 151 :1809 – 1818.

[339] Sujatha S Salgado, Pathmeswaran A. Effects of placental infarctions on the fetal outcome in pregnancies complicated by hypertension *J Coll Physicians Surg. Pak* Apr - Apr 2008; 18(4): 213 - 216.

[340] Taylor RN, Davidge ST, Roberts JM. Endothelial cell and oxidative stress. In Chesley's Hypertensive Disorders in Pregnancy, Lindheimer MD, Cunningham F G Joberts JM. Eds, Elseviser, Amsterdan The Netherlands 3rd edition 2009.

[341] R. J. Levine, S. E. Maynard, C. Qian et al., "Circulating angiogenic factors and the risk of preeclampsia,"*The New England Journal of Medicine*, 2004; 350; 7: 672 – 683.
[342] C. J. Robinson, D. D. Johnson, E. Y. Chang, D. M. Armstrong, and W. Wang, "Evaluation of placenta growth factor and soluble Fms-like tyrosine kinase 1 receptor levels in mild and severe preeclampsia,"*American Journal of Obstetrics & Gynecology*, 2006; 195 (1): 255–259.
[343] H. Siddiqui, R. A. Irani, S. C. Blackwell, S. M. Ramin, R. E. Kellems, and Y. Xia, "Angiotensin receptor agonistic autoantibody is highly prevalent in preeclampsia: correlation with disease severity,"*Hypertension*, 2010; 55: (2): 386 – 393.
[344] G. Wallukut, V. Homuth, T. Fisher, et al., "Patients with preeclampsia develop agonistic autoantibodies against the angiotensin AT1 receptor," *The Journal of Clinical Investigation*. 1999; (103): 945 – 952.
[345] Bharathi K N , Prasad Kvsrg ,Jagannath P, Nalini ks . A Comparison of nifedipine with methyldopa for control of blood pressure in mild to moderate pregnancy induced hypertension. *Journal of Clinical and Diagnostic Research*. 2010; 4(3): 2406 – 2409.
[346] Cockburn J, Moar VA, Ounsted M, Redman CW. Final report of study on hypertension during pregnancy: the effects of specific treatment on the growth and development of the children. *Lancet*. 1982;18273:647–9.
[347] Montan S, Anandakumar C, Arulkumaran S, Ingemarsson I, Ratnam SS. Effects of methyldopa on uteroplacental and fetal hemodynamics in pregnancy-induced hypertension. *Am. J. Obstet Gynecol*. 1993;1681 pt 1:152 – 156.
[348] Kasper Meidahl Petersen, Espen Jimenez-Solem , Jon Traerup Andersen , Morten Petersen, Kasper Brødbæk, Lars Køber, Christian Torp-Pedersen, Henrik Enghusen Poulsen. β-Blocker treatment during pregnancy and adverse pregnancy outcomes: a nationwide population-based cohort study. *BMJ Open* 2012;2:e001185 doi:10.1136/bmjopen-2012-001185
[349] Task Force on the Management of Cardiovascular Diseases During Pregnancy of the European Society of Cardiology. Expert consensus document on management of cardiovascular diseases during pregnancy. *Eur Heart J*. 2003; 24: 761–781.
[350] Sushrut D, Girij A. Labetalol - An Emerging First-line Drug for Pregnancy-induced Hypertension. *Indian Journal of Clinical Practice,* Vol. 23, No. 10 March 2013
[351] Subhedar V, Inamdar S, Hariharan C, Subhedar S. Comparison of efficacy of labetalol and methyldopa in patients with pregnancy-induced hypertension. *Int. J. Reprod Contracept Obstet Gynecol*. (2013), [cited February 15, 2015]; 2(1): 27-34. doi:10.5455/2320-1770.ijrcog20130205
[352] Gruppo di studio Ipertensione in Gravidanze. Nifedipine versus expectant management in mild to moderate hypertension in pregnancy. *Br. J. Obstet Gynaecol* 1998; 105: 718 - 722.
[353] Cooper WO, Sonia Hernandez-Diaz S, Arbogast PG, et al. major congenital malformations after first-trimester exposure to ACE inhibitors. *N. Engl. J. Med*. 2006; 354: 2443 - 2451.
[354] Lloyd-Sherlock P, Beard J, Minicuci N, Ebrahim S, Chatterji S. Hypertension among older adults in low-and middle-income countries: prevalence, awareness and control. *International journal of epidemiology*. 2014; 1-13. Doi:10.1093/ije/dyt215
[355] Feng-Hwa Lu, Shiung-Janp Tang, Jin-Shang Wu, Yi-Ching Yang, Chih-JenChang. Hypertension in elderly persons:Its prevalence and associated cardiovascular risk

factors in Tainan City, Southern Taiwan. Journal of gerontology: *Medical Sciences*. 2000. Vol. 55A; 8; M463 - M468.

[356] Donald M. Lloyd-Jones, Jane C. Evans, Daniel Levy. Hypertension in Adults Across the Age Spectrum: Current Outcomes and Control in the Community. *JAMA*. 2005; 294(4):466-472. doi:10.1001/jama.294.4.466

[357] Peter Weidmann, Sylvianne De Myttenaere-Bursztein, Morton H Maxwell and José de Lima. Effect of aging on plasma renin and aldosterone in normal man Kidney International (1975) 8, 325–333; doi:10.1038/ki.1975.120

[358] Palmer RM, Osterweil D, Loon-Lustig G, Stern N. The effect of dietary salt ingestion on blood pressure of old-old subjects. A double-blind, placebo-controlled, crossover trial. *J. Am. Geriatr. Soc*. 1989; 37: 931– 936.

[359] Centre for Disease Control. NHANES III. Prevalence of overweight among children and adolescents. United States 1999. Atlanta, GA Centres for Disease Control; 2001.available at: http:/www.cdc.gov/produts/pubs/pubd/hestats/overeght99.htm.

[360] Oduwole AA, Ladapo TA , Fajolu IB, Ekure EN, Adeniyi OF. Obesity and elevated blood pressure among adolescents in Lagos, Nigeria: a cross sectional study. *BMC Public Health* 2012. 12:616.

[361] Agyemang C, Redekop WK, Owusu-Dabo E, Brujinzeels MA. Blood pressure patterns in rural, semi-urbanand urban children in the Ashanti region f Ghana,West Africa. *BMC Public Health2005*, 5:114. doi :10.1186/1471-2458-5-1140.

[362] Sinaiko AR. Hypertension in children. *N. Eng. J. Med*. 1996; 355:1968- 1973.

[363] Bartosh SM, Aronson AJ. Childhood hypertension. An update on etiology, diagnosis, and treatment. *Pediatr Clin. North Am*. 1999; 46:235–52.

[364] Freedman DS, Dietz WH, Srinivasan SR, Berenson GS. The relation of overweight to cardiovascular risk factors among children and adolescents: the Bogalusa Heart Study. *Pediatrics*. 1999; 103 (6 pt 1): 1175 – 1182.

[365] de Jonge LL, van Osch-Gevers L, Willemsen SP, Steegers EAP, Hofman A, Helbing WA et al. Growth, Obesity and cardiac structure in early childhood. The Generation R study. *Hypertension*. 2011; 57:934 - 940.

[366] Mitchell BM, Gutin B, Kapuku G, Barbeau P, Humphries MC, Owens S, et al. Left ventricular structure and function in obese adolescents: relations to cardiovascular fitness, percent body fat, and visceral adiposity, and effects of physical training. *Pediatrics*. 2002;109:E73–3.

Index

A

D

E

H

I

J

K

L

M

Q

R

S

T

U

V

W

X

Y

β